Companion Animal Ethics

D1275379

The Universities Federation for Animal Welfare

UFAW, founded in 1926, is an internationally recognised, independent, scientific and educational animal welfare charity that promotes high standards of welfare for farm, companion, laboratory and captive wild animals, and for those animals with which we interact in the wild. It works to improve animals' lives by:

- Funding and publishing developments in the science and technology that underpin advances in animal welfare;
- Promoting education in animal care and welfare;
- Providing information, organising meetings and publishing books, videos, articles, technical reports and the journal Animal Welfare;
- Providing expert advice to government departments and other bodies and helping to draft and amend laws and guidelines;
- Enlisting the energies of animal keepers, scientists, veterinarians, lawyers and others who care about animals.

Improvements in the care of animals are not now likely to come of their own accord, merely by wishing them: there must be research...and it is in sponsoring research of this kind, and making its results widely known, that UFAW performs one of its most valuable services.

Sir Peter Medawar CBE FRS, 8 May 1957

Nobel Laureate (1960), Chairman of the UFAW Scientific Advisory Committee (1951–1962)

UFAW relies on the generosity of the public through legacies and donations to carry out its work, improving the welfare of animals now and in the future. For further information about UFAW and how you can help promote and support its work, please contact us at the following address:

Universities Federation for Animal Welfare
The Old School, Brewhouse Hill, Wheathampstead, Herts AL4 8AN, UK
Tel: 01582 831818 Fax: 01582 831414 Website: www.ufaw.org.uk
Email: ufaw@ufaw.org.uk

UFAW's aim regarding the UFAW/Wiley-Blackwell Animal Welfare book series is to promote interest and debate in the subject and to disseminate information relevant to improving the welfare of kept animals and of those harmed in the wild through human agency. The books in this series are the works of their authors, and the views they express do not necessarily reflect the views of UFAW.

Companion Animal Ethics

Peter Sandøe
Professor of Bioethics,
University of Copenhagen, Denmark

Sandra Corr
Reader in Veterinary Surgery,
University of Nottingham, UK

Clare Palmer
Professor of Philosophy,
Texas A&M University, USA

WILEY

Contents

Foreword   *vii*
Acknowledgements   *ix*

    Introduction   1
1 History of Companion Animals and the Companion Animal Sector   8
2 The Development and Role of the Veterinary and Other Professions in
    Relation to Companion Animals   24
3 Human Attachment to Companion Animals   41
4 Companion Animal Welfare   58
5 Theories of Companion Animal Ethics   73
6 Breeding and Acquiring Companion Animals   89
7 Selective Breeding   103
8 Feeding and the Problem of Obesity   117
9 Companion Animal Training and Behavioural Problems   132
10 Routine Neutering of Companion Animals   150
11 Performing Convenience Surgery: Tail Docking, Ear Cropping, Debarking
    and Declawing   169
12 Treating Sick Animals and End-of-Life Issues   186
13 Unwanted and Unowned Companion Animals   201
14 Ethics and Broader Impacts of Companion Animals   217
15 Other Companions   235
16 Companion Animals and the Future   252

Index   *269*

Foreword

Humans have been domesticating animals and keeping some of them as companions for thousands of years. Over the past century, the industrialized Western world has seen a huge increase in the number of companion animals, especially dogs and cats; and this increase has been accompanied by a number of ethical and welfare issues specific to those companion animals. Those who keep animals as companions usually have no wish to harm the animals in their care, but the way we treat companion animals is, whether we like it or not, affected by both tradition and culture, and because humans and animals have for the most part evolved separately, compromises sometimes have to be struck between the best interests of the animal and those of the owner. So, how should individuals and society address these compromises? What ethical principles should we use to determine how to interact with companion animals? How do we decide what really matters and how we should treat companion animals? How do we decide whether new and sometimes painful or stressful treatments developed for humans should be used on companion animals? How do we deal with issues where a decision in the best interests of one companion animal impacts adversely on other animals whether in our control or in the wild?

The science of animal welfare has proven extraordinarily useful in providing the evidence to help us with such questions, but decisions on appropriate behaviour are ultimately dependent on society reaching a consensus on what should be done. This is where ethics helps make clear what the issues are, alerts us to the dangers of relying on custom and past behaviour and helps us to work through the implications of adopting a particular ethical position. This is the first book that has set out to provide a comprehensive ethical analysis of this topic, and the authors are admirably placed to guide the reader through this forest, being eminent and respected in the fields of both ethics and the science of animal welfare. We are very grateful to them for undertaking the task and for providing us with this excellent and very readable account combining a synthesis of the existing literature and the authors' original perspectives on the issues. It will be an excellent addition to the UFAW/Wiley Series.

Robert Hubrecht

January 2015

Acknowledgements

In this book, we explore the important ethical questions and problems that arise as a result of humans keeping animals as companions who live with us in our homes. These ethical issues are not only important but also highly complex. To do justice to this complexity, we draw on a wide range of disciplines to underpin our arguments, including history, psychology, ethical and political theory, and the veterinary, behavioural and social sciences. In addition to incorporating a significant body of published research, we have also been greatly helped by our colleagues.

Four of these colleagues, Brenda Bonnett, Andrew Gardiner, Iben Meyer and James A. Serpell, have contributed so much, through advice and written input, to certain chapters that we have acknowledged them as co-authors of those chapters. We are immensely grateful for their contributions.

Many other friends and colleagues have given advice and/or have commented on specific chapters. In particular, we would like to thank Charlotte Reinhard Bjørnvad, Stine B. Christiansen, Lise Lotte Christensen, Björn Forkman, Merete Fredholm, Gail Golab, Ayoe Hoff, T. J. Kasperbauer, Sara Kondrup, Vibeke Knudsen, Helle Friis Proschowsky and Cecilie Agnete Thorslund. Special thanks are due to Geir Tveit for helping us to check the references and to Sara Kondrup for helping us make the index.

About 4 years have passed since we made the first outline for the book. Since then, working on the book has taken up a significant part of our time. While it has been enjoyable, it was also at times a struggle, due to conflicting commitments. Much of the work has been conducted at odd hours, in evenings, on weekends and during vacations; this has been a strain on our family and friends, and we are grateful for their patience.

Finally, Peter would like to thank the Department of Food and Resource Economics at the University of Copenhagen for financial and other kinds of support that, among other things, enabled him to go to University of Pennsylvania for two research visits; he would also like to thank James A. Serpell for hosting him during these visits. Clare would like to thank Texas A&M University for a Faculty Development Leave in Autumn 2012 that allowed her some time to work on the book. Sandra would like to thank Professor Christopher Wathes (OBE) for encouraging and developing her interest in ethics.

Peter Sandøe
Sandra Corr
Clare Palmer

Introduction

I.1   Introduction   1
I.2   Companion Animal Ethics   2
I.3   Why We Use The Terms 'Companion Animals' and 'Owners'   4
I.4   The Structure of This Book   7

I.1 Introduction

Companion animals can be a source of pleasure, fun, exercise, comfort, fascination and consolation. Choosing to live with animal companions can be life enriching, even when it comes with some expense and inconvenience. Most of those who live with animal companions believe this to be a two-way relationship: as well as being fed and cared for, the animal companions also derive pleasure, satisfaction and comfort from living with people.

This seems, therefore, to be a win–win situation: what is good for people is also good for the animals; the animals are cared for, and they help to create human happiness. Put like this, there does not seem to be much need for a book on companion animal ethics. But things are not that simple. For instance, it is not always clear what is good for animal companions, and what is good for animals may be in conflict with what is good for the people with whom they live. Animal companions can also be the source of very different human responses than pleasure and consolation, such as anxiety, fear or distress. So, there is a need for ethical reflection regarding our relationship with companion animals.

In this short introductory chapter, we first elaborate on why we think there is a need for ethical reflection about companion animals and then explain our ethical approach. In the following section, we will try to explain what we mean by 'companion' animals and

Companion Animal Ethics, First Edition. Peter Sandøe, Sandra Corr and Clare Palmer.
© Universities Federation for Animal Welfare 2016.

why we have chosen to focus on them, rather than on the wider group of pet animals. Finally, we will briefly outline the structure of the book.

I.2 Companion Animal Ethics

Even those who are well informed about veterinary and animal science and who have kept animals as companions for many years are sometimes unsure about what is in the best interests of their animals. Those without such knowledge and experience may be even more uncertain. For example, someone may be doubtful as to whether neutering is in the best interests of their male dog or whether their cat should be let out to roam. To complicate matters, popular ideas about companion animals' interests may not reflect the findings of current behavioural and veterinary research.

People may also find it difficult to balance potentially conflicting concerns for the well-being of their animals. If a dog or a cat is seriously ill, for example, due to a malignant type of cancer, an owner may find it difficult to weigh the interest of the animal in living (and their own desire for the animal to remain alive) against a concern to prevent their companion from suffering. This may lead to a dilemma between continuing veterinary treatment and euthanasing the animal. The owner may ask the vet for advice, but she or he may have similar doubts.

In other cases, different people may have strong and conflicting views about the significance of companion animals and how we should treat them. These conflicting views are often rooted in different ideas about animals' moral status, whether there is something special about companion animal species and what we do and do not owe to them. For example, some people consider painlessly killing stray and feral cats and dogs to be ethically unproblematic. Others claim that healthy dogs and cats have a right to life, whether owned or not. Similarly, some people see no moral problem in docking dogs' tails to make their appearance meet breed standards, whereas others find tail docking a morally unacceptable violation of the dog's bodily integrity.

Thus, living with companion animals gives rise to *uncertainties* about what is in the animals' best interests, *moral dilemmas* in weighing different human and animal well-being concerns and *ethical disagreements* concerning the moral significance and appropriate treatment of companion animals. These uncertainties, dilemmas and disagreements are the subject of this book (Figure I.1).

Despite the millions of cats, dogs and other animals kept as companions around the world, the ethical aspects of this unique relationship have not previously been the subject of a comprehensive ethical analysis. As a result, although the ideas of animal welfare and the approaches to ethics that we discuss here are well established, the present book breaks new ground. In particular, previous work on animal ethics has tended to focus on higher-level theoretical questions, rather than on the more practical ethical issues that arise from our day-to-day engagement with the animals in our homes.

We believe that thinking through some of these everyday ethical issues – issues that can be incredibly important in individual animal lives, as well as our own human lives – is a critical step in developing and applying animal ethics. Partly because much of this material is new and cannot be taken for granted, and also for practical reasons of space,

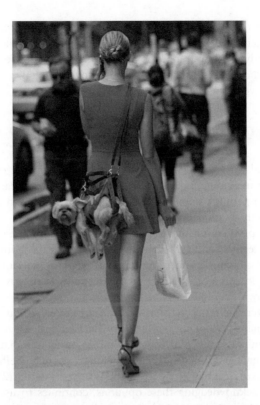

Figure I.1 A 1-year-old cross-breed dog being carried in a 'Pooch Pouch'. In an accompanying article, the owner claimed that the dog loves it and it keeps him safe on the busy streets of New York; but critics claim the pouch is a 'fashion statement', which causes distress to the animals. (*Alberto Reyes/Wenn*)

we have been selective in terms of the topics and frameworks we discuss. Consequently, there are omissions and places where we are, of necessity, somewhat brief. However, we hope that what is included will provide a useful resource and a starting point for future work.

This book, unlike many in the field of animal ethics, does not advocate any particular ethical position, beyond the widely accepted idea that the lives and experiences of sentient animals should count for something in our ethical decision making. We take a pluralist perspective, presenting a variety of approaches to human and animal welfare, to animal ethics and to particular ethical problems raised by companion animals. Although we, as the authors of this book, have our own (often divergent) views, we have attempted to present the arguments in a balanced way, though there may be places where we have not always succeeded in putting our sympathies to one side. We hope to show that at least some disputes about our ethical relations with companion animals may flow from different understandings of animal welfare or different approaches to ethics, but that – considered from those perspectives – they are at least comprehensible and rational.

This book draws on a wide range of supporting scientific material, particularly from psychology and veterinary, behavioural and social sciences. In order to ensure that this book is as informative and up to date as possible, we invited experts in relevant fields to join us in co-authoring several chapters, to improve the quality and accuracy of the empirical material we discuss.

1.3 Why We Use The Terms 'Companion Animals' and 'Owners'

Humans use animals in various ways, mostly linked to tangible outputs or services, such as for food or fur, riding, guarding or modelling human diseases. However, some animals are kept in people's homes where they appear to serve a less clearly defined purpose – typically these animals are referred to as 'pets'.

As Grier (2006: p. 8) comments, the term 'pet' has 'a complex history and obscure origins'. In the sixteenth century, 'pet' was used to describe both people who were indulged or treated as favourites and tamed animals kept for pleasure or companionship (Grier 2006: p. 9). In some cases, the term 'favourite' was also used for animals kept for human company.

Recently, however, the term 'pet' has become controversial, on the grounds that it fails to respect animals' own dignity or integrity. For instance, Linzey and Cohn (2011) argue that calling animals 'pets' is derogatory and insulting and that we should instead use the term 'companion animals'. The Companion Animal Welfare Council in the United Kingdom takes a similar perspective (CAWC, n.d.). Grier (2006: p. 10), on the other hand, while acknowledging these opinions, continues to use the term 'pet' on the grounds that 'it is in wide use' and that people have a 'practical understanding of its meaning'.

In thinking about this book, we recognised the arguments on both sides: while 'pet' is the most widely used and understood term, we also accept that it may have demeaning connotations. However, we were persuaded by another set of arguments – that 'pet' and 'companion animal' are not straightforwardly interchangeable terms, but rather that we should think of 'companion animals' as a subset of those animals commonly called 'pets'. We take the term 'pet' to encompass a very broad range of animals alongside whom people choose to live and consider 'companion animals' to be a subset of 'pets', with whom we have a special interactive bond.

Let us consider this more systematically. Although the term 'pet' can be used in different ways, some features seem to be widely accepted as characterising the human/pet relationship. Grier (2006: p. 10) draws on Keith Thomas' characterisation of pets in England between 1400 and 1800: pets were distinguished by being allowed in the house, being given individual names and never being eaten. This is a useful starting point, although some animals widely regarded as pets, for example, fish in a tank, may well not be given individual names. Varner (2002) drawing on Barnbaum (1998) suggests a further set of characterisations, with which it is worth engaging.

First, Varner suggests, we expect a pet's owner to regard it affectionately. He seems right that this is normally the case – a 'pet' is not usually an object of hate, fear or disgust to its owner (in the way that, say, an invading cockroach may be regarded). Still, it would presumably be possible to keep a pet – say, a snake or a stick insect – because one is fascinated by it or curious about it, rather than because one felt affection for it.

Second, Varner suggests, a pet should live in or close to the home (this was also part of Thomas' characterisation of a pet). To rule out plants, Varner adds that for something to be a pet, it should be mobile, and thus, either voluntarily choose to remain in the home or be prevented from leaving. We decided to restrict our definition of 'pet' still further, to animals that actually live *in* the home, thereby ruling out horses.

We recognise that some readers will see the exclusion of horses as a significant omission from the book. While some people do regard horses as pets or companion animals, and they can be kept near to (though very rarely in) one's home, they also to a very large degree have other roles. Firstly, for many people, horses are primarily kept for sport. Secondly, the keeping of horses is still in many respects linked to an agricultural context. For example, in many places, even in industrial Western nations, often *the very same* horses that are kept by private individuals are eventually slaughtered and used for human or animal food. So, although there is much to be said about horses and ethics, we will not say it here.

Third, Varner proposes, a pet must be the kind of being that lives a life different in kind from the owner, in terms of its capacities, occupations and so on; this rules out keeping another human as a pet.

Fourth, a pet should have interests – its life can go better or worse for it; it has a welfare or a good of its own – and it should depend in significant ways on its owner to help fulfil those interests. So, a pet cannot be a robot, such as a Tamagotchi, which cannot, for instance, have 'poor welfare'.

Although this characterisation of a pet rules out plants, pests, human beings and robots, it includes most animals voluntarily kept by people in their homes: mammals, birds, fish, reptiles, amphibians, insects and arachnids. While keeping such animals as pets certainly does raise ethical issues, the focus of this book is narrower: we are interested in animals kept primarily as companions. Even if one has affection for one's pet tarantula, it is, as Varner (2002) notes, a stretch to call it a companion. Insects and fish, likewise, may be kept for many reasons, but rarely primarily for their companionship. As argued by Varner (2002: p. 452), while a companion animal has all the characteristics shared by pets, it has additional characteristics that make it more than a pet.

However, this raises questions about what we mean by 'companionship'. Likewise, there is no generally accepted definition of 'companion animal'. The US-based animal welfare organisation, the ASPCA (n.d.) somewhat circularly defines companion animals as 'domesticated or domestic-bred animals whose physical, emotional, behavioural and social needs can be readily met as companions in the home, or in close daily relationship with humans'.

What seems critical to this definition is the emphasis on relationship and reciprocal engagement. Varner (2002) takes the term 'companion' to imply a 'significant degree of social interaction' between the owner(s) and the animal. Although somewhat vague, this involves humans and animals recognising and responding to one another as specific individuals (rather than, for instance, a fish swimming to the top of the tank to pick up food thrown in by anyone). For humans, companionship normally includes seeking out the company of the particular animal for comfort, consolation, play and so on, and this is likely to be reciprocal in the case of companion animals.

We take this kind of reciprocal engagement to be the hallmark of human/animal companionship, and as the vast majority of the animals with whom we have such mutual relations are dogs and cats, they are the main focus of this book. However, other animals may be companions, and these are discussed in Chapter 15.

Some readers may think it an omission that we do not discuss in detail the relations between humans and working animals kept in the home, such as guide dogs, guard dogs and some hunting dogs. Although much of what we say about dogs kept as companions also applies to working dogs, we concluded that they raise special ethical questions beyond the scope of this book. For similar reasons, we decided to exclude companion animals used for various forms of animal-assisted therapy.

Another important terminological question relates to what we should call those people who live with and look after companion animals. Again, the terms used here have recently become controversial. Linzey and Cohn (2011) reject the term 'owners' in favour of 'carers'. 'The Guardian Campaign' run by the international animal rights and rescue organisation, In Defense of Animals (IDA), promotes a switch to the language of guardianship from the language of ownership. IDA (n.d.) argues that 'since other animals, whether domesticated or wild, are living beings, they ought not to have owners, only guardians, friends, caretakers, protectors, family or respectful observers'. The popularity of the term 'guardian' is slowly growing in the United States at least; a few US cities and Rhode Island have now incorporated the term into their animal-related ordinances.

While we have no objections to either 'carer' or 'guardian' and are sympathetic to the arguments, we were reluctant to use terms not currently in widespread use. Legally speaking, companion animals *are* the property of the people who look after them. While many of those who defend animal rights, in particular, find the idea of companion animals as property offensive and immoral, changing the terminology does not change the legal situation. So, we decided to use the more traditional term, 'owners', in this book.

We also recognise that relations people have with their animal companions, and the kinds of animals they keep as companions, vary significantly across cultures. In some cultures, for instance, dogs are regarded as belonging to an entire human community and are fed by a number of different households. For example, this often seems to be the case for unowned street dogs in India, which are also legally protected (see, for instance, Srinivasan 2013). Some cultures tame and keep members of local wild species as companions – for instance, long-tailed macaques on Angaur Island in Polynesia. These relationships, while clearly important, raise their own ethical issues. We did not want to deal superficially with such issues, nor to attempt to tackle them without sufficient cultural knowledge. So, we decided to limit the scope of this book to the keeping of animal companions in what we (very roughly) call the industrialised West, focusing on Europe, Australasia and North America. This is where all the authors are located, and *Companion Animal Ethics* reflects this location.

Finally, we decided not to make either serious cruelty towards or neglect of companion animals a focus of this book (although we do say a little about this in Chapters 3 and 4). Serious cruelty and neglect of companion animals are, virtually universally, ethically condemned and, in many places, are already illegal. We wanted instead to discuss the ongoing ethical uncertainties, dilemmas and disagreements about living with companion animals, rather than issues about which everyone already agrees and to which we could make little new ethical contribution.

1.4 The Structure of This Book

The book begins with three chapters that establish the context and background for thinking about ethics and companion animals. Chapter 1 provides a brief history of the development of human relations to companion animals. Chapter 2 outlines the development of the veterinary and other animal-related professions with a focus on how these professions influence and deal with ethical issues relating to companion animals, and Chapter 3 explores the nature of the human–companion animal bond, including the ways in which humans are psychologically attached to companion animals, and the effects of keeping companion animals on human health. The next two chapters examine two essential concerns for companion animal ethics: ideas of animal welfare (Chapter 4) and different approaches to thinking about ethics (Chapter 5). Chapters 6–13 then consider particular ethical issues raised by breeding and rearing, pedigree selective breeding, diet, training and behaviour, convenience surgeries and neutering. We also consider ethical issues raised by unwanted animal companions, including the euthanasia of healthy animals; and by the veterinary treatment of sick animals. Chapter 14 considers how to deal with broader negative impacts of animal companions in terms of zoonoses, environmental effects and the use of resources. Chapter 15 considers special ethical issues raised by companion animals other than cats and dogs. Finally, in Chapter 16, we speculate on the future of the companion animal sector in terms of ethics, law, policy and the market.

References

ASPCA (n.d.) *Definition of companion animal*. The American Society for the Prevention of Cruelty to Animals. [Online] Available from: http://www.aspca.org/about-us/aspca -policy-and-position-statements/definition-of-companion-animal [Accessed 9 July 2014].

Barnbaum, D. (1998) Why Tamagotchis are not pets. *Thinking: The Journal of Philosophy for Children* 13 (4), 41–43.

CAWC (n.d.) *Companion: what are companion animals?* Companion Animal Welfare Council. [Online] Available from: http://www.cawc.org.uk/companion-animals [Accessed 9 July 2014].

Grier, K. (2006) *Pets in America: a history*. Durham, NC, The University of North Carolina Press.

IDA (n.d.) *The guardian campaign*. In Defense of Animals. [Online] Available from: http://www.idausa.org/campaigns/the-guardian-campaign/ [Accessed 30 May 2014].

Linzey, A. & Cohn, P. (2011) Terms of discourse. *Journal of Animal Ethics* 1 (1), vii–ix.

Srinivasan, K. (2013) The biopolitics of animal being and welfare: dog control and care in the UK and India. *Transactions of the Institute of British Geographers* 38 (1), 106–119.

Varner, G. (2002) Pets, companion animals and domesticated partners. In: Benatar, D. (ed.) *Ethics for everyday*. New York, McGraw-Hill, pp. 450–475.

History of Companion Animals and the Companion Animal Sector

1

Co-author: James A. Serpell, PhD

Marie A. Moore Professor of Animal Ethics and Welfare, Director, Center for the Interaction of Animals and Society, School of Veterinary Medicine, University of Pennsylvania, Philadelphia, PA, USA

1.1	Introduction	8
1.2	Early Human Relations to Companion Animals	10
1.3	Animal Companions in Medieval and Early Modern Europe	11
1.4	Europe and North America 1600–1950	13
	1.4.1 Breeding	15
	1.4.2 Diet	16
	1.4.3 Training	17
1.5	From the 1950s to the Present	17
1.6	Are Companion Animals Benefactors or Social Parasites?	20

1.1 Introduction

Many households in the industrialised Western world own companion animals. The American Veterinary Medical Association (AVMA, 2012) reported that just over a third of US households kept one or more dogs in 2011, and just under a third kept one or more

Companion Animal Ethics, First Edition. Peter Sandøe, Sandra Corr and Clare Palmer.
© Universities Federation for Animal Welfare 2016.

cats (AVMA, 2012: p. 1). Figures are similar, though somewhat lower, in the European Union (EU) where, in 2010, just over 25% of households had at least one dog, and just under 25% had at least one cat, according to the European Pet Food Industry (FEDIAF, 2010). In most Western countries, the number of households keeping dogs and cats has been steadily growing for decades.

The AVMA (2012) also gives us information on people's attitudes to the animals in their homes. Two-thirds of US dog owners see their dogs as members of the family; most of the rest, according to the survey, view them as 'companions' or 'pets'. Over half the owners see cats as family members. For both species, the younger the owners, the more likely they are to view their animals as family members (AVMA, 2012: p. 14). According to a survey prepared for a pet food company in 2000, nearly half of American dog owners have taken their dog on vacation, and a similar number have celebrated their dog's birthday (Ralston Purina, 2000). Thus the general trend is not only to allow dogs and cats into the family home but also – in these respects, at least – to treat them as members of the family.

Many owners of companion animals put their money where their mouth is. Thus they both demand, and can access, a growing supply of expensive products and services, including organic dog and cat food, elaborate day-care facilities, special overnight hotels, and advanced veterinary care. It's difficult to pin down the exact sums involved here, as different surveys produce different figures; but all show that animal companions are costly. According to the AVMA (2012: p. 57) in 2011, the average US dog owner spent $378 on veterinary services alone. The American Pet Products Association puts expenditure much higher: $655 on routine and surgical veterinary visits, $254 on food, $274 on kennel boarding and $359 on other products and services, in total more than $1500 per year. The amount spent by the average cat owner is smaller, but not by much according to the American Pet Products Association (APPA, n.d.). Although there may be significant local variations, it is reasonable to claim that the trend to spend increasing amounts on dogs, cats and other companion animals is representative of the industrialised Western world as a whole.

Yet this, surely, raises interesting questions. The number of animal companions is growing, while the costs of keeping them are increasing. Why would so many contemporary households – in particular, urban and suburban households in industrial societies – decide to spend their scarce resources on sharing their lives and homes with members of other species? How did our relationship with animal companions develop such that this could come about, and why? Could companion animals be some kind of substitute for the animals that people formerly lived alongside in rural, agriculturally based societies? Is keeping animal companions a symptom of changing family and household structures, and perhaps increasing loneliness? Or is it, instead, a way of expanding relations to nature that has been made possible by growing wealth? Are companion animals giving their owners tangible benefits or are they, rather, a diversion from other, more important, things?

In this chapter we will try to address these questions in two ways: first, we will sketch an outline of some key historical developments that led to current Western attitudes to animal companions. Second, from the perspective of evolutionary biology, we will consider whether animal companions do benefit their owners, and if so, in what ways and how much.

As we noted in the Introduction, the scope of this book is limited to the Western nations, in particular to Europe, Australasia and North America. Although living with animals as companions is practiced globally, the practice takes so many different forms internationally that – unfortunately – we do not have space to discuss them all in sufficient detail.

1.2 Early Human Relations to Companion Animals

There is sound evidence to show that humans have lived alongside domesticated animals for more than 10,000 years. But there is still considerable dispute about how, when and why animal domestication first occurred (and even what we should take domestication to mean). It is widely agreed, however, that dogs were the first animals to be domesticated, though even here there is uncertainty over whether dogs as opportunistic scavengers 'domesticated themselves' or whether they were deliberately drawn in or captured by people (see Cassidy, 2007: p. 7).

However domestication began, it is likely that dogs soon became useful to people in a practical sense, in particular by warning of intruders, tracking down prey animals, and finding wounded animals that escaped during hunts. But we do not know whether dogs were more than this; not just helpers and guards, but also objects of human affection. There is some archaeological evidence that prehistoric humans had affectionate feelings for dogs. In 1978, at a late Paleolithic site in northern Israel, for instance, a tomb was uncovered where about 12,000 years ago a person had been buried with a dog or wolf puppy. The hand of the dead person, who was around 50 years old, was placed on the animal's shoulder. It is likely that the dog was sacrificed when the person died in order that it could accompany the person onwards in his or her spiritual journey (Davis & Valla, 1978). There are many other cases, across the globe, where dogs appear to have been buried after death, a practice that was rarely adopted with other animals, with the exception of the mummification of cats in Egypt. In fact, the archaeologist Morey notes that, across many cultures, dead dogs seem to have been treated rather like dead people (Morey, 2006: p. 164).

The history of the emergence of cats as human companions is even less clear than that of dogs, in part because of uncertainty over whether and how cats could have been useful to people. Genetic evidence suggests that all current housecats come from *Felis s. lybica* wildcat populations in the Middle East, and there is some archaeological evidence to suggest that they became human companions as long as 10,000 years ago (Driscoll *et al.*, 2009). It's likely that certain human-tolerant cats came to live near humans to feed on small rodents and trash, that humans in turn tolerated them, and that gradually these bolder cats diverged from their wild relatives (Driscoll *et al.*, 2009). However, it was in Egypt around 3700 years ago that cat domestication really seems to have spread, with cats living in homes, being represented in art, and being bred (Driscoll *et al.*, 2009). From Egypt, the practice of living with domesticated cats seems to have spread across the world.

From ancient times it has also been common to keep other animals, not least birds, as companions. For example, there is ample evidence from ancient Greece that people kept a number of bird species in cages for company, and according to Kitchell (2011: p. 19) next to dogs, birds 'may have been the second most common type of pet in ancient Greece'.

Living affectionately with animals also seems to have been common in many hunter-forager societies across the globe. Evidence for this can be found in reports from early European explorers, missionaries and, later, anthropologists, who describe the affection with which dogs and other animals in the households of peoples living as hunters, gatherers and horticulturalists were regarded (Serpell, 1996: Chapter 4). Among these peoples, keeping some animals for company, not food, seemed to be the norm rather than the exception; humans were unwilling to sell or give away their animals, and became distraught with grief when the animals were taken away from them by force (Serpell, 1996: Chapter 4). These attachments are seen as strange by the European authors who write about them, and who express amusement or astonishment at the degree of affection so-called primitive peoples expressed towards animals (Serpell, 1996: Chapter 4). These accounts themselves suggest, however, that while attachments to animals were not widely accepted in Europe, they were nonetheless widespread elsewhere. Keeping animals as companions seems to be a widely practiced part of human life; it may be the European failure to do so until relatively recently that requires explanation.

1.3 Animal Companions in Medieval and Early Modern Europe

Christian theology shaped Europe's cultural and political climate from medieval times, and its influence was persistent. Prior to 1600, at least, a dominant view held within Christian orthodoxy was that close relations between humans and animals were theologically and morally troubling, and were best avoided. Of course, different theological traditions had somewhat divergent approaches here, and there were some notable exceptions. The best known of these is St Francis of Assisi, who famously called animals his brothers and sisters, and as Hughes (1996: p. 313) notes, friendships with animals were not unusual among religious ascetics.

A key idea that strongly influenced the dominant Christian tradition of keeping animals at a distance was the belief that humans had a unique status in nature. This idea was supported in multiple ways. One of the most influential was Aristotle's argument that humans, like other animals, have a nutritive and sensitive soul, but that they differ from animals by also having an intellectual or a rational soul. Medieval theologians linked this idea with a second powerful concept of separation, drawn from the Judaeo-Christian tradition, that man is created in God's image:

> Let us make mankind in our image, in our likeness, so that they may rule over the fish in the sea and the birds in the sky, over the livestock and all the wild animals, and over all the creatures that move along the ground.
>
> (Genesis 1: 26)

This idea of separation was reflected and revitalised in early modern philosophy in the work of René Descartes (1596–1650). Descartes divided the world into souled and soulless beings, arguing that animals lacked souls while humans possessed them. Since Descartes equated the soul with the mind and consciousness, his view entailed the conclusion that animals lack consciousness and rational thought, and that their actions and responses were purely the result of mechanistic processes. Although Descartes' work is open to more subtle interpretation (see Cottingham, 1978) the claim that animals are essentially mechanisms, lacking both agency and feelings (including the capacity to feel pain) was influential not only in terms of reinforcing the existing view of human supremacy, but also serving as a licence to deny that animals could have morally relevant needs.

That humans have a unique status vis-à-vis the animals does not, by itself, imply anything about whether or not humans should enjoy their company – just as the assumption that flowers lack sentience should not debar us from enjoying their beauty. The claim that humans ought to maintain a clear boundary between themselves and other animals follows from a different aspect of a Christian view of human nature: the idea that to get close to God, humans should suppress and forsake the animal sides of their natures. The historian Keith Thomas maintains that humans were taught 'to regard their bodily impulses as "animal" ones, needing to be subdued' (Thomas, 1984: p. 38). Lust, in particular, was seen as belonging to human's problematic nature; and one of Thomas's sixteenth-century sources is quoted as saying that lust made men 'like … swine, goats, dogs and the most savage and brutish beasts in the world' (Thomas, 1984: p. 38). A tacit premise here seems to be that by enjoying the company of animals, a human being will excite his or her 'animal side'. Bestiality therefore was a particularly heinous sin, since it 'was the sin of confusion; it was immoral to mix the categories' (Thomas, 1984: p. 39).

However, the idea of 'mixing the categories' of human and animal was regarded as more broadly problematic, beyond having sex with them. According to Thomas 'in early modern England even animal pets were morally suspect, especially if admitted to the table and fed better than the servants'; and he quotes a moralist from the early seventeenth century as saying: 'Over-familiar usage of any brute creature is to be abhorred' (Thomas, 1984: p. 40).

Thomas reproduces the following story of a pious woman from the sixteenth century who on her deathbed regrets the way she and her husband have privileged their female dog:

> She … said "Good husband, you and I have offended God grievously in receiving many a time this bitch into our bed; we would have been loathe to have received a Christian soul … into our bed, and to have nourished him in our bosoms, and to have fed him at our table, as we have done this filthy cur many times. The Lord give us grace to repent it" … and afterwards she could not abide to look upon the bitch any more.
>
> (Thomas, 1984: p. 40)

Being too close to dogs, or treating them better than some people, was seen as problematic. Occasionally, dogs were even demonised, although in this respect, the dog's situation during the Middle Ages seems to have been better than that of cats.

There is considerable uncertainty as to the roles cats played in medieval Europe. We have evidence that they were skinned, though this may not mean that they all were kept for their skins; many may have led essentially feral lives, while others were kept as companions (O'Connor, 1992). It is clear, though, that cats were sometimes portrayed as the personification of the devil, and this served as a justification for their persecution. Serpell notes that on feast days, cats were tortured and killed in violent ways as a way of symbolically driving out the Devil:

> By associating cats with the Devil and misfortune, the medieval Church seems to have provided the superstitious masses of Europe with a sort of universal scapegoat; something to blame and punish for all of life's numerous perils and hardships.

> (Serpell, 2000: p. 12)

Of course, some people still had close relations with cats, although especially for women, this could be seen as evidence of involvement with witchcraft. The cat typically was ascribed the role of the witch's 'familiar', that is, as a demonic companion that the witch sends out to do her evil deeds in return for protection and nourishment. In some cases it was also assumed that the witch transformed herself into the shape of a cat (Serpell, 2000). Although 'official' Christian views in medieval and early modern times required animals to be kept at a distance, in practice, Thomas suggests, 'human relations with domestic animals were closer than official religion implied' (Thomas, 1984: p. 93). Among the aristocratic social elite, for instance, dogs were frequently kept for companionship or as status symbols (Swabe, 1999: p. 161). There were clear differences between these dogs and the dogs used by working people for pulling, guarding and herding. The dogs owned by aristocrats were different breeds – typically very large breeds such as mastiffs, so-called hounds, including beagles, spaniels, setters and greyhounds, used by the men for hunting, or 'lapdogs' used as company for the ladies (Figure 1.1).

While working people may have felt some attachment and admiration for their dogs, they 'seem to have been regarded unsentimentally; and they were generally hanged or drowned when they had outlived their usefulness' (Thomas, 1984: p. 102). So, although there may have been many different individual relations to the animals with whom people lived, attitudes of affection and closeness towards animal companions were not widespread.

1.4 Europe and North America 1600–1950

Gradually during the seventeenth and eighteenth century, the habits of the wealthy trickled down to the members of the expanding middle classes, especially in towns. Dogs and caged birds became increasingly popular companions. In the eighteenth century, it also became common to keep cats as companion animals; and in the nineteenth century, children often kept small pets such as rabbits, white mice and guinea pigs (Grier, 2006: p. 32).

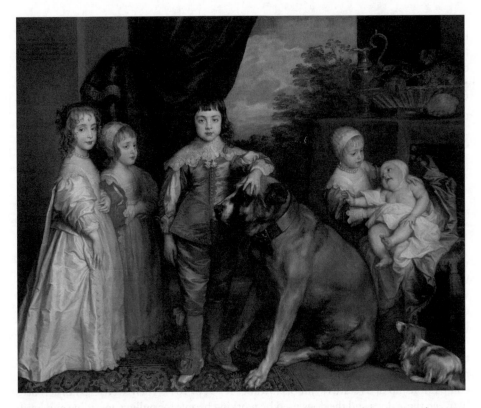

Figure 1.1   Five eldest children of King Charles 1 of England, by Sir Anthony van Dyck (1637). In the picture are two dogs of breeds typically owned by aristocrats at the time, a mastiff and a toy spaniel. (Royal Collection Trust, UK)

There seem to have been several parallel reasons for this development. First, the influence of the church gradually diminished, particularly in Northern Europe following the Reformation. Second, during this period many people became wealthier, and a growing urban middle class seems to have supported the expanding numbers of dogs, birds and cats kept as companions. The shift towards urban life also distanced increasing sectors of the population from any direct involvement in farming and livestock exploitation, and this may have helped to promote less use-oriented, more anthropomorphic attitudes and feelings towards animals (Serpell, 1996; Thomas, 1984). Clearly there are significant local differences in the speed with which these developments took place. Most of the sources we use here concern the United Kingdom and, for the later part of the period, also North America. In the United Kingdom particularly, urbanisation and the expansion of the middle classes set in very early; it followed somewhat later in other parts of the Western world.

A further factor that may have played a role in the development of the companion animal sector was a growing interest in biology and, in particular, in breeding. This interest took the shape of an expansion in breeding so-called purebred dogs, and later cats, and the establishment of breeding institutions or 'fancies'. Breeding – along with the development of specialised diets, and the growth of dog training – was one of the major structural changes in human–animal relations during this period; we will look briefly at each of these factors.

1.4.1 Breeding

The systematic breeding of dogs emerged in the middle of the nineteenth century. Although there were already clearly distinguishable breeds of dogs and other domestic animals before this, the new trend was characterised by conscious efforts to 'improve' domestic animals through controlled breeding. These efforts were combined with a sporting element in which people competed for prizes at shows, and this was typically linked to social status. In 1859, the world's first dog show was held in Newcastle-upon-Tyne, England. The 60 dogs showed were confined to pointers and setters, and a group of judges was appointed to assess the dogs and find a winner in each class (Sampson & Binns, 2006: pp. 21–22). This was the beginning of a trend; subsequent dog shows were organised in Birmingham and Manchester (where they still occur annually) and in other European countries.

While dog shows emphasised the form and appearance of dogs, later 'field trials' were established in which hunting dogs competed with one other for their ability to solve practical tasks such as finding and retrieving a 'lure'. In the early years the same dogs would typically appear both in dog shows and field trials. Later these activities became specialised, and dogs were divided into show or field trial types (Sampson & Binns, 2006: p. 22).

These new purebred dogs had a documented pedigree. This meant that their breed ancestors were documented in stud books. Stud books were established by including particular animals that were thought at the time to represent the best specimens of their breed, after which the stud book was typically closed. This meant that only offspring of those original dogs would count as purebred. So all purebred dogs of a certain breed could be traced back to a limited number of founders. In some cases, a dog's favourable performance at a dog show could also be set as an additional requirement for its offspring to qualify as purebred.

The potential for conflicts to arise concerning whether a dog should qualify as purebred, along with the management of stud books, led to the establishment of kennel clubs. The first was (and still is) simply called the Kennel Club, established in England in 1873. The first *Kennel Club Stud Book* was published in 1874. Other kennel clubs followed suit, including the French Société Centrale Canine in 1882, the American Kennel Club in 1884, and an international umbrella organisation, the Fédération Cynologique Internationale, in 1911.

Many factors drove this early enthusiasm for dog breeding. Apart from the sporting element, and an obsession with exhibitions and shows, there seems to have been a wider, underlying idea of eugenics at play:

> The Victorians were clearly fascinated by the ideas of breed purity and genetic improvement. Indeed, there was widespread concern about the concept of degeneration, the progressive ill health in succeeding generations of a family, and the need to actively reverse this trend. This in turn probably lay behind early ideas of eugenics … that also advanced in parallel with the ideas of breed purity in dogs and other species.
>
> (Sampson & Binns, 2006: p. 27)

It is ironic, as we shall see in Chapter 6, that the same breeding system concerned about generational *ill* health, set up in the nineteenth century, is to blame for much of the current health and welfare problems of modern pedigree dogs and cats.

In addition, engaging in dog breeding may have allowed people to maintain their own social status. As Harriet Ritvo (1987: p. 104) argues, the structures evolving around the breeding and showing of pedigreed dogs 'figuratively expressed the desire of predominantly middle-class fanciers for a relatively prestigious and readily identifiable position within a stable, hierarchical society'.

The first Kennel Club stud book identified 40 different breeds of dogs. This number has been growing steadily over the years; in 2003, the Kennel Club recognised 201 breeds. Some of these were types of dogs that already existed as geographic 'landraces', but were then transformed into breeds through genetic isolation; others were the results of the creative efforts of passionate and entrepreneurial individuals. The English Golden Retriever, for instance, was produced by hybridizing a yellow wavy-coated retriever over a number of generations with a spaniel, a setter, a Labrador Retriever and a Bloodhound. It is, therefore, essentially the product of deliberate line breeding involving a range of different breeds (Sampson & Binns, 2006: pp. 27–29). Eventually, dogs not typically owned by the aristocracy, such as the Staffordshire Bull Terrier in 1935, were recognised as breeds by the Kennel Club.

Cat breeding and cat shows also became established in parallel with dog shows; the late nineteenth-century 'cat fancy' was extremely popular both in England and on the European continent (Kete, 1994: p. 131), and successful cat breeders made good profits. However, although certain fine breeds of cats became reasonably popular, the interest in cat shows declined, and the majority of cat owners, unlike dog owners, stuck with ordinary domestic cats that were not purebred or pedigree, nor the subject of planned breeding (Hartwell, 2003–2014).

1.4.2 Diet

Alongside selective breeding for pedigree, a second area in which substantial changes took place during the nineteenth and early twentieth century was in the diet of companion animals. As far back as the eighteenth century, books on dogs began to provide recipes for proper feeding; and in the nineteenth century, the first commercial dog food was developed in the form of so-called Meat Dog Biscuits. Later came granulated and canned versions of ready-made dog food. These products were marketed through relentless advertising, in the beginning aimed primarily at the high-end market. Thus the first main producer of dog food, Spratt's, targeted their advertisements at dog shows. Later these products gradually gained a wider uptake:

> Dog food, both wet and dry, gradually became part of the middle-class grocery list because of its convenience and availability, its gradually decreasing cost, changes in cooking practices, and changing beliefs about the needs of dogs.
>
> (Grier, 2006: p. 377)

The new dog foods were marketed as providing dogs with a more balanced and healthy diet than that which could come from table scraps; the importance of meat in dogs' diet was also emphasised. By the 1930s, commercialised canned cat food also became available – although the availability of specialised food for animal companions was severely restricted during World War II. One factor influencing the development of this market was the improvement in human food quality. This led to by-products becoming available, particularly from the slaughter and fisheries industries, for which the dog and cat food industry provided a good outlet. By the later part of the twentieth century, as we will discuss in Chapter 8, commercial cat and dog food came to constitute virtually the entire diet of dogs and cats in the industrialised West. Commercial feed for birds, guinea pigs and other small companion animals also proliferated and became standard stock in supermarkets.

1.4.3 Training

A final development we should note here was an increased focus on obedience training of dogs during the first half of the twentieth century (Cats by tradition have been regarded as being 'untrainable', though as we will see in Chapter 9, this is not necessarily true). Of course, dogs used for tasks such as herding and hunting were always trained to perform these functions. But the early twentieth century saw the broader propagation of dog training.

At the beginning of the twentieth century, programs for systematic training of the dogs used by the military and the police were established. Dog trainers, who had worked in these contexts, began to extend dog training into the civilian world, so that the training of police dogs spilled over to the rest of society (Johnson n.d.). For example, in Denmark, a club for people training police dogs was established in 1909; and this club also allowed 'civilians' to participate in training. However, the non-police members decided to break away and establish their own Civilian Club for Dog Handlers in 1937, now the largest Danish dog-handling club (Hansen, 2012).

The main focus in dog training clubs was, and still is, on obedience training as a sport. However, increasingly, many clubs opened their doors to ordinary dog owners who wanted to train their newly acquired puppies to become well-behaved members of a modern suburban family. More recently, training became necessary to enable owners to follow requirements to control dogs in public, and, in particular, to walk them on a leash.

By the mid-twentieth century, then, the companion animal sector had changed and expanded dramatically. The lives of animal companions had become considerably more structured and heavily influenced by people in terms of breeding, training and diet. While the hardships and shortages of World War II put many of these processes on hold, the end of the war and the growth and prosperity that followed led to an unprecedented boom in the companion animal sector.

1.5 From the 1950s to the Present

The most striking post-war trend was the major growth in the number of dogs and cats kept as companions. Other animals, especially birds, became much less popular. This trend can be seen in the following graph mapping ownership of dogs, cats and budgerigars (also known as common pet parakeets – a common type of caged bird in the United Kingdom) (Figure 1.2).

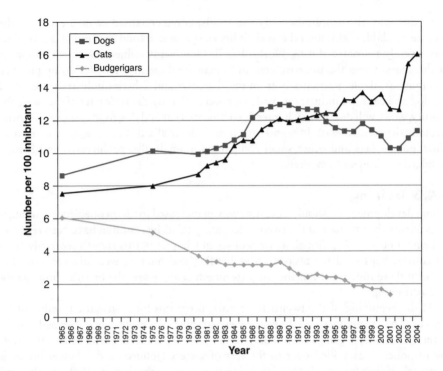

Figure 1.2   Dogs, cats and budgerigars per 100 inhabitants in the UK. Based on information from the Pet Food Manufacturers Association (n.d.) and from the UK Office for National Statistics (2012).

The graph also shows a trend for an uneven, and roughly parallel, increase in the number of dogs and cats kept as companions until the 1990s, followed by an increase in cats and a temporary decline in dogs. This seems to be a general phenomenon across the Western world, apparently driven by socio-economic and demographic changes. First, there has been an unprecedented growth in wealth, and an expansion in urban and suburban development. The growing number of middle-class families living in suburban areas has been an ideal background for an expansion in the number of family dogs and cats. More recently, changes in the family structure, in particular more working women and more singleton and single-parent households, have made cats a more manageable option than dogs, because they are generally less demanding companions.

In the following chapters, we will discuss significant ethical issues raised by developments since the mid-twentieth century in how companion animals are kept, bred, cared for and thought of. Here, we will just briefly mention some of these developments:

The growth of animal professionals: A number of professions have arisen or developed to cater for the perceived needs of companion animals. The veterinary profession has transformed since the 1940s, to include companion animals as a key area of work. This transformation coincided with the gradual disappearance of horses associated with the rise of motorised transport. Alongside vets, there has been a significant growth in other animal professionals including nurses, therapists, trainers and shelter workers. The growth in companion animal professionals has led to a corresponding expansion in services available to companion animals, from vaccinations and spaying, to complex surgeries, to grooming and kennelling.

Control over animal companions' lives: Following the pattern from the early twentieth century, animal companions' lives have become increasingly controlled, in a variety of ways. Freedom of movement is curtailed: in most Western countries, dogs must be leashed, exercised in controlled areas, and must undergo at least basic training; most are also neutered. Cats' movements are controlled even more, particularly in North America, where they are routinely confined indoors, and are also, in most places, routinely neutered, unless they are used for breeding; and (again, especially in North America) may undergo declawing surgery, in order to make them better indoor companions – an issue that will be discussed in Chapter 11.

Expansion in numbers of purebred dogs: Today most dogs in the Western world are of a specific breed, although far from all of them have a pedigree. Those that are not of a specific breed are mostly crosses between dogs of specific breeds. Mixed-breed dogs are increasingly acquired from shelters. The increase in purebred and pedigree dogs has led to an increase in genetically related health problems in dogs (see Chapter 7). Among cats, only a minority are of any specific breed; most are shorthair domestic cats, although recently there have been a number of experiments in creating new cat breeds, including crosses with wild cats.

Commercial pet food: Most animals are fed a standardised diet of commercial pet food produced according to legally defined nutritional standards. However, recently there has been movement towards more 'natural' forms of commercial food for both dogs and cats (see Chapter 14).

Higher moral significance: Most people value companion animals more highly than was usual in the past. This concern has underpinned legislation aimed at protecting companion animals in a number of countries. While the world's first anti-cruelty law, which came into force in the United Kingdom in 1822, only covered horses and cattle and did not even mention dogs and cats, current animal welfare legislation in many European countries now has special provisions protecting dogs and cats. In the United States, the first federal animal law that was passed in the 1960s focused mainly on the protection of family dogs and cats from being stolen and used in research.

Furthermore, it seems clear (though we lack documented evidence of this) that the many organisations aiming to promote animal welfare or animal rights have, over the last 50 years or so, increasingly focused on dogs and cats. This is particularly true of issues that have a strong emotional appeal, including cases of cruelty, commercial breeding of puppies and kittens (puppy and kitten mills), the selective breeding of animals with extreme phenotypes, and dealing with stray or relinquished dogs and cats. While this development reflects a greater public concern about dogs, cats and other companion animals, these welfare organisations have also contributed to raising public awareness about such issues (many of which will be discussed in detail in the following chapters).

So, the dogs have moved out of the kennel and the cats have moved out of the barn; both have instead moved into the family home. Here, the average Western dog or cat owner, as we have noted, lavishes money on special food, veterinary care, boarding kennels and so on – often taken for granted as part of a normal life of a family dog or cat. In addition, the typical owner spends not only his or her *money* on the companion animal, but also his or her *time*. These are significant costs. Yet, despite this, numbers of companion animals have increased.

How can this be explained? In the following section, we try to situate this historical discussion within a wider biological discussion about the role of animal companions in human life.

1.6 Are Companion Animals Benefactors or Social Parasites?

One opening thought here is this: if people spend their precious time and hard-earned money on caring for dogs and cats, they must feel that they get something in return that is worth the investment. As there is no sign of this process stopping, this appears to be a good indication that the animals make a positive contribution to people's lives.

However, in an influential paper, the British psychologist Archer (1997) questioned whether people are right to claim that dogs and cats really make a positive contribution to their lives. Are they instead really being conned by clever social parasites? Archer's provocative answer is that companion animals or pets, as he calls them, are indeed social parasites that divert time and energy away from what should, from a biological point of view, be our highest priority – that is, to look after our own offspring and other close relatives.

Archer reviews the literature on the benefits conferred by pet ownership, and concludes that indeed there are some benefits. The average dog or cat owner will, according to him, have better health and a higher quality of life, compared to the average person who does not own a companion animal. Archer does not want to deny this: rather his claim is that the resources spent achieving these benefits would, from the point of view of promoting the owners' 'biological fitness', be better spent on people's next of kin.

Archer also does not seek to deny that companion animals have strongly appealing features that motivate us to care for them. Quite the contrary – his claim is that the appeal of a puppy or a kitten serves as a very strong motive, what evolutionary biologists call a *proximal mechanism*, through which dogs and cats trick us into looking after them.

Archer neatly summarises his argument in the following way:

> Why do people love their pets? In answering this question, we had to separate the ultimate Darwinian explanation from the proximal mechanism through which people develop attachments to their pets. As we have seen, these attachments are often strong ones when judged by the standards of human attachments. I argued that, in evolutionary terms, humans are manipulated by pets: they are cuckoos in our nests, albeit not as destructive to our own offspring as are cuckoo chicks.

(Archer, 1997: p. 253)

So, Archer's claim is that dogs and cats appeal to dispositions and instincts that developed in humans through evolution, 'to care for their children, to form relationships with mates and kin, and to show empathy with other human beings'; and that dogs and cats divert our attention away from alternative ways of spending our time and resources which would be more useful from a biological point of view.

There are at least two ways in which someone who wants to claim that living with companion animals is nonetheless worthwhile for us may try to respond to Archer. One way is to grant Archer's point, but to say that it is merely a biological point that does not cut any ice in an ethical discussion about how to lead our lives. So, even if it is true that, biologically speaking, humans could be more successful if they turned energy and spending away from companion animals and instead directed it at their relatives, it does not follow that this is the right thing to do from an ethical perspective. There is no ethical imperative to spread our genes more effectively than we already do – perhaps rather the opposite.

The other way in which one may try to answer Archer is by arguing that the reason why he cannot see significant benefits in terms of biological fitness from keeping pets is that he has not looked hard enough. Archer himself would be sympathetic to this reply, since he clearly admits that the available evidence on the matter is incomplete. And he suggests that there may be some 'additional benefits that are hard to quantify, such as the contribution to children's psychological development, longer-term effects on self-esteem and well-being, and the facilitation of social interactions with other humans' (Archer, 1997: p. 254).

There are a number of other hypotheses about how keeping of companion animals may possibly affect the biological fitness of their owners. One is that keeping companion animals serves as a social buffer against the negative health effects of psychosocial stress. Another is that looking after a companion animal gives future parents experience that will be useful in caring for their own offspring. (See Serpell and Paul (2011) for more on this.) In Chapter 3, we will review some of the literature concerning the potential benefits of keeping companion animals.

From the perspective of biological fitness, it is not, at present, possible to give a final verdict on the value to humanity of keeping companion animals. However, there is no doubt that, throughout history, dogs and cats living with human beings as companions have found an important biological niche. How well they are looked after is another question that will occupy us in many of the following chapters.

Key Points

- Keeping animals as companions is a widely practiced part of human life found throughout most human history and across the globe.
- A possible exception to this is medieval and early modern Europe, where attitudes of affection and closeness towards animal companions were less accepted; this gradually changed in Europe and other parts of the Western world from the seventeenth century onwards.

- By the mid-twentieth century, the companion animal sector had expanded significantly, and the lives of animal companions had become considerably more structured and heavily influenced by people in terms of breeding, training and diet.
- Over the last 50 years, we have witnessed a further dramatic expansion of the companion animal sector, with substantial increases in numbers of dogs and cats kept as companions (though declines in some other pets) and the typical owner not only spending a significant part of his or her *money* on commercial food and veterinary and other services, but also investing more *time* in their companion animals.
- Whether companion animals benefit their owners or whether they are effectively social parasites is still the subject of debate, but from the perspective of biological fitness, it is not, at present, possible to give a final verdict on the value to humanity of keeping companion animals.
- However, there is no doubt that, through history, humans have created an important new biological niche for companion dogs and cats.

References

APPA (n.d.) *Pet industry market size & ownership statistics*. American Pet Products Association. [Online] Available from: http://www.americanpetproducts.org/press_industrytrends.asp [Accessed 6 June 2013].

Archer, J. (1997) Why do people love their pets?, *Evolution and Human Behavior* 18 (4), 237–259.

AVMA (2012) *U.S. pet ownership & demographics sourcebook*. 2012 edition. Schaumburg, IL, American Veterinary Medicine Association.

Cassidy, R. (2007) Introduction. In: Cassidy, R & Mullin, M. (eds) *Where the wild things are now: domestication reconsidered*. Oxford, Berg, pp. 1–25.

Cottingham, J. (1978) A brute to the brutes? Descartes' treatment of animals. *Philosophy* 53 (206), 551–559.

Davis, S.J.M. & Valla, F.R. (1978) Evidence for domestication of the dog 12,000 years ago in the Natufian of Israel. *Nature* 276, 608–610.

Driscoll, C.A., Clutton-Brock, J., Kitchener, A.C. & O'Brien, S.J. (2009) The taming of the cat. *Scientific American* 300, 68–75.

FEDIAF (2010) *FEDIAF facts & figures 2010*. Brussels, European Pet Food Industry Federation.

Grier, K.C. (2006) *Pets in America: a history*. Orlando, FL, Harcourt.

Hansen, M. (2012) Danmarks civile Hundeførerforening har 75 års jubilæum. *DCH Bladet* 74 (04), 21–24.

Hartwell, S. (2003–2014) *A history of cat shows in Britain*. [Online] Available from: http://messybeast.com/showing.htm [Accessed 10 July 2014].

Hughes, J.D. (1996) Francis of Assisi and the diversity of creation. *Environmental Ethics* 18, 311–320.

Johnson, J. (n.d.). *A brief history of dog training*. [Online] Available from: https://k9densolutions.com/History_of_Dog_Training.html [Accessed 10 July 2014].

Kete, K. (1994) *The beast in the boudoir: petkeeping in nineteenth-century Paris*. Berkeley, CA, Los Angeles, CA & London, University of California Press.

Kitchell, K. (2011) Penelope's geese: pets of the ancients Greeks. *Expedition* 55 (3), 14–23.

Morey, D.F. (2006) Burying key evidence: the social bond between dogs and people. *Journal of Archaeological Science* 33, 158–175.

Pet Food Manufacturer's Association (n.d.) Pet data (1965–2004). [Online] Available from: http://www.pfma.org.uk/historical-pet-ownership-statistics/ [Accessed 21 March 2015].

O'Connor, T.P. (1992) Pets and pests in Roman and edieval Britain. *Mammal Review* 22 (2), 107–113.

Office for National Statistics. (2012) UK Population Totals 1851–2010 [Online] Available from: http://www.ons.gov.uk/ons/about-ons/business-transparency/freedom -of-information/what-can-i-request/published-ad-hoc-data/pop/june-2012/index.html [Accessed 21 March 2015].

Ralston Purina (2000) *The state of the American pet: a study among pet owners*. Ralston Purina, St. Louis, MO.

Ritvo, H. (1987) *The animal estate: the English and other creatures in the Victorian age*. Cambridge, MA, Harvard University Press.

Sampson, J. & Binns, M.M. (2006) The Kennel Club and the early history of dog shows and breed clubs. In: Ostrander, E.A., Giger, U. & Lindblad-Toh, K. (eds) *The dog and its genome*. Cold Spring Harbor, NY, Cold Spring Harbor Laboratory Press, pp. 19–30.

Serpell, J. (1996) *In the company of animals: a study of human-animal relations*. 2nd edition. Cambridge, UK, Cambridge University Press.

Serpell, J. (2000) Domestication and history of the cat. In: Turner, D.C. & Bateson, P.P.G.B. (eds) *The domestic cat: the biology of its behaviour*. 2nd edition. Cambridge, UK, Cambridge University Press, pp. 1–19.

Serpell, J.A. & Paul, E.S. (2011) Pets in the family: an evolutionary perspective. In: Salmon, C. & Shackleford, T.K. (eds) *The Oxford handbook of evolutionary family psychology*. Oxford, Oxford University Press, pp. 297–309.

Swabe, J. (1999) *Animals, disease and human society: human-animal relations and the rise of veterinary medicine*. London & New York, Routledge.

Thomas, K. (1984) *Man and the natural world: changing attitudes in England 1500-1800*. Harmondsworth, Penguin.

The Development and Role of the Veterinary and Other Professions in Relation to Companion Animals

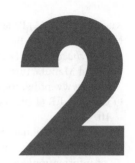

Co-author: Andrew Gardiner, BVM&S, Cert SAS, MSc, PhD, MRCVS,
Senior Lecturer

Royal (Dick) School of Veterinary Studies, The University of Edinburgh, Scotland, UK

2.1	Introduction	25
2.2	The Veterinary Profession	25
	2.2.1 Development of veterinary treatments	26
	2.2.2 Early development of companion animal veterinary practice	28
	2.2.3 Development of the veterinary profession and the rise of companion animal veterinary practice	30
	2.2.4 Role of the veterinary profession in setting ethical standards	32
2.3	Development and Role of Other Professions in Relation to Companion Animals	35
	2.3.1 Veterinary nurses and Veterinary technicians	36
	2.3.2 Behaviour therapists	37

Companion Animal Ethics, First Edition. Peter Sandøe, Sandra Corr and Clare Palmer.
© Universities Federation for Animal Welfare 2016.

2.1 Introduction

In Chapter 1 we saw how it became possible for many people in industrialised Western nations to keep cats, dogs, and other animals as companions. In this chapter, we consider how the veterinary profession evolved alongside these changes, and how these developments affected the lives of companion animals, and shaped emerging ethical concerns.

Take, for example, an issue such as the neutering of dogs. That people have their dogs neutered is to some extent driven by demand. However, this demand is enabled and encouraged by the availability of veterinary services and the activities of animal welfare organisations; across nations (e.g. United States vs. Sweden), the level of neutering of dogs is influenced by the different policies of the respective national veterinary associations (see Chapter 10).

The chapter also briefly considers two of the other most significant professions dealing with companion animals: veterinary nurses/technicians and behaviour therapists.

2.2 The Veterinary Profession

As an intellectual discipline and empirical practice, veterinary medicine arose from three factors that came together in the late eighteenth century: the idea of comparative anatomy, the pursuit of livestock improvement, and the commercial, military, and social role of horse power.

Human anatomy had been intensively studied in Europe from the fourteenth century. The similarity of humans to other animals was evident to very few people in 1600, but by 1700 'nearly everybody recognised it' (Fraser, 2008: p. 33). This new, comparative way of looking at human and animal bodies generated the same degree of intense interest and speculation throughout society that, for example, gene technology does today. However, the major stimulus for building and opening most European veterinary schools in the late eighteenth and nineteenth centuries was a devastating livestock disease that regularly wreaked havoc with national economies: cattle plague (also known as rinderpest and steppe murrain). Another major influence on the emergence of veterinary education was the wish to develop an improved approach to the health and productivity of the horse, whose labour kept society, industry and armies moving.

Against the background of these intellectual and economic drivers, different political regimes also shaped the development of veterinary education. In France and many other European countries, veterinary schools were mostly public institutions, founded and funded by the state; in Britain, they were initially private enterprises; in the United States, a mix of private and university-based schools developed, the latter mainly being associated with Land Grant universities in rural areas (Jones, 2003: pp. 49, 55). Nearly all European veterinary schools started in towns or cities, where many horses and cows (in large urban dairies) were to be found. There were also a great many dogs, and archival research into the caseloads of nineteenth-century veterinary schools shows that surprising numbers of dogs were treated at a time well before the main 'rise' of canine medicine in the 1930s (Gardiner, 2010: pp. 83–90).

However, until relatively recently, for a vet to focus exclusively on dogs suggested an unhealthy (even unmanly) sentimentality. Even by the middle decades of the twentieth century, to call someone 'a mere dog doctor' was a professional insult (Anon, 1947). Cats did not fully appear on the veterinary radar as a species in their own right (rather than as 'small dogs') until the 1960s. What changed, then, such that the majority of time spent by practising vets in the industrialised Western nations today is directed towards ensuring the health of companion animals, in what is now regarded as a highly prestigious field within clinical veterinary medicine?

Part of the answer, as we saw in Chapter 1, has to do with demographic changes, with middle-class families moving into suburban areas, and later with changes to the traditional family structure. Companion animals moved into homes and took up a place in human families and domestic life (Fudge, 2008). As people became wealthier after World War II, they were prepared (and able) to pay for more elaborate medical interventions to maintain the health of these new additions to the family, and as a result, companion animal medicine flourished (Swabe, 1999).

However, there are also other drivers behind this development; we will consider two of these here. First, technological developments allowed vets to do things to dogs and cats that were previously unheard of. We will consider two examples, one surgical (limb prostheses for dogs) and the other medical (the treatment of diabetes mellitus with insulin). Second, there were important developments in animal welfare and protection: various charities that cared about those in poverty and their companion animals adopted practices with much broader ramifications for companion animal veterinary care. We will illustrate this by discussing the pivotal role played by the British charity, the People's Dispensary for Sick Animals (PDSA).

2.2.1 Development of veterinary treatments

Although currently considered 'cutting edge', and the subject of some ethical debate (see Chapter 12), the fitting of limb prostheses to dogs has a long medical history. The procedure was originally described in a textbook first published in 1900 (Hobday, 1900a). As general anaesthesia (with chloroform) was being used more often and was proving safe and practicable (Hobday, 1900b), dogs with crippling leg problems could have their damaged limbs removed. Fitting a prosthesis after limb amputation was a straightforward example of translational medicine – treating canine orthopaedic patients like human ones. And, just as in people, the quality and cosmetic appearance of the prosthesis depended on the socioeconomic status of the animal's owner (Hobday, 1906: pp. 343–347).

However, the fashion for canine prosthetic limbs declined as vets realised that dogs appeared to cope well without one, and occasionally even two, legs. Recently, interest in canine limb prostheses has re-emerged, and advanced prosthetics (intra-osseous transcutaneous amputation prostheses, or ITAPs) are being developed for both dogs and cats, and human beings (see Chapter 12 for an ethical discussion of 'novel' treatments and 'overtreatment').

The development of limb prostheses for dogs may sound like a fairly straightforward example of a development or discovery (safer anaesthesia in this case) making a new form of treatment possible (the ability to amputate a dog's damaged leg and subsequently fit a prosthesis). However, the process by which clinical signs become recognized as a 'disease' that should be 'treated' is actually rather complex, involving social, economic, political and cultural factors. Diseases such as rabies in dogs and foot-and-mouth disease in cattle are interpreted through political, economic and cultural lenses that make them much more than simply physical signs of illness and pathologies (Pemberton and Worboys, 2007; Woods, 2004). Seen from this perspective, diseases are not simply 'discovered' but are the results of a social process – a kind of 'framing' of a group of clinical signs as a disease that can and should be treated in particular ways.

One of the important consequences of calling something a 'disease' is that it may imply a prospect for treatment or intervention where none existed before, potentially generating new ethical issues. Either withholding a treatment, or administering one that is experimental or has unpleasant side effects, may raise ethical questions. For example, does the ability to fit complex limb prostheses to dogs and cats mean that it is right to do so? Given the availability of a preventive vaccine for parvovirus, should an owner be castigated for electing *not* to have their dog immunised?

The transfer of technology and procedures from human to veterinary medicine is an important and recurring theme in the development of the profession. But the direction of transfer from human to animal often turns out to be more complex than it first appears. This is illustrated in the second brief case study.

Diabetes mellitus, caused by lack of the pancreatic hormone insulin, was first treated in 1922, when a seriously ill 14-year-old boy, Leonard Thompson, was injected with a crude substance derived from bovine pancreases (Bliss, 1984). A few days previously, a small crossbreed dog called Marjorie had received the same treatment for her own diabetes (although Marjorie's diabetes had been created experimentally by removing part of her pancreas). Leonard initially received a 'dog dose' of the extract based on comparison of his and Marjorie's weights. In this sense, Leonard was treated 'like a dog' and the translation of medical treatment was the opposite of that seen with limb prostheses, that is, dog → human (insulin), rather than human → dog (prosthetic limb). The discovery of insulin became one of the iconic discoveries of modern medicine, and Marjorie became a 'canine heroine', featuring on stamps and other memorabilia across the world (Gardiner, 2006a,b).

In the development of insulin, the dogs (Marjorie was just one of many) were models and research tools rather than patients in their own right. However, the distinction was sometimes blurred: Marjorie became a companion animal to the lead researcher Frederick Banting, who was reportedly deeply upset when she had to be euthanased. The first dog to receive insulin as a patient (rather than an experimental subject) was probably treated in Ithaca in 1923, around 14 months after insulin's discovery: she survived for 5 months, before being euthanased because of complications (Milks, 1932).

The introduction of insulin therapy into clinical veterinary medicine was, therefore, more complicated than the simple unidirectional movement of the new technology of prosthetics. It followed a pattern of: animal model in human medicine → clinical treatment established in human medicine → clinical treatment moves across to veterinary medicine. Transfer back into clinical veterinary medicine presupposes the demand for advanced medical treatment of animals; this demand was generated through the development of companion animal veterinary practice as a major branch of veterinary medicine, to which we shall now turn.

2.2.2 Early development of companion animal veterinary practice

It is often assumed that the rapid expansion of companion animal practice in Britain and in other Western countries was a post-war activity, associated with economic recovery and urbanisation. The formation of the British Small Animal Veterinary Association (BSAVA) in 1957 fits with this chronology. However, in another important sense, there was a great deal of companion animal practice taking place in the United Kingdom earlier, in the 1920s and 1930s. This activity is largely ignored in 'official' histories of the British profession (e.g. BSAVA, 2007) because it happened outside the veterinary profession itself, in charity animal clinics staffed by unqualified practitioners, that is, individuals who were not members of the Royal College of Veterinary Surgeons (RCVS). Nevertheless, the emergence of this activity, and the profession's response to it, was central in defining what companion animal practice would later become.

Clinical activity by individuals who were not veterinary surgeons was possible because, until the second Veterinary Surgeons Act of 1948 in Britain, the veterinary profession did not have a legal monopoly on the treatment of animal disease, only on the use of the specific title 'veterinary surgeon'. In fact, many individuals without veterinary qualifications were successfully treating animal disease. They were free from prosecution as long as they were careful in how they described their animal-curing activities (a similar situation had existed in other health professions, e.g. dentistry). Some of these individuals were undoubtedly very skilled. In 1926, Captain R. Cornish-Bowden MRCVS, reporting to a committee of the RCVS, described an unqualified practitioner he had seen working at premises at Commercial Street, London, belonging to the People's Dispensary for Sick Animals (PDSA). On the day of his visit, more than 100 people and their animals were waiting to be seen:

> The gentleman I saw alleviating the suffering of these animals was a 'quack', but he had a better means of studying the sickness of animals than was ever accorded to me at the Royal Veterinary College. He had 30 years' experience attending small animals; the work he was doing was excellent; he handled his animals with a great deal more care and skill than many veterinary surgeons I have seen.
>
> (Cornish-Bowden, 1926)

Some animal charities had a policy of employing vets, but the largest organisation that focused on treatment of companion animals, the PDSA, established in 1917, initially had a policy of *not* employing them. This arose from the very poor relations between the charity's founder, Maria Dickin, and the British veterinary establishment. Dickin was frequently outspoken in the press and never held back from criticising what she saw as the veterinary profession's poor response to the treatment of animals whose owners could not afford to pay. She felt there was a need for a large-scale social programme to treat the animals of the poor. In 1931, she criticised both the RSPCA and the veterinary profession for failing to respond to this need and, instead, attacking her own organisation:

> If you are so concerned about the proper treatment of Sick Animals of the Poor, open your own dispensaries; open them everywhere for there are vast factory, mining, manufacturing and dockland areas where nothing at all exists to help the Sick Animal. [...] Live among it as we do. [...] Do the same work we are doing. Instead of spending your energy and time in hindering us, spend it in dealing with this mass of misery.
>
> (Dickin, 1931)

Maria Dickin's uncompromising stance towards employing non-vets undermined veterinary professional expertise and authority. When the charity was very small, this was not very significant, but the situation became more problematical for the veterinary profession in the light of the charity's hugely successful fundraising efforts and increased exposure within society throughout the 1920s and 1930s, when it became affectionately known as the 'Poor Doggers Salvation Army' and was supported by many prominent figures in politics, the aristocracy and the British royal family (Figure 2.1).

The PDSA challenged the mainstream veterinary profession, not only by using unqualified staff in its clinics, but also by defining a form of veterinary medicine that the

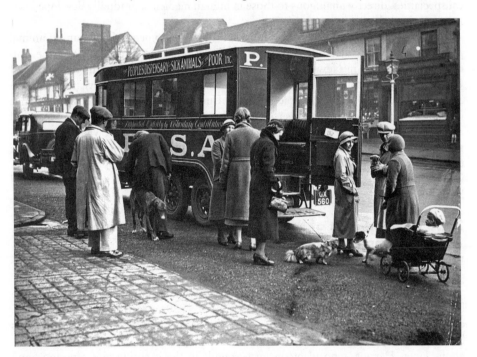

Figure 2.1 Pet owners awaiting treatment from the PDSA Caravan in the 1940s. (*PDSA. Reproduced with permission from the PDSA.*)

veterinary profession itself had not yet fully envisaged: one modelled on the ideals of the human voluntary hospital, focusing on urban, companion animals, and operating on a very large scale indeed, treating up to 750,000 animals per year. It must be remembered that, in terms of professional focus, dogs and cats were ranked far below the animal at the centre of the eighteenth- and nineteenth-century veterinary universe – the horse. In a very real sense, the veterinary profession used horses to help forge a professional identity. This happened to such an extent that, when horse transport went into decline, the profession faced an identity crisis because no other species was thought to match up to the superior qualities of this animal. Some predicted that the profession would itself cease to exist. In this regard, the mainstream profession underestimated the potential of companion animal practice as a worthy professional activity and, for a time, there became a risk that it would remain outwith the profession's control, in unqualified practitioners' hands (Gardiner, 2014).

The change of focus in the veterinary profession towards the small companion animal required a cognitive shift, whereby the profession stopped seeing small animal work as a peripheral activity, based on over-sentimentality and 'pandering', and instead recognized it as a specialty of considerable potential and prestige. The dog – and later the cat – became viewed as patients whose treatment need not be limited by the harsh economic constraints of the agricultural sector, and science and sentiment became linked in a promising new future for veterinary medicine. As a result, a host of veterinary clinical specialties, directly analogous to those in human medicine, gradually developed (see more on this below).

Animal protection societies also influenced the development of companion animal practice in other countries. The Angel Memorial Animal Hospital in Boston, the Animal Medical Centre in New York, and the San Francisco Society for the Prevention of Cruelty to Animals (SPCA) – all highly prestigious institutions which have helped set the agenda for companion animal practice in the United States – had strong backgrounds in charitable provision, analogous to that of the PDSA in Britain. The Angel Memorial and the Animal Medical Centre are now world-renowned academic veterinary hospitals, but their origins were in the charitable movements dating from the first half of the twentieth century, treating animals belonging to the urban poor. Similarly, the PDSA is now a highly respected animal welfare charity with a network of modern pet aid hospitals and clinics across Britain.

2.2.3 Development of the veterinary profession and the rise of companion animal veterinary practice

In the second half of the twentieth century, the veterinary profession underwent some significant changes in all industrialised Western countries.

One major change was that companion animal veterinary practice expanded to become the largest area of veterinary activity. In the 1930s, practices were often mixed, combining companion animals, farm animals and horses. However, gradually practices became more specialized and the traditional multi-species vet, as portrayed in books about James Herriot, who went on farm rounds in the morning and afternoon and attended to dogs and cats in the evening, became far less common. Vets who want to go into practice now typically focus on particular species fairly early in their careers, the majority of them going into companion animal practice. That said, traditional mixed practices are still found in more rural areas.

There has also been a substantial change in the structure and organisation of veterinary practices. Before 1950, most UK and North American veterinary practices were small, either single-handed, or with just one or two vets. In 2009, in the United Kingdom, the average practice employed a mean of 4.2 full-time veterinary assistants or employees, and far fewer practices were owned by sole principals – this figure had nearly halved in the United Kingdom since 2002 (Tartan Business Solutions, 2009). The number of corporate practices (i.e., owned by a company rather than an individual or group of individuals) was small, estimated to be 6% in United States and 11% in United Kingdom in 2009, but was predicted to grow (Tartan Business Solutions, 2009). This indeed seems to be occurring: By the beginning of 2015, Banfield, for example, the largest of these corporate practices, owned more than 900 clinics and employed more than 3200 vets in the United States and Puerto Rico (Banfield 2015).

Another significant change was demographic: the profession changed from being mainly male and rural to become mainly urban and female. Since 2004, applications to veterinary schools in the United States have been around 80% female; Lincoln (2010) lists possible explanations for this (beyond reduced admission discrimination), including technological improvements such as in animal restraint, more flexible working hours, and more female role models. A similar situation exists in the United Kingdom. According to a 2010 RCVS survey of the profession, only 24% of students who started their degree, and 21% who obtained their degree in 2009 were male (RCVS, 2011).

A third significant change has been the development of specialization within the companion animal field. In most countries, governing bodies accredit or register vets, to allow them to practice legally. In the United Kingdom, the RCVS plays this role. In the United States, accreditation is regulated state-by-state through veterinary practice acts, and corresponding departments of professional regulation and state boards. Within the profession, there are also associations reflecting different clinical or species interests. For example, in the United Kingdom, the vets working with companion animals often belong to the BSAVA. The BSAVA was founded in 1957 by a group of London-based vets who were interested in developing and promoting the field of dog and cat treatment. In the United States, formal professional organisation around small animals started earlier – the American Animal Hospital Association was founded in 1933.

Within UK companion animal practice, clinical specialization developed from the 1950s to 1960s in areas such as radiology and small animal orthopaedics (Vaughan, 2007). More recently, an expanding range of postgraduate qualifications has been established and is administered by bodies such as the European College of Veterinary Surgery and the American College of Veterinary Internal Medicine. So-called Board-certified Diplomates of these colleges act as specialist consultants and may work in referral-only practices, seeing more complex cases. Data from the AVMA show that there were 11,761 active board-certified Diplomates in 2014 (an increase of 38.36% since 2006), which, they suggest, responds to the demand for a higher level of care by animal owners (Gail Golab, AVMA, Personal Communication).

The growing importance of small animal practice, and the development of specializations within the field, paralleled the increasing perception that veterinary practices are, or should be, profitable businesses. Within veterinary education, elements of business training are now increasingly provided as part of a new subject group called 'professional skills', taught alongside more traditional subjects such as anatomy and pathology. For example, students at Nottingham Veterinary School in the United Kingdom are introduced to the concepts of the veterinary business early in year 1, and during their fourth year, they have a 2-week module covering key concepts of veterinary business and management including strategy, finances, the veterinary team, and clinical governance. This type of approach is replicated at the other veterinary schools around the world, reflecting how the core veterinary curriculum has changed in response to perceived future needs (Gardiner & Rhind, 2013).

The development of veterinary specializations leading to new, complex animal treatments raises some ethical questions about appropriate treatment, and potential overtreatment (see Chapter 12). The role of veterinary practices as profit-making businesses inevitably raises the possibility of conflict between the interests of the practices' human clients and their animal patients, and the success of the business. This, in turn, highlights the need for professional regulation, particularly with respect to professional ethics (Figure 2.2a and b).

2.2.4 Role of the veterinary profession in setting ethical standards

As noted above, in order to practice, a vet must not only hold a veterinary degree (obtained by university examination), but also be accredited or registered by a professional governing body (e.g. the RCVS in the United Kingdom or departments of state governments that are responsible for professional regulation in the United States). Gaining – and maintaining – a license to practice requires that a vet meets certain professional and ethical standards. Declarations, which are often made upon graduation, typically include language that is broadly descriptive of the expectations underlying such standards. In the United States, the veterinarian's oath currently (2015) has the following wording:

> Being admitted to the profession of veterinary medicine, I solemnly swear to use my scientific knowledge and skills for the benefit of society through the protection of animal health and welfare, the prevention and relief of animal suffering, the conservation of animal resources, the promotion of public health, and the advancement of medical knowledge.
>
> I will practice my profession conscientiously, with dignity, and in keeping with the principles of veterinary medical ethics.
>
> I accept as a lifelong obligation the continual improvement of my professional knowledge and competence.
>
> (AVMA, 2010)

This oath, drafted by the AVMA, expresses the ethos of the profession, and is a core part of professional identity. A similar declaration is signed as part of registration by the RCVS in the United Kingdom, and many other national veterinary associations.

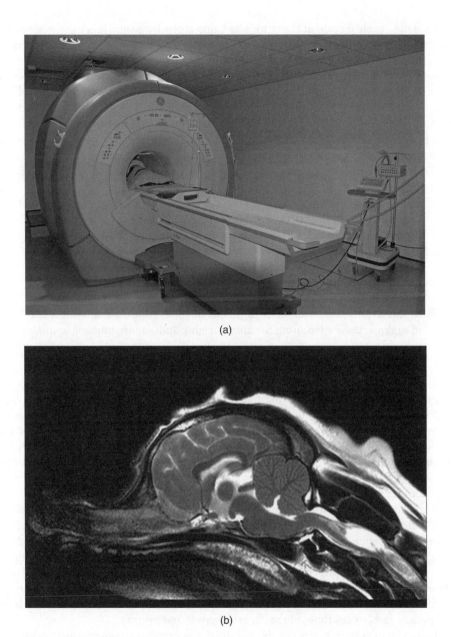

(a)

(b)

Figure 2.2 (a) An anaesthetized dog undergoes an MRI scan of its brain in a modern Veterinary Hospital. (b) MRI of a Cavalier King Charles Spaniel with Chiari malformation and secondary syringomyelia. Due to the abnormally shaped skull in this breed, there is an increased risk of pressure building up causing an abnormal flow of cerebrospinal fluid; affected dogs often have neck pain, and frequently scratch the neck and shoulder areas. (Images used courtesy of Sandra Corr.)

One noticeable feature of the oath is its value-laden language. It is clearly not just a contract defining what vets are obliged to do in return for the social privileges they have, such as to be permitted to treat other people's animals. It is the statement of a morally defined mission: vets are not just here to make a living, but are expected to benefit society through the scientific knowledge and skills they have acquired, to protect animal welfare and to adhere to 'the principles of veterinary medical ethics' – a multifaceted code of professional conduct, defined by the AVMA. The requirement to protect animal welfare was new to the version of the oath agreed in 2010, clearly reflecting both a shift in what society expects from vets, and how vets understand their own profession.

This shift is clearly recognized in the official history of the AVMA, published on the occasion of AVMA's 150th year anniversary in 2013:

> Until the late 1970s, veterinarians and the AVMA were considered author-
> ities on the acceptable uses and treatment of animals. However, activists
> inside and outside the veterinary profession began challenging the notion
> that veterinarians alone could speak about animal welfare, as they pressed
> for reforms in the treatment of animals by the research and agricultural
> industries. This dissent would evolve into ever increasing public criticism
> of the AVMA for a lack of engagement in these issues, along with a rise
> in organizations advocating for animal rights and a more humane animal-
> use ethic.
>
> (AVMA, 2012)

Such external pressures, shifting public attitudes, and the changing demographics and focus of the profession itself, led the veterinary profession in the United States to move away from a more anthropocentric view, according to which the sole role of the profession was to protect human interests linked to animal use, towards a view where animals mattered in their own right. A number of factors played a role in this movement, one of which was a shift in focus in the veterinary profession from agricultural animals kept for use, to animals kept as companions.

The US veterinary oath contains a reference to 'principles of veterinary ethics' to which the vet must adhere. The first principle in the current version issued by the AVMA states that "A veterinarian shall be dedicated to providing competent veterinary medical care, with compassion and respect for animal welfare and human health." Annotations are used to clarify the principles and, in this case, an annotation indicates 'Veterinarians should first consider the needs of the patient: to prevent and relieve disease, suffering, or disability while minimizing pain or fear' (AVMA, n.d.). Here, clearly, the needs of the patient rather than those of the client are given first priority.

However, of course, this is not the full story. Annotations to other principles clearly set limits to the obligations that vets have towards patients. For example, one of those annotations clarifies that even though vets have an ethical obligation to help critically ill animals, 'such emergency care may be limited to euthanasia to relieve suffering, or to stabilization of the patient for transport to another source of animal care'. The point of this annotation is to protect the interests of the vet by limiting the amount of unpaid work that she or he will have to deliver to help a critically ill animal when there is no client who is willing or able to pay for it.

The preferences of human clients are also given considerable weight in the principles and policies of the AVMA. For example, relevant AVMA policies do not condemn vets who conduct and make an income from so-called convenience surgeries, such as the declawing of cats, even though these surgeries do not directly benefit the animals but rather are undertaken to satisfy the preferences of their human clients (see Chapter 11). This suggests that although the AVMA is moving towards an emphasis on animal welfare, it still acknowledges the preferences of the animals' owners, and the economic interests of vets themselves, which can lead to dilemmas in terms of animal treatment (something common to members of veterinary associations internationally).

However, as will become apparent in later chapters, there are clear differences between different national veterinary associations with respect to issues such as convenience surgery, neutering and limits to veterinary treatment. For example, kidney transplantation in cats, where a kidney is taken from a healthy donor animal, is accepted in the United States, but so far has been resisted by the veterinary profession in the United Kingdom (see Chapter 12).

Such principles and other policy statements also serve as a form of self-regulation. Members of the veterinary profession now have the privilege of being the only ones allowed to provide medicine, surgery and other forms of veterinary treatment to other people's animals. Given this, potential clients should reasonably expect competent and fair treatment when they visit a vet. To avoid external state regulation by those who do not really understand the profession and may undermine professional autonomy, it is clearly in the interest of the profession to try to self-regulate (Rollin, 2006: p. 13; also see Chapter 16). So, many principles and policies set up by AVMA and veterinary organisations in other countries are created to ensure consistent high standards in veterinary practice, and either encourage (in the USA) or require (in the UK) practising vets to regularly update their knowledge and skills. These policies include systems for formal complaints about issues such as malpractice and for the sanction of vets who do not comply.

Traditionally, most of what was found in the ethical principles and policies defined by veterinary organisations dealt with questions of etiquette (Rollin, 2006: p. 12) and mainly served to protect veterinary practitioners from inappropriate behaviour by colleagues. While some of this remains, the focus more recently has been on responsibilities towards animal patients and human clients.

Although the veterinary profession clearly has its own, vested interests, it has been centrally important in developing companion animal ethics, both in terms of generating new ethical questions about living with companion animals, and in thinking about how to address those questions.

2.3 Development and Role of Other Professions in Relation to Companion Animals

Vets form a profession by sharing certain key characteristics: they have the same higher education; they are organised in national organisations; they have exclusive privilege to deliver certain services, including veterinary treatment of companion animals; and as a group, they have a more or less well-defined set of professional norms. Furthermore, they are also viewed and recognised by the public as professionals along with medical doctors and lawyers.

There are no other professions dealing with companion animals as old, coherent and well-defined as the veterinary profession. However, after World War II, a number of other groups delivering assistance to companion animals and their owners have gradually emerged with a profession-like profile such as veterinary nurses/veterinary technicians, behaviour therapists, animal physiotherapists and dog groomers. We here focus on the first two of these.

2.3.1 Veterinary nurses and Veterinary technicians

In the early male-dominated profession of largely single-handed practitioners, nursing assistance was often provided by the vet's wife. This began to change in the 1920s when several British vets focused on canine patients, mostly practising in London, employed 'canine nurses'. However, these were unusual and elite metropolitan practitioners, probably not very representative of the profession as a whole.

Additionally, there was resistance from within the RCVS to formal recognition of the title 'Canine Nurse', probably because the veterinary profession itself was still fighting to attain a legal monopoly on animal treatment, and facing stiff competition from the PDSA. Only after World War II, was there a gradual formalisation and expansion of veterinary nursing. One of the first indicators of this was the addition of a short nursing chapter to the fifth edition of *Hobday's Surgical Diseases of the Dog and Cat* (McCunn, 1947: pp. 410–415). The author, Phyllis Peake, was uniquely qualified to write this, being both a human nurse and a veterinary surgeon. There was, however, no formal qualification in the United Kingdom until the RCVS set up the Animal Nursing Auxiliary (ANA) training scheme in 1961. The term 'veterinary nurse' was in use from 1984, but it was not until 1991 that the Veterinary Surgeons Act 1966 was amended and the role of the veterinary nurse became formally recognised in British law (Pullen, 2006).

Both the role of veterinary nurses, and their professional organisation and career options, have evolved in line with the rest of the veterinary profession, and specialisation within nursing by species (equine/small animal) and discipline (medicine/surgery) is well established. A non-statutory register of veterinary nurses in the United Kingdom was begun in 2007, and in 2012, their new code of professional conduct included a declaration to be made upon registration which begins with the words: 'Veterinary nurses must make animal health and welfare their first consideration when attending to animals' (RCVS, 2014). A professional disciplinary system, as with vets, is also in place.

In the United States, the North American Veterinary Technician Association (NAVTA) was formed in 1981 (NAVTA, n.d.), and in 1992, it was recognised by the AVMA as the national association representing veterinary technicians. Broadly similar ethical guidelines apply to the role of veterinary technicians as to veterinary nurses (NAVTA, 2007). Similar developments have taken place in other industrialised Western countries, including Australia and New Zealand.

Much of the content of the codes and declarations relating to the veterinary nursing and technician professions is very similar to relevant parts of the veterinary profession. However, some small differences do seem to emerge. The nursing and technician professions, to a greater extent than the veterinary profession, emphasise care and emotional support to animals and their owners. The NAVTA code for animal technicians, for example, states that 'veterinary technicians shall strive to understand, support, and promote the human-animal bond', signalling an ethical approach based on relations rather than solely on consequences for animal welfare (see Chapter 5).

2.3.2 Behaviour therapists

Those who help owners of companion animals to deal with behavioural problems on a commercial or semi-commercial basis constitute by far the youngest and the most heterogeneous of the professions we consider here. While professional dog training began in the early twentieth century (see Chapter 9), it was not initially focused on solving behaviour problems. In fact, professional activity aimed specifically at dealing with behaviour problems in dogs and cats does not seem to have begun until the 1970s. According to one account, 'the profession of "pet behaviour counsellor", or "companion animal behaviour therapist", and similar titles, first appeared in the UK in the late 1970s' (ASAB, 2001).

From the outset, three groups were involved in developing the field: those with an academic background in comparative psychology or zoology, those who developed an interest in behaviour therapy out of dog training, and, finally, vets with a special interest in animal behaviour (Hecht, n.d.). These three groups developed organisational structures, certification schemes and professional identities more or less in parallel. However, unlike vets and veterinary nurses, there is no required certification: the title 'behaviour therapist' is not protected.

There are some potential and real dividing lines between these groups. One concerns the role of science and evidence. An expert in the field nicely describes this in the following way:

> The practice of animal behaviour therapy is both an art and a science. It has become a popular area of employment, with a caché rather like that of some affluent people hiring a personal fitness trainer. Many of those who offer behavioural services have no formal biological or clinical training, yet are free in describing themselves as "behaviourists", "behaviour consultants", "dog listeners", etc. There is conflict between veterinary and scientifically trained practitioners versus those who come to the field as a vocation or as a pleasant, profitable route to self-employment.
>
> (Mugford, 2007: p. 232)

One important difference between the veterinary behaviour therapists and the other groups is that only the vets are allowed to prescribe drugs. This may be linked to another dividing line concerning whether behaviour problems are primarily viewed as illnesses or as normal forms of behaviour that are inconvenient or harmful to the owners (Hart, Hart & Bain, 2006). However, it is important to stress first that some behaviour problems clearly are rooted in illnesses, and secondly that many vets who specialise in behaviour problems share the view that most behaviour problems are not signs of disease, and are not primarily to be treated with medication.

So, behaviour therapy as a profession is still in its very early stages, and according to Mugford, the big challenge ahead:

> ... lies in integrating this young discipline with everyday education and practice of veterinarians and to 'professionalize' the quality, conduct and content of services provided by behaviour therapists who do not have veterinary qualifications... Most professions have agreed, tried and tested approaches, for example to cardiac surgery, dentistry or even car repair. However, the practice of animal behaviour therapy is remarkable for the diversity of methods and their underlying theoretical assumptions.
>
> (Mugford, 2007: p. 233)

So, while it seems as though professional standards for people acting as behaviour therapists are necessary, these are not likely to be forthcoming for the profession as a whole. Rather they will emerge within the different groups here described, and common professional standards will have to await the emergence of a more unified profession.

Key Points

- The first veterinary schools became established in the eighteenth century, mainly to treat agricultural animals and working horses.
- Animal welfare charities were instrumental in shaping the development of companion animal treatment in the early twentieth century.
- In the second half of the twentieth century, the focus of the veterinary profession changed dramatically and vets began to treat companion animals in large numbers.
- In the twenty-first century, a number of other professions, including veterinary nursing/ technicians, physiotherapy, animal behaviour therapy, and dog grooming, are developing, with varying degrees of regulated membership and ethical requirements.
- Increasing specialisation within the veterinary profession and the availability of advanced treatments for animals raises novel ethical questions about treatment decisions.
- The perception of veterinary practice as a business similarly raises ethical challenges.

References

Anon (1947) The clinician is important. *Veterinary Journal* 103, 155.

ASAB (2001) *Working Party on the certification of clinical animal behaviourists: final report.* Association for the Study of Animal Behaviour. [Online] Available from: http://asab. nottingham.ac.uk/downloads/certificationreport.pdf [Accessed 14 September 2014].

AVMA (2010) *Veterinarian's oath.* [Online] Available from: https://www.avma.org/KB /Policies/Pages/veterinarians-oath.aspx [Accessed 14 September 2014].

AVMA (2012) *The AVMA: 150 years of education, science, and service (Volume 4).* Schaumburg, IL, American Veterinary Medical Association.

AVMA (n.d.) *Principles of veterinary medical ethics of the AVMA*. [Online] Available from: https://www.avma.org/KB/Policies/Pages/Principles-of-Veterinary-Medical-Ethics-of-the-AVMA.aspx [Accessed 22 February 2015].

Banfield (2015) *Banfield Pet Hospital® Announces Vincent Bradley as New President and Chief Executive Officer*. [Online] Available from: http://www.banfield.com/about-us/news-room/news-archives/banfield-pet-hospital®-announces-vincent-bradley-a [Accessed 26 February 2015].

Bliss M. (1984) *The discovery of insulin*. Toronto, McClelland and Stewart.

BSAVA (2007) *British Small Animal Veterinary Association: supporting, representing and leading the profession for fifty years*. Gloucester, BSAVA.

Cornish-Bowden, R. (1926) The veterinary profession and poor people's clinics. *Veterinary Record* 6, 530–531.

Dickin, M. E. (1931) *The PDSA, the RCVS and the RSPCA. To the Supporters of the PDSA*. London, PDSA.

Fraser, D. (2008) *Understanding animal welfare: the science in its cultural context*. Oxford, Wiley-Blackwell.

Fudge, E. (2008) *Pets*. Stocksfield, Acumen.

Gardiner, A. (2006a) The canine history of diabetes mellitus: part 1 diabetes before insulin. *Veterinary Times* 36, 10–12.

Gardiner, A. (2006b) The canine history of diabetes mellitus: part 2 diabetes after insulin. *Veterinary Times* 36, 12–15.

Gardiner, A. (2010) *Small animal practice in British veterinary medicine: 1920–56*. PhD thesis. Manchester, University of Manchester.

Gardiner, A. & Rhind, S. (2013) Taking a history on veterinary education. *Veterinary Record* 173, 388–393.

Gardiner, A. (2014) The 'dangerous' women of animal welfare: how British veterinary medicine went to the dogs. *Social History of Medicine* 27(3): 466–487. doi: 10.1093/shm /hkt101 [Accessed 14 September 2014].

Hart, B.L., Hart, L.A. & Bain, M.J. (2006) *Canine and feline behavior therapy*. 2nd edition. Ames, IA, Blackwell Publishing.

Hecht, J. (n.d.) *So, you want to become an animal behaviourist?* [Online] Available from: http://www.patriciamcconnell.com/sites/default/files/So%2C%20you%20want%20to%20become%20an%20animal%20%20behaviorist%3F.pdf [Accessed 14 September 2014].

Hobday, F. (1900a) *Surgical diseases of the dog*. London, Baillière Tindall & Cox.

Hobday, F. (1900b) The choice of general anaesthetic for surgical purposes. *Veterinary Record* XII(64), 599–601.

Hobday, F. (1906) *Surgical diseases of the dog and cat and anaesthetics*. London, Baillière Tindall & Cox.

Jones, S.D. (2003) *Valuing animals: veterinarians and their patients in modern America*. Baltimore, MD, Johns Hopkins University Press.

Lincoln, A.E. (2010) The shifting supply of men and women to occupations: feminisation in veterinary education. *Social Forces* 88(5), 1969–1998

McCunn, J. (1947) *Hobday's surgical diseases of the dog and cat*. 5th edition. London, Baillière Tindall & Cox.

Milks, H.J. (1932) Some cases of diabetes in dogs. *Journal of the American Veterinary Medical Association* 34 (5), 620–626.

Mugford, R.A. (2007) Behavioural disorders of dogs. In: Jensen, P. (ed.) *The behavioural biology of dogs*. Wallingford & Cambridge, UK, CABI, pp. 225–242.

NAVTA (n.d.) *About NAVTA*. The National Association of Veterinary Technicians in America [Online] Available from: https://www.navta.net/about-navta/about [Accessed 14 September 2014].

NAVTA (2007) *Veterinary technician code of ethics*. [Online] Available from: http://www.navta.net/files/navta_vt_code_of_ethics_07.pdf [Accessed 14 September 2014].

Pemberton, N. & Worboys, M. (2007) *Mad Dogs and Englishmen. Rabies in Britain 1830–2000*. Basingstoke, Palgrave Macmillan.

Pullen, S. (2006) Veterinary nursing: the road to professionalism. In: Pullen, S. & Gray, C. (eds) *Ethics, law and the veterinary nurse*. Philadelphia, PA, Elsevier, pp. 1–10.

Rollin, B. (2006) *An introduction to veterinary medical ethics: theory and cases*. Oxford, Blackwell.

RCVS (2011) *RCVS survey of the veterinary professions 2010*. Royal College of Veterinary Surgeons. [Online] Available from: http://www.rcvs.org.uk/document-library/rcvs-survey-of-the-veterinary-professions-2010/ [Accessed 14 September 2014].

RCVS (2014) *Code of professional conduct for veterinary nurses*. Royal College of Veterinary Surgeons. [Online] Available from: http://www.rcvs.org.uk/advice-and-guidance/code-of-professional-conduct-for-veterinary-nurses/ [Accessed 14 September 2014].

Swabe, J.M. (1999) *Animals, disease and human society: human-animal relations and the rise of veterinary medicine*. London, Routledge.

Tartan Business Solutions (2009) *Corporate veterinary practice in the UK, the Netherlands and Switzerland*. [Online] Available from: http://www.fve.org/members/uevp/pdf/working_documents/presentations/UK%20corporate%20veterinary%20practices_ross_tiffin.pdf [Accessed 14 September 2014].

Vaughan, L.C. (2007) A review of the history of small animal orthopaedics: 1950-2006. *Veterinary History* 13 (4), 310–338.

Woods, A. (2004) *A manufactured plague. The history of foot and mouth disease in Britain*. London, Earthscan.

Human Attachment to Companion Animals

3

Co-authors: Iben Meyer, DVM, PhD[1] and James A. Serpell, PhD[2]

[1] Postdoctoral Fellow, Department of Large Animal Sciences, University of Copenhagen, Copenhagen, Denmark
[2] Marie A Moore Professor of Animal Ethics and Welfare, Director, Center for the Interaction of Animals and Society, School of Veterinary Medicine, University of Pennsylvania, Philadelphia, PA, USA

3.1 Introduction   41
3.2 What People Do with Their Companions   42
3.3 Relating to Companion Animals   46
3.4 Effects on Human Health   52

3.1 Introduction

Companion animals are distinctive by virtue of their relationship with their human owners and other co-habitants. Although they may have other roles too, dogs, cats and other companion animals play a part in the personal and emotional lives of the humans with whom they live and interact. The relationship is often described by using expressions such as 'friends' or 'family', terms otherwise reserved for important relations between human beings.

The relationship between humans and companion animals is sometimes understood in terms of a special bond between the human and the animal; the 'human-companion animal bond'. While it is very difficult to know how the companion animal experiences this bond (Prato-Previde *et al.*, 2003), much more is known about how the human attaches to the companion animal – which is the focus of this chapter. We will try to understand the ways in which people interact with, and become attached to their companion animals, and we will also look at how this affects their well-being and health. In passing, we will also consider some of the consequences for the well-being of the animals. However, our main discussion of companion animal welfare and how to assess it is in Chapter 4.

The main focus of this chapter is on human attachment to dogs and cats. Of course, people also keep other species such as guinea pigs, rabbits or various birds for companionship. However, it is fair to say that dogs and cats are the typical companion animals. Unlike the other animals that fill the role of companions, dogs and, to a lesser extent, cats, are highly domesticated and a key part of their domestication has been to fit into the niche of co-habiting with humans.

Dogs and cats, unlike most other types of companion species, are usually allowed to move freely around – at least within the house – because they can relatively easily be housetrained and, in the case of dogs (and to a lesser degree cats), they can also be trained to obey instructions. Together with their highly expressive natures, and sensitivity to human nonverbal communication signals, this enables these animals to easily achieve particularly close bonds with their human co-habitants.

In the following section, we outline the diversity of activities through which people bond with their animal companions. Then, we survey the psychological literature on human attachments to companion animals, to try to gain a deeper understanding of how companions matter to their human owners. Finally, we briefly review the potential beneficial, or harmful, psychological and other health effects that humans may experience as a result of their relation to companion animals.

3.2 What People Do with Their Companions

Attachment typically develops through doing things together, so an overview of the ways in which people engage with their companion animals is a useful starting point for this chapter.

As already mentioned, the dog was the first animal to be domesticated, and historically, human relations to dogs have developed through very practical shared activities. Evidence suggests that people used dogs for guarding and hunting more than 8000 years ago (Miklósi, 2007: p. 56). With the emergence of agricultural societies, dogs' roles diversified, and there is evidence that different strains of dogs were then bred for different tasks, such as hunting, herding, guarding, warfare and providing companionship (Brewer, Clark & Phillips, 2001; Miklósi, 2007).

Many of these classic tasks are still performed by working dogs, but some dogs primarily kept as companions also carry out similar tasks. For example, companion dogs are used in recreational hunting, for herding by those with hobby farms, in competitive sports, or are trained for police or military-type work as a sport. Many people take their young dogs or puppies to obedience training as part of their upbringing, and then continue to other types of competitive activities, such as agility. Finally, owners may enter their dog in shows, where they are assessed both for how well they meet breed standards, and how they behave when presented in the show ring.

A dog sport can develop into a 'culture of commitment' which, according to one study,

> shapes such life realms as how time is used, how money is spent, how kin are defined, and how profit is viewed. Sometimes it generates strong behavioural expectations for participants, expectations that clash with those of the "real world".
>
> (Gillespie, Leffler & Lerner, 2002: p. 285)

Like any sport or hobby, dog sports can absorb the participants to a degree where it is difficult to balance other demands, for example, from family, work and the like. The following is an example, quoted in the previously mentioned study, of how much a dog sport can affect the life of even a newcomer:

> My best friend adopted a young Border Collie from the Humane Society last year. She thought "just for fun" she would try some herding. Well, that adopted dog and that "just for fun" herding experience has [sic] prompted a move to the country so she could have her own sheep, a new Border Collie puppy (you can't have just ONE Border Collie if you also have sheep!), and a new van to haul the Border Collies around. That adopted Border Collie also turned out to have tremendous obedience and agility potential as well, so of course the new place has to have an adequate area for obedience and agility training!
>
> (Gillespie, Leffler & Lerner, 2002: pp. 289–290)

Cats are much less often used in recreational and training activities, with the exception of the competitive showing of purebred pedigree cats. Although there are more companion cats than dogs (as we saw in Chapter 1), fewer are purebred. Since all animals entering shows organised by breed clubs must be purebred (see more on this in Chapter 7), a much lower proportion of cats are used for showing, compared to dogs.

Most companion animals, however, are not involved in a hobby or sport – their role is to be part of the family or the household. Even within this role, dogs and cats may serve a number of different functions.

Some family dogs take on the traditional role of guardian: having a dog in the house may make people feel safer (Serpell, 1990). For the same reason, some people may acquire dogs, such as Dobermans or Rottweilers, that appear intimidating. Typically, however, the main role of a dog or a cat in the home is to provide company. This is especially the case for people who live on their own, childless couples or those whose children have left home (empty nesters). A dog or a cat may provide an opportunity to have another being to look after and care for. Care giving is rewarding in its own right for some people (Julius *et al.*, 2013: p. 139) and the dog or cat is likely to reward the owner by showing affection and thereby making her or him feel needed. It is common for people to refer to their companion animal as their child, and to refer to companion dogs and cats as members of the family (cf. e.g. Greenebaum, 2004; Hirschman, 1994; Marinelli *et al.*, 2007; Power, 2008). Even parents with children commonly acquire dogs or cats to provide company, not only for themselves but also for their children. According to one American study,

Pet ownership is particularly high among families with grammar-school-age and teenage children… The motivation for owning a pet among families at the "middle" stage of the life cycle is rooted in the belief that pets perform beneficial functions for children. Data obtained in the home interviews reveal that parents view the activities involved in caring for a pet as useful in teaching children desirable attributes such as independence and responsibility. Parents also stress the companionship roles that pets play for children.

(Albert & Bulcroft, 1988: p. 547)

However, in contrast to this, an Australian study found that a majority of dog owners did not think that, 'to teach children about responsibility' and 'to provide children with companionship' were important reasons to acquire a dog (Bennett *et al.*, 2007). Similarly, a report from Statistics Sweden shows that the number of households with both dogs or cats and children had decreased from 2006 to 2012, whereas the number of households with dogs or cats and two adults had increased in the same period (Statistics Sweden, 2012). This may indicate that the role of dogs and cats in the family is undergoing change so that dogs and cats are increasingly not just being seen as companions for children (Figure 3.1). Below, more is said about how the animal's role in a family structure may affect human attachment.

Dogs (much more than cats) typically also have other functions than to provide company. Walking a dog may be intrinsically rewarding, but it also offers other more indirect benefits. First, walking may be good for the walker's general well-being and long-term health – we will return to this later in the chapter. Second, being with a dog in a public space can facilitate social contact with, and help from, other people (Guéguen & Ciccotti, 2008; McNicholas & Collis, 2000). Furthermore, the presence of dogs and other companion animals may have a general positive 'ripple' effect within a neighbourhood, for example by 'fostering of a "visible people presence" in the community' or because 'pet owners are more likely to be interested in local issues and to engage in civic activities' (Wood *et al.*, 2007). Of course, a high number of large dogs that are not well controlled may have the opposite effect.

Research also suggests that dogs, in particular, may be used as means for their owners to portray themselves as they want to be seen by others (Hirschman, 1994; Mosteller, 2008). So, for instance, owners may acquire dogs that are viewed as loyal and affable, thereby displaying family values; or they may choose more extreme dog types, such as Rottweilers or Chihuahuas, that are sometimes associated with masculine or feminine stereotypes, respectively. Companion animals with extreme and endearing features such as Shar Peis, Bulldogs, Pugs or Persian cats may also focus interest on the people who own them. Here we start to move away from animals as companions towards animals viewed as toys, status symbols or brands – what some authors term 'the dark side of pet ownership' (Beverland *et al.*, 2008).

Finally, companion animals may give people with whom they interact the opportunity to try to view the world and their surroundings from new perspectives. For example, when walking with a dog, one may become aware of a multifaceted olfactory dimension of reality of which we, as humans, with our limited and culturally suppressed sense

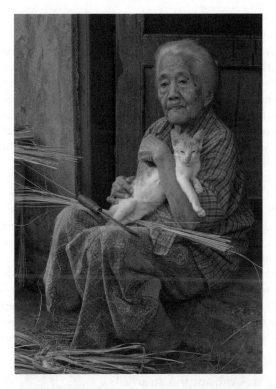

Figure 3.1 Centenarian lady with her pet cat. Companion animals are increasingly viewed as family members, to spend time and do enjoyable things with, confide in, love and take care of. (*Olyniteowl/Getty Images.*)

of smell are normally not aware. One author (Timmins, 2008) links this to the alleged need to be in touch with nature (cf. Wilson's (1984) idea of *biophilia*). Thus according to Timmins, 'companion animals may serve as transitional objects that satisfy this innate urge to interact with the natural world' (p. 540).

There is no doubt that these activities normally improve the quality of life of the owners who live with them. But how do they impact on the animals? Some of the activities will likely affect animals' welfare positively, with two particular potential benefits from the companionship relation: dogs and cats gain from being fed and looked after, and they typically seem to enjoy engaging with their human owners.

Many companion dogs seem to prefer human company to the company of conspecifics. For example, the smell of a familiar human is associated with more positive expectations than the smell of a familiar dog (Berns *et al.* in press), and humans have been shown to have a greater stress-reducing effect on shelter dogs than conspecifics (Tuber *et al.*, 1996). This may be one of the reasons why many cases of separation-related behaviour problems in dogs are not solved by the acquisition of a second, companion dog.

Successful human–animal interactions will, therefore, often also benefit the animal. For example, a dog used by an owner for hunting or training will probably gain positive experience from the activity. A cat pampered by an elderly owner will very likely enjoy the attention the owner gives it.

However, there are also potential problems of at least four sorts, which will be dealt with in more detail later in the book. First, sometimes a bond is not successfully created, or something damages it, resulting in frustration for the owner and potentially in welfare problems and relinquishment for the animal (see Chapter 13). Second, there can be welfare dilemmas, for example, animals with an extreme conformation that can help to generate deep bonds with people, but which at the same time leads to breed-related welfare problems (see Chapter 7). Third, some owners are too busy, and do not manage to make time for their animals. This may result in boredom, lack of care and other welfare problems for the animal, but may also potentially reduce the owner's welfare, by generating guilt about not being able to look after the animal well, and because the perceived costs of keeping the animal (vet bills, reduced freedom, etc.) exceed the perceived benefits. Finally, there are owners who acquire animals for reasons that make developing a bond with them less likely – for instance, as a pure status symbol – and others that have unrealistic expectations of what living with an animal involves.

Despite these not uncommon problems, companion animals are both highly significant and, as we saw in Chapter 1, hugely popular – with between a fifth and a third of all households in most Western countries having dogs and similar proportions with cats. They affect how people organise their lives, and spend their time and money; they also have the potential to significantly impact the quality of the lives of their human owners.

3.3 Relating to Companion Animals

In this section, we look at attempts to conceptualise and measure the ways people relate to companion animals, in terms of the relations that characterise typical human–human family relations. A widely used approach to the characterisation of the human–companion animal relation is the psychological framework of attachment. The concept of attachment was originally used to describe the degree of emotional bonding between an infant and its caregiver (Bowlby, 1958) and was later broadened to also include other types of human relationships (Hazan & Shaver, 1987; Trinke & Bartholomew, 1997) as well as human–dog relationships (Julius et al., 2013).

Although it seems that dogs, and perhaps also other companion animals, can function as attachment figures for their owners, the use of measures from human–human attachment models to characterise human attachment to animals has been questioned, as it does 'not necessarily encompass the entirety of attachment theory as it has been applied in human–human relationships' (Crawford, Worsham & Swinehart, 2006: p. 100). In addition, attachment models only look at the positive aspect of forming bonds with a companion animal. This could result in bias when assessing the value of human relations to companion animals, which should be seen as depending on the balance between perceived benefits and costs. Relationship models that incorporate both positive and negative aspects include the Monash Dog Owner Relationship Scale (MDORS) (Dwyer, Bennett & Coleman, 2006) and the Network of Relationships Inventory (NRI) (Furman & Buhrmester, 1985).

The NRI is used in a study that we will take as our starting point in the description of the human bond to companion animals. The study was undertaken in Britain, where 90 participants belonging to 40 households with dogs, cats and other companion animals were asked to fill out a questionnaire originally developed to measure relations between humans in their functions as family members, friends and the like (Bonas *et al.*, 2000). The study is interesting because it compares human–human and human–companion animal relations, and it looks at both positive and negative aspects of these relations.

The questionnaire separates the relations that people have with companion animals and other humans into the following seven components: *companionship* (spending time or doing enjoyable things together), *instrumental aid* (the other is providing help), *intimacy* (confiding in or sharing private thoughts with), *nurturance* (taking care of the other), *affection* (love and care, both ways), *admiration* (the other showing respect for or approving the actions of the person), and *reliable alliance* (the person's belief that the relationship will last). Each of these components was measured by means of three questions with five possible answers linked to a five-point scale (Bonas, McNicholas & Collis, 2000: p. 215).

One important result of the study is that it seems possible to measure human–animal relations on roughly the same scale as that normally used for measuring human–human relations. According to the authors, this 'adds empirical weight to the view that human–pet relations are similar in nature to human–human relationships' (Bonas, McNicholas & Collis, 2000: p. 219). (For another study reaching a similar conclusion, see Kurdek (2008).)

Another important result is that the same scale allows for a comparison between the social support provided by humans and different companion animals. The study showed that the subjects generally received more support from other humans in their household than from their companion animals. However, the support provided by dogs was only slightly less than from other humans, and although cats provided less again, it was still much higher than the relatively limited support provided by other pets (Bonas, McNicholas & Collis, 2000: pp. 219–221) (an empirical argument supporting, we think, our focus on dogs and cats as typical companion animals).

Conflict and antagonism in both directions were also measured. Not surprisingly, it was found that the relative level of negative interactions was very similar to the overall level of support: thus, most negative interactions are found between humans, less between human and dog, less between human and cat and much less between human and other pets (Bonas, McNicholas & Collis, 2000: p. 223). So, positive attachment and problems in relations seem to be two sides of the same coin.

Interestingly, whereas humans are better than dogs at providing some elements of support, dogs are better at providing other elements, as can be seen in Figure 3.2.

Dogs provide better support than humans in three ways: through more lasting relationships ('reliable alliance'); as a better outlet for providing care for another individual; and as a better source of companionship. It is, however, important to note that only humans who choose to live with companion animals have been studied; and it is, therefore, not possible to say anything about whether those who choose to live *without* animals would have experienced similar benefits.

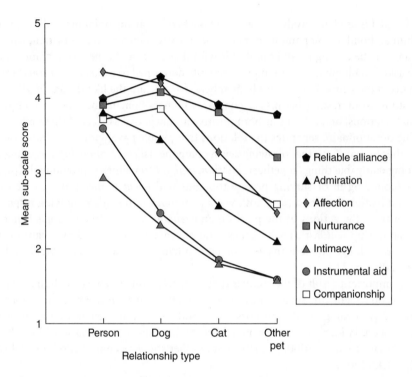

Figure 3.2 For explanation of components, see preceding text. (*Bonas et al.,* 2000 p. 222. *Reproduced with permission of Cambridge University Press.*)

Cats do nearly as well in terms of providing the first two kinds of social support, but not in terms of companionship (described here as spending time or doing enjoyable things together). The latter result is no surprise based on the previous discussion of what people do with dogs and cats and is in line with findings made by other scholars according to which people tend to be more strongly attached to dogs than to cats (Albert & Bulcroft, 1988; Smolkovic, Fajfar & Mlinaric, 2012). However, one author claims that the scales typically used to study the attachment of humans to their companion animals are biased in favour of dogs. She argues that the scales measure things typically done with dogs, and not cats, and that when this bias is corrected, there is no basis for saying that people are typically more attached to a dog than to a cat (Zasloff, 1996).

Fewer studies have been conducted concerning the relationships that humans have with other animal companions, such as birds. According to one study however, birds and owners can form strong bonds, 'similar in many ways to those shared by dogs and cats and their owners' (Loughlin & Dowrick, 1993).

These comparative studies of attachment also provide interesting information about the connection between attachment to companion animals and attachment to humans. For example, Bonas, McNicholas & Collis (2000) found that 'subjects reporting low levels of provision of support from humans also report low levels of provision from pets'

(p. 229); these authors, therefore, do not find support for the idea that, 'owners use provisions from pets to compensate for shortcomings in other human relationships' (p. 233).

However, even though at the individual level it may be the case that people who get along well with companion animals also find it easy to get along with other humans, there are some interesting demographic variations. For example, one study based on a survey conducted in an urban US context showed that attachment to companion animals, 'is highest among never-married, divorced, widowed and remarried people, childless couples, newlyweds, and empty-nesters' (Albert & Bulcroft, 1988: p. 543).

According to the same study, adults with children in the home show a lower degree of attachment to their animals. The attachment is particularly low in families with infants. Thus, 'young mothers report that, since the arrival of the baby, they have little time for the family pet. In addition, young mothers express feelings of guilt about "neglecting" the pet and they reveal that the pet became less important in the family after the baby was born' (p. 550). Paradoxically, according to the same study, the highest level of ownership of companion animals is found in families where there are children.

So, when companion animals have to compete with children, their owners, at least, typically feel that the animal companions are losing out. In support of this, a study looking at dog and owner characteristics affecting the dog–owner relationship, as measured by the previously mentioned MDORS, found that dog owners with children felt less emotionally close to their dog than dog owners without children (Meyer & Forkman, 2014).

However, companion animals may do better in other family situations. For example, in families without children or where the children have left home, as noted earlier in this chapter, dogs and cats may assume the role of children (Hirschman, 1994). Sometimes they may even outcompete a human partner (Gillespie, Leffler & Lerner, 2002). But there need not always be competition: sometimes the two kinds of relationship may complement each other. Thus, Beck & Madresh (2008) speculate that companion animals:

> … are not merely substitutes for human interaction, but fill a specific role by providing a consistent, and relatively controllable, sense of relationship security. A dependable source of security may help to cushion the uncertainty of more complex relationships with humans, making it easier for pet owners to cope with the ups and downs of daily life.
>
> (Beck & Madresh, 2008: p. 53)

Similarly, companion animals can play an important role for children; it has been shown that levels of attachment to dogs are higher for children in single-parent families, than for those in two-parent families (Bodsworth & Coleman, 2001). The same study refers to other studies showing 'that having an attachment bond with a dog can provide emotional support to people in families where there is limited access to significant other humans' (p. 221). Other studies have also demonstrated stronger attachments for companion animals among 'only' (singleton) children and the youngest children in families (Melson & Fogel, 1996; Paul & Serpell, 1992), suggesting that dogs and cats may sometimes substitute for a lack of younger siblings.

In relation to human attachment to companion animals, it is also relevant to mention extreme attachment styles in humans and how these can affect the human–animal relationship (Figure 3.3). A person's attachment style is developed in childhood mainly as a function of the person's attachment experiences with primary caregivers (Julius *et al.*, 2013). Extreme attachment styles are highly correlated with personality disorders and have also been linked to pathological keeping of companion animals in large numbers; so-called animal hoarding (Patronek & Nathanson, 2009; Williams, 2014).

Different kinds of animal hoarding have been described; common to all of them is that the humans are unable to take care of the large number of animals that they have accumulated, and unable or unwilling to recognise the welfare-related problems for the animals and themselves (Patronek, 2006; Williams, 2014). In some cases, the animal hoarder is exploitative, 'controlling and lacking in empathy with animals or humans' (Williams, 2014: p. 201), but in many cases, the animal hoarder has no intention to do harm, feels very attached to the animals and shows self-neglect and neglect of others and of the surroundings. These characteristics have resulted in animal hoarding being described as a deviant form of the human bond to companion animals that actually

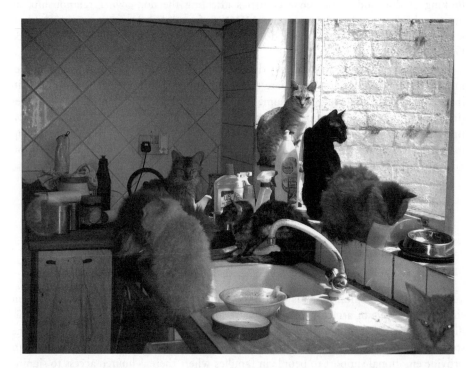

Figure 3.3 Human attachment to animals can become extreme, as seen with animal hoarding. Many individuals who accumulate large numbers of animals often have good intentions, but become overwhelmed; in other cases, hoarding can be exploitative, and associated with a lack of empathy. (*Image used courtesy of the RSPCA.*)

represents a separate dimension of animal abuse, different from deliberate abuse and neglect (Patronek, 2008).

So far, we have been looking at attachment mainly as a function of the needs and expectations of the people who live with animal companions. However, it is clear that individual differences between animals will also affect how successfully they bond with the people who look after them. (We will take a closer look at extreme cases of this, in terms of behavioural problems, in Chapter 9.)

In one study conducted by Serpell (1996), the owners of dogs and cats sourced from shelters were questioned about both their attachment to their animals and on how well the animal's actual behaviour matched their ideal expectations. Marked differences were found between the expected and actual behaviours. With dogs, 'the main discrepancies were associated with nervousness/fearfulness, excitability, lack of obedience, hyperactivity, and separation-related anxiety' (Serpell, 1996: p. 57); similar discrepancies were found for cats. As regards attachment, 'actual' behaviour of dogs, as assessed by their owners, appeared to be a poor predictor of the owner's level of attachment to the dog, whereas discrepancies between owner ratings of the dog's 'actual' and 'ideal' behaviour appeared to predict levels of owner attachment: actual-ideal differences were consistently higher among less attached owners.

The study found no relation between owners' attachment level and their ratings of their dogs' ideal behaviour, and therefore, according to Serpell, it is 'unlikely that the less strong attachments developed by some owners were a consequence of them having exaggerated or unrealistic behavioural expectations of the pet' (p. 57). The explanation for the findings could be that less attached owners perceive the behaviour of their dogs less positively and thereby further from the ideal, but it could also be that less attached owners had been matched up with dogs that fitted less well with their expectations of a dog. A similar effect was not found for cats. It is speculated by Serpell that the difference between the two species may be due to the fact that the behaviour of dogs is typically more intrusive than that of cats and/or that people expect less, or have more realistic expectations of their cats.

Later studies have found that a high degree of matching between a large set of owner and dog characteristics does not necessarily result in the owner being more satisfied with the dog. Matching the dog and owner on very specific characteristics, such as 'enjoyment of running outside', is, however, positively associated with owner satisfaction, and certain dog behaviours, such as level of territorial behaviour and the desire to destroy objects, also seem to have a direct negative effect on the level of owner satisfaction (Curb et al., 2013). Similarly, certain dog traits have been found to affect the strength of human attachment, for example, according to Hoffman et al. (2013) 'the strength of owners' attachments to their dogs was associated with dog trainability and separation problems'. However, according to the same study, there may be clear demographic differences in which traits matter for a person's attachment. For example, dog excitability was negatively associated with owner attachment to the dog for Caucasians, but not for non-Caucasians.

It appears then that the mechanisms by which owner attachment and companion animal characteristics correlate are complex. In a study on the effect of dog and owner characteristics on dog–owner relationship quality (measured by the aforementioned

MDORS scale), it was found that a fairly large set of the characteristics investigated only had a small impact on relationship quality, supporting the notion that the owner's attachment to the dog is a complex matter. Interestingly, it was also found that factors related to the owner, for example, presence of children and amount of activity with the dog, seemed to influence the relationship more than factors related to the dog (Meyer & Forkman, 2014).

It seems reasonable to conclude that in general, dogs and cats matter significantly to the humans who live with and interact with them. These animals are typically viewed as family members. However, it may seem irrational to other people to view members of other species as kin (cf. the discussion in Chapter 1 about whether companion animals are social parasites). As a result, there have been a number of studies that have looked for more tangible benefits that companion animals may give their human owners. We will now briefly consider these studies.

3.4 Effects on Human Health

Since the early 1980s, studies have been undertaken concerning the effects of keeping companion animals on human physical and mental health. Some of the studies have shown significant positive results that have been widely publicised and received much popular attention. One example is a study based on focus group interviews with 65, mainly elderly, dog walkers in England, in which 'all participants agreed that having a dog was good for their health' and also saw huge psychological benefits (Knight & Edwards, 2008). However, while some later studies supported this positive view of companion dogs, others did not; and some have even shown negative effects both in terms of physical and psychological health (Chur-Hansen, Stern & Winefield, 2010; Siegel, 2011). In addition, these and other reviews comment on the lack of rigour in some aspects of the research in this field.

Perhaps the most striking example of a positive health effect of living with animals was found in two longitudinal studies of survival after a cardiac event published in 1980 (Friedmann *et al.*, 1980) and 1995 (Friedmann & Thomas, 1995). These studies reported longer survival for heart attack survivors who owned pets, with greatest effect found among dog owners. However, a third study published in 2010 (Parker *et al.*, 2010) was not able to replicate the results of the first two studies and found that owners of companion animals, particularly cat owners, did less well after a cardiac event than those without companion animals (Siegel, 2011). Nonetheless, in a recent scientific statement, the American Heart Association cautiously concluded that dog ownership is probably associated with decreased risk of cardio-vascular disease (Levine *et al.*, 2013).

Recently, there has also been a growing interest in considering the role of companion animals in child development and long-term health (see for example McCardle *et al.*, 2011a, 2011b), but this is still work in progress.

As it is difficult to document a robust correlation between physical health and just owning companion animals, it seems more promising to look at some mechanisms through which companion animals may enable their owners to lead more healthy lives. The most obvious mechanism is through dog walking; and a number of studies have been able to document a positive correlation between having a dog and getting exercise from walking, which in turn is likely to have an effect in the prevention of a number of lifestyle-related diseases (Coleman *et al.*, 2008; Hoerster *et al.*, 2011; Lentino *et al.*, 2012; Serpell, 1991); similar effects, in terms of reducing lifestyle-related diseases have also been documented for children (Owen *et al.*, 2010).

In terms of the effects of living with companion animals on *psychological* health, a number of studies report a positive effect. These studies seem to be backed up by physiological studies that show how both humans and companion animals, through contact, will typically experience elevated levels of oxytocin and other neurochemicals associated with positive affiliative emotions (Julius *et al.*, 2013; Odendaal & Meintjes, 2003).

Two recent studies from Australia (Peacock *et al.*, 2012) and Canada (Antonacopoulos & Pychyl, 2010) assessed correlations between attachment to companion animals and levels of psychological problems. However, these two studies failed to demonstrate a simple positive correlation between attachment to a cat or a dog, and reduced levels of, for example, loneliness and depression. Instead, they found some negative correlations.

According to the first study, 'attachment to a companion animal was a significant positive predictor of psychological distress in the form of depression, anxiety, and somatoform symptoms' (Peacock *et al.*, 2012: p. 299). The authors suggest that their results differ from those of other studies for two main reasons. First, they compare actual attachment to (not just ownership of) a companion, to levels of psychological stress. Second, they look at a broader age range of owners, unlike previous studies that have primarily focussed on elderly owners of companion animals. According to their study, attachment to a companion animal can be a mixed blessing. Close attachment to a dog or a cat could, for people with psychological health issues, be a sign of problems with establishing attachment to other humans. Also, they show that attachment to a companion animal may prevent people from going to hospital for necessary treatment because they are not able to find someone to look after their animals while they are away.

Antonacopoulos & Pychyl (2010) focussed on people living alone, and found that psychological benefits of being attached to a companion animal were only seen in dog owners who already had a well-functioning social life. They suggested that the emotional support provided by a dog

> may not be sufficient to compensate for insufficient human social support, which may explain why they do not differ from non-owners with low levels of human social support in terms of loneliness levels (p. 49).

Furthermore they argue that,

> individuals with low levels of human social support, if they choose to spend time with their pet rather than socializing with other people, may begin to feel somewhat socially isolated. Furthermore, if these individuals decline social invitations in order to be with their pet, they may end up in a vicious cycle, whereby the number of social invitations extended to them decreases (p. 50).

While it may be tempting to try to rationalise human attachment to dogs and cats by claiming benefits to physical and mental health, the scientific evidence has not yet delivered a clear verdict on the existence of such benefits, or the extent to which they are generalisable. At the same time, it should be recognised that studying the health effects of pet ownership is extremely challenging, and it may not in fact be possible to design and conduct the definitive study that will finally settle this debate. In the meantime, it is probably wise in all discussions about the effects of human–companion animal relations on human health to distinguish between the different types of human–animal interactions, the different motivations for acquiring and keeping companion animals, and the different human and animal personalities involved.

Key Points

- Humans engage in a wide range of activities with their companion animals, particularly with dogs.
- Companion animals, therefore, have the potential to significantly impact the quality of the lives of their human owners.
- Humans form attachments to companion animals that are similar in many ways to those formed with fellow humans.
- Although there are significant differences in levels of attachment depending on breed and individual differences, it seems that in general, people attach themselves most strongly to dogs and cats.
- Relations to dogs and, to a lesser extent, to cats can in some respects matter at least as much as relations to other humans.
- Attempts have been made to understand human attachment to companion animals in terms of potential benefits to physical and psychological health. However, the current literature provides conflicting evidence in this regard.

References

Albert, A. & Bulcroft, K. (1988) Pets, families, and the life course. *Journal of Marriage and Family* 50 (2), 543–552.

Antonacopoulos, N.M.D. & Pychyl, T.A. (2010) An examination of the potential role of pet ownership, human social support and pet attachment in the psychological health of individuals living alone. *Anthrozoös* 23 (1), 37–55.

Beck, L. & Madresh, E.A. (2008) Romantic partners and four-legged friends: an extension of attachment theory to relationships with pets. *Anthrozoös* 21 (1), 43–56.

Bennett, P.C., Cooper, N., Rohlf, V.I. & Mornement, K. (2007) Factors influencing owner satisfaction with companion-dog-training facilities. *Journal of Applied Animal Welfare Science* 10, 217–241.

Berns, G.S., Brooks, A.M. & Spivak, M. (2015) Scent of the familiar: an fMRI study of canine brain responses to familiar and unfamiliar human and dog odors. *Behavioural Processes* 110, 37–46.

Beverland, M.B., Farrely, F. & Lim, E.A.C. (2008) Exploring the dark side of pet ownership: status- and control-based pet consumption. *Journal of Business Research* 61 (5), 490–496.

Bodsworth, W. & Coleman, G.J. (2001) Child–companion animal attachment bonds in single and two-parent families. *Anthrozoös* 14 (4), 216–223.

Bonas, S., McNicholas, J. & Collis, G. (2000). Pets in the network of family relationships: an empirical study. In: Podberscek, A., Paul, E.S. & Serpell, J.A. (eds) *Companion animals and us: exploring the relationships between people & pets.* Cambridge, UK, Cambridge University Press, pp. 209–236.

Bowlby, J. (1958) The nature of the child's tie to his mother. *The International Journal of Psychoanalysis* 39, 350–373.

Brewer, D., Clark T. & Phillips, A. (2001) *Dogs in antiquity: Anubis to Cerberus: the origins of the domestic dog.* Warminster, Aris & Phillips.

Chur-Hansen, A., Stern, C. & Winefield, H. (2010) Gaps in the evidence about companion animals and human health: some suggestions for progress. *International Journal of Evidence-based Healthcare* 8 (3), 140–146.

Coleman, K.J., Rosenberg, D.E., Conway, T.L., Sallis, J.F., Saelens, B.E., Frank, L.D. & Cain, K. (2008) Physical activity, weight status, and neighborhood characteristics of dog walkers. *Preventive Medicine* 47 (3), 309–312.

Crawford, E.K., Worsham, N.L. & Swinehart, E.R. (2006) Benefits derived from companion animals, and the use of the term "attachment". *Anthrozoös* 19 (2), 98–112.

Curb, L.A., Abramson, C.I., Grice, J.W. & Kennison, S.M. (2013) The relationship between personality match and pet satisfaction among dog owners. *Anthrozoös* 26 (3), 395–404.

Dwyer, F., Bennett, P.C. & Coleman, G.J. (2006) Development of the Monash Dog Owner Relationship Scale (MDORS). *Anthrozoös* 19 (3), 243–256.

Friedmann, E., Katcher, A.H., Lynch, J.J. & Thomas, S.A. (1980). Animal companions and one-year survival of patients after discharge from a coronary care unit. *Public Health Reports*, 95 (4), 307–312.

Friedmann, E. & Thomas, S.A. (1995). Pet ownership, social support, and one-year survival after acute myocardial infarction in the Cardiac Arrhythmia Suppression Trial (CAST). *American Journal of Cardiology* 76, 1213–1217.

Furman, W. & Buhrmester, D. (1985) Children's perceptions of the personal relationships in their social networks. *Developmental Psychology* 21 (6), 1016–1024.

Gillespie, D.L., Leffler, A. & Lerner, E. (2002) If it weren't for my hobby, I'd have a life: dog sports, serious leisure, and boundary negotiations. *Leisure Studies* 21, 285–304.

Greenebaum, J. (2004) It's a dog's life: elevating status from pet to "fur baby" at yappy hour. *Society & Animals* 12 (2), 117–135.

Guéguen, N. & Ciccotti, S. (2008) Domestic dogs as facilitators in social interaction: an evaluation of helping and courtship behaviors. *Anthrozoös* 21 (4), 339–349.

Hazan, C. & Shaver, P. (1987) Romantic love conceptualized as an attachment process. *Journal of Personality and Social Psychology* 52 (3), 511–524.

Hirschman, E.C. (1994) Consumers and their animal companions. *Journal of Consumer Research* 20 (4) 616–632.

Hoerster, K.D., Mayer, J.A., Sallis, J.F., Pizzi, N., Talley, S., Pichon, L.C. & Butler, D.A. (2011) Dog walking: its association with physical activity guideline adherence and its correlates. *Preventive Medicine* 52 (1), 33–38.

Hoffman, C.L., Chen, P., Serpell, J.A. & Jacobson, K.C. (2013) Do dog behavioral characteristics predict the quality of the relationship between dogs and their owners? *Human-Animal Interaction Bulletin* 1 (1), 20–32.

Julius, H., Beetz, A., Kotrschal, K., Turner, D. & Uvnäs-Moberg, K. (2013) *Attachment to pets: an integrative view of human-animal relationships with implications for therapeutic practice*. Cambridge, MA & Göttingen, Hogrefe.

Knight, S. & Edwards, V. (2008) In the company of wolves: the physical, social, and psychological benefits of dog ownership. *Journal of Aging and Health* 20 (4), 437–455.

Kurdek, L.A. (2008) Pet dogs as attachment figures. *Journal of Social and Personal Relationships* 25 (2), 247–266.

Lentino, C., Visek, A.J., McDonnell, K. & DiPietro, L. (2012) Dog walking is associated with a favorable risk profile independent of moderate to high volume of physical activity. *Journal of Physical Activity & Health* 9 (3), 414–420.

Levine, G.N., Allen, K., Braun, L.T., Christian, H.E., Friedmann, E., Taubert, K.A., Thomas, S.A., Wells, D.L. & Lange, R.A. (2013) Pet ownership and cardiovascular risk: a scientific statement from the American Heart Association. *Circulation* 127, 2353–2363.

Loughlin, C.A. & Dowrick, P.W. (1993) Psychological needs filled by avian companions. *Anthrozoös* 6 (3), 166–172.

Marinelli, L., Adamelli, S., Normando, S. & Bono, G. (2007) Quality of life of the pet dog: influence of owner and dog's characteristics. *Applied Animal Behaviour Science* 108 (1–2), 143–156.

McCardle, P., McCune, S., Griffin, J.A., Esposity, L. & Freund, L.S. (eds) (2011a) *Animals in our lives: human-animal interaction in family, community, and therapeutic settings*. Baltimore, London & Sydney, Paul H. Brookes Publishing Co.

McCardle, P., McCune, S., Griffin, J.A. & Maholmes, V. (eds) (2011b) *How animals affect us: examining the influence of human-animal interaction on child development and human health*. Washington, DC, American Psychological Association.

McNicholas, J. & Collis, G.M. (2000) Dogs as catalysts for social interactions: robustness of the effect. *British Journal of Psychology* 91, 61–70.

Melson, G.F. & Fogel, A. (1996) Parental perceptions of their children's involvement with household pets: a test of a specificity model of nurturance. *Anthrozoös* 9, 95–105.

Meyer, I. & Forkman, B. (2014) Dog and owner characteristics affecting the dog-owner relationship. *Journal of Veterinary Behavior: Clinical Applications and Research* 9 (4), 143–150.

Miklósi, Á. (2007) *Dog behaviour, evolution, and cognition*. Oxford & New York, Oxford University Press.

Mosteller, J. (2008) Animal-companion extremes and underlying consumer themes. *Journal of Business Research* 61 (5), 512–521.

Odendaal, J.S. & Meintjes, R. (2003) Neurophysiological correlates of affiliative behaviour between humans and dogs. *The Veterinary Journal* 165 (3), 296–301.

Owen, C.G., Nightingale, C.M., Rudnicka, A.R., Ekelund, U., McMinn, A.M., van Sluijs, E.M.F., Griffin, S.J., Cook, D.G. & Whincup, P.H. (2010) Family dog ownership and levels of physical activity in childhood: findings from the Child Heart and Health Study in England. *American Journal of Public Health* 100 (9), 1669–1671.

Parker, G.B., Gayed, A., Owen, C.A., Hyett, M.P., Hilton, T.M. & Heruc, G.A. (2010) Survival following an acute coronary syndrome: a pet theory put to the test. *Acta Psychiatrica Scandinavica*, 121, 65–70.

Patronek, G. (2006) Animal hoarding: its roots and recognition. *Veterinary Medicine* 101, 520–530.

Patronek, G. (2008) *Animal hoarding: a third dimension of animal abuse*. In: Ascione, F.R. (ed.) *The international handbook of animal abuse and cruelty: theory, research and application*. West Lafayette, IN, Purdue University Press, pp. 221–238.

Patronek, G.J. & Nathanson, J.N. (2009) A theoretical perspective to inform assessment and treatment strategies for animal hoarders. *Clinical Psychology Reviews* 29, 274–281.

Paul, E.S. & Serpell, J.A. (1992) Why children keep pets: the influence of child and family characteristics. *Anthrozoös* 5, 231–244.

Peacock, J., Chur-Hansen, A. & Winefield, H. (2012) Mental health implications of human attachment to companion animals. *Journal of Clinical Psychology* 68 (3), 292–303.

Power, E. (2008) Furry families: making a human–dog family through home. *Social & Cultural Geography* 9 (5), 535–555.

Prato-Previde, E., Custance, D.M., Spiezio, C., Sabatini, F., Psicologia, I., Milano, U. & College, G. (2003) Is the dog-human relationship an attachment bond? An observational study using Ainsworth's strange situation. *Behaviour* 140, 225–254.

Serpell, J.A. (1990) Evidence for long-term effects of pet-ownership on human health. In: Burger, I.H. (ed.) *Pets, benefits and practice*. London, British Veterinary Association Publications, pp. 1–7.

Serpell, J.A. (1991) Beneficial effects of pet ownership on some aspects of human health and behaviour. *Journal of the Royal Society of Medicine* 84, 717–720.

Serpell, J.A. (1996) Evidence for an association between pet behavior and owner attachment levels. *Applied Animal Behaviour Science* 47 (1–2), 49–60.

Siegel, J.M. (2011) Pet ownership and health. In: Blazina C., Boyraz G. & Shen-Miller D. (eds) *The psychology of the human-animal bond*. New York, Heidelberg, Dordrecht & London, Springer, pp. 167–177.

Smolkovic, I., Fajfar, M. & Mlinaric, V. (2012) Attachment to pets and interpersonal relationships. *Journal of European Psychology Students* 3, 15–23.

Statistics Sweden (2012) *Hundar, katter och andra sällskapsdjur 2012*. Statistiska centralbyrån. [Online] Available from: http://www.skk.se/Global/Dokument/Om-SKK /SCB-undersokning-Hundar-katter-och-andra-sallskapsdjur-2012.pdf [Accessed 11 July 2014].

Timmins, R.P. (2008). The contribution of animals to human well-being: a veterinary family practice perspective. *Journal of Veterinary Medical Education* 35 (4), 540–544.

Trinke, S. & Bartholomew, K. (1997) Hierarchies of attachment relationships in young adulthood. *Journal of Social and Personal Relationships* 14 (5), 603–625.

Tuber, D.S., Hennessy, M.B., Sanders, S. & Miller, J.A. (1996) Behavioral and glucocorticoid responses of adult domestic dogs (*Canis familiaris*) to companionship and social seperation. *Journal of Comparative Psychology* 110 (1), 103–108.

Williams, B. (2014) Animal hoarding: recognition and possible interventions. *Practice* 36 (4), 199–205.

Wilson, E.O. (1984) *Biophilia*. Cambridge, MA, Harvard University Press.

Wood, L.J., Giles-Corti, W, Bulsara, M.K. & Bosch, D. (2007) More than a furry companion: the ripple effect of companion animals on neighborhood interactions and sense of community. *Society and Animals* 15 (1), 43–56.

Zasloff, R.L. (1996) Measuring attachment to companion animals: a dog is not a cat is not a bird. *Applied Animal Behaviour Science* 47 (1–2), 43–48.

Companion Animal Welfare

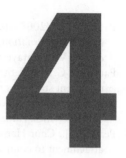

4.1 Introduction   58
4.2 Theories About Animal Welfare   60
4.3 From Farm Animal Welfare to Companion Animal Welfare   65
4.4 Assessing the Welfare of Companion Animals   67

4.1 Introduction

As we saw in the previous chapter, keeping dogs, cats and other companion animals fulfils a number of roles in people's lives. Generally, companion animals contribute to the quality of the lives of their owners or keepers, and so in most cases, keeping companion animals is an activity that people find fulfilling and pleasurable. However, the fact that people keep companion animals because they enjoy doing so does not necessarily mean that they care about or prioritise the animals' welfare. Certainly, most owners of companion animals probably think of their relationship to their animal(s) as win-win: a well cared for and thriving animal improves the owner's quality of life. However, compromises sometimes have to be made between what is good for animal companions and what is in the interests of their owners.

For example, many owners of cats and dogs put them in boarding facilities when they go on holiday, even though they believe it would be better for their animals' welfare if they all stayed home. In such cases, owners prioritise their need for a holiday over their animals' welfare. Even so, most owners typically try to find out which boarding facility will look after the animals in the best way – ideally where they will be provided with enough space, and cared for by people who pay attention to their needs.

However, owners of dogs and cats can be faced with choices where they are genuinely in doubt about what is best for the animal. A number of such choices will be discussed

Companion Animal Ethics, First Edition. Peter Sandøe, Sandra Corr and Clare Palmer.
© Universities Federation for Animal Welfare 2016.

later in this book; for example, the choice about whether or not to neuter a companion animal, or to treat a severely ill animal rather than to euthanase it ('put it to sleep').

In addition to areas of uncertainty, there are also disagreements about what constitutes an animal's welfare. We will use the case of indoor versus outdoor cats as an example. Many cat owners have to choose between sometimes allowing their cat(s) to go outdoors, or keeping them indoors all the time; many people have strong views about this choice. Often these views are based on claims about what matters most from the point of view of the affected cats.

An illustrative exchange of views can be found on the website of the US animal rights organization PETA (People for the Ethical Treatment of Animals). Under the heading 'Why all cats should be indoor cats', the organization argues that for the welfare of cats, it is better never to allow them to go out and roam:

> [There are] … several deadly diseases that cats who roam outdoors can catch. Unattended cats also face dangers posed by dogs, wildlife, and the scariest predator of all, humans. Thieves, or "bunchers", cruise neighbourhoods for friendly dogs and cats who can easily be picked up and sold to dealers, who in turn sell them to laboratories. Cats are often poisoned, shot, set on fire, or trapped and drowned by intolerant neighbors or bored juveniles. They are hit by cars, accidentally poisoned by spilled antifreeze, or maimed by fan blades when they crawl into warm engines on winter days. "But he wants to go outside." "We live on a very quiet street." "It's cruel to keep her in." These are things said by people who would never dream of opening the door and sending toddlers to wander down the street on their own… Today's concrete jungles are far too dangerous for vulnerable, trusting little animals.
>
> (PETA, 2013)

This argument is followed by a list of things that a cat owner can do to enrich the indoor environment to keep her or his cat active and engaged without letting it out.

However, a number of readers have posted comments on PETA's argument; some of these are highly critical about the idea that good cat welfare requires keeping cats indoors. Here are two examples:

> I believe cats should be free to roam; that is one of the wonders of owning cats. I have 2 very happy healthy cats who have a great life. I don't believe in house cats. It's no different to keeping a rabbit in a hutch with a run in the garden – completely unnatural. That may suit the owner but not the creature. I do, though, keep them in at night so they are safe. If there is lots of traffic or you don't have a suitable home then you should not have a cat. Let's not go the way we have with children where people are scared to let them play in the street when in fact a child is more likely to be harmed by a family member than a stranger. (Victoria 30 January 2013 [punctuation and spelling corrected by authors])

> 'Yes it is more dangerous for cats to go outdoors. Same applies to people. But we don't lock ourselves away because the outside world is such a dangerous scary place … Cats are independent creatures…. It is cruel to keep cats indoors'. (Vicky 22 January 2013)

Thus, there can be clear disagreement between people who all seem genuinely to care about the welfare of cats. However, the two sides of the discussion cannot both be right. So, how can someone who is genuinely in doubt decide what constitutes 'good welfare' for cats? Can animal welfare science help?

These are the kinds of question that we will consider in this chapter. In the next section, we begin by outlining different philosophical theories about what counts as a 'good life'. In the following section, we discuss the role of science in finding out about what is optimal welfare for companion animals.

4.2 Theories About Animal Welfare

Achieving good welfare is equivalent to having a good life. If we agree that some action or resource helps to give an animal a good life, then – assuming that it is appropriate to assist the animal in question – we have a reason to act, or to help the animal to access the resource. But how can we know what actually does contribute to giving an animal a good life – for example, whether it is good for a cat to be let out to roam?

Scientific studies may help us find out how animals are affected by the way we treat them. For example, epidemiologists can try to find out how allowing a cat to roam may affect its risk of getting certain diseases, and how this may be relevant to its survival. Behavioural scientists may study how living indoors can affect a cat's behaviour, and whether being indoors causes behavioural disturbances or signs of frustration. But although such information would inform the discussion, the results, unless they are very extreme, are unlikely to settle the debate. For the parties engaged in the indoor/outdoor cat debate not only disagree about the likely consequences for cats, they also appear to disagree about how to define a 'good' or 'bad' life for a cat. While typical proponents of keeping cats confined indoors seem to focus on safety as a key feature of cat welfare, opponents focus on other aspects of a 'good life' such as freedom and naturalness. It seems that clarification is required on what, in principle, matters in a cat's life.

Debates about what constitutes a 'good life' have a long history. One influential thinker here is the English lawyer and philosopher Jeremy Bentham (1748–1832). Bentham is famous for saying that animals – like humans – matter morally because they are able to *suffer*. According to Bentham, the avoidance of suffering contributes to making a good life.

However, avoidance of serious pain, intense fear, depression and other forms of suffering cannot be the only thing that matters in life. If it were, the safest goal in life would be to die, painlessly, as soon as possible: suffering seems to be an unavoidable part of life, and death seems to be the only safe route to total avoidance of it. There must also be something of positive value that makes life worth living; this positive element Bentham identifies as *pleasure*. In this category, he collects a whole range of mental states, all of which are positive or pleasant. These states include various forms of joy, fulfilment and comfort. According to Bentham, the good life consists of getting the optimal balance between, on the one hand, pain and other forms of suffering, and on the other hand, joy and pleasure (Bentham, 1789/1989).

The theory that Bentham endorses is usually called *hedonism*.

The best life, according to hedonism, is one in which there are as many stimulating, comfortable and joyful experiences, and as few frustrating, unpleasant or painful experiences, as possible. The more positive experiences relative to negative ones there are (i.e. the higher the net level of positives), the better the quality of the life is.

Returning to the example of outdoor cats, a defender of hedonism would claim that for the cat, the best option will depend on how many negative or positive experiences are either lost or gained by going out. So, the specific situation is important, for example, the kind of risks the cat actually faces outdoors, in terms of level of traffic, presence of potential predators, diseases, and hostile humans. Equally, the quality of the alternative indoor environment also matters, including the availability of enrichments that allow the cat to engage in indoor behaviours that are equally as rewarding or pleasurable as the missed outdoor behaviours (Figure 4.1).

For the hedonist, there is no *a priori* answer as to what is best for cats in general – it will depend on how the chances of pleasure and risks of pain add up in the specific circumstances, and to the particular individual (because what gives pleasure to one cat may cause fear to another). To try to calculate this would be difficult, in terms of weighing different kinds of states against each other and assessing risks. How, for example, should the potential pleasure of being allowed to roam outdoors be weighed against (say) a 5% risk of becoming infected with an unpleasant disease that will cause an early death?

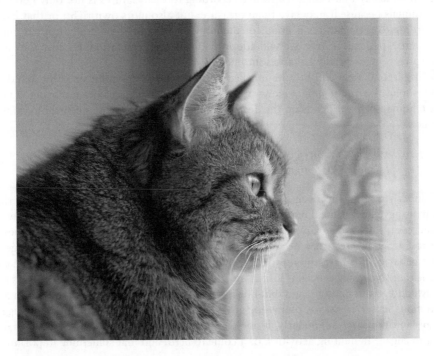

Figure 4.1 Cats kept indoors: a safe but frustrated life? (*Maria Sbytova/Shutterstock.com.*)

In addition, welfare, on a hedonist account, may not be a simple additive function of positive and negative states. If, for example, an animal experiences mild pain, its welfare may not be significantly affected if it is able to cope with the pain. However, beyond a certain threshold, the animal may no longer be able to cope, and may start to suffer.

Setting these problems of measurement and aggregation aside, some people challenge the hedonist position on the grounds that things other than positive and negative experiences matter. They say that it also matters whether the animal is allowed to lead a full and natural life:

> Animals, too, have natures – the pigness of the pig, the cowness of the cow, "fish gotta swim, birds gotta fly" – which are as essential to their well-being as speech and assembly are to us.
>
> (Rollin, 1993a: p. 11)

and:

> Not only will welfare mean control of pain and suffering, it will also entail nurturing and fulfilment of the animals' natures, which I call *telos*.
>
> (Rollin, 1993b: p. 48)

In these two excerpts, the American philosopher, Bernard Rollin, seems to be suggesting that it is good for animals to be free to live in accordance with their natures. Reading Rollin, and philosophers who hold similar views, it can be unclear whether they wish to say that being free to live according to their natures is not only good for the animals because it may give them pleasure, but also in its own right; or that living according to their natures is good for the animals, because it generally leads to more pleasant experiences. Here, we will adopt the former interpretation, because the latter interpretation essentially collapses into hedonism.

This second view will here be labelled *perfectionism*. Perfectionism is the standard philosophical term for similar views in the human case, which maintain that a good life for a human being depends on the development of certain capacities central to human nature:

> *According to the perfectionist, being able to realise significant natural or species-specific potentials is a precondition of a good life.*

Underlying this approach is the common, but also controversial, assumption that animals have well-defined natures (a perfectionist uses these to define criteria for living a successful life). For example, it may be claimed that it is the nature of a domestic cat to engage in predatory behaviours, and that having the opportunity to engage in such behaviours is part of a normal cat life. So, adopting a perfectionist view, one can argue that something crucial is lost in the life of a cat when it is kept indoors and is not allowed to go out hunting; and that this is so even if an indoor cat would not in (in any conscious sense) 'be aware' of missing anything because the indoor life does not trigger its predatory instincts. Similarly, it could be argued that it is the nature of a retriever dog to engage in hunting activities, or a collie to herd, and that something important is lost in the life of such dogs if it they are kept purely as family pets – even if they show no signs of frustration.

A related view of a 'good life' for an animal has been developed by the philosopher Martha Nussbaum, in what is known as her 'capabilities' approach. Nussbaum maintains that 'animals are entitled to a wide range of capabilities to function, those that are most essential to a flourishing life, a life worthy of the dignity of each creature' (Nussbaum, 2006: p. 392). If we are to ensure that an animal – such as a companion animal – has a good life, we need to identify which capabilities are most important to animals to ensure their flourishing, based on what's normal for the species. Once we have identified these core capabilities, we should recognise both that companion animals can be harmed if prevented from fulfilling their core capabilities (even if they are not aware of the harm) and that, where necessary, we should assist animals to fulfil their core capabilities. So, to return to the cat example: on Nussbaum's view, if we can establish that running, hunting and jumping are core capabilities for cats, and required for a cat's flourishing, then we should endeavour to make sure that the cat has the freedom to perform those behaviours. However, if these behaviours could be satisfactorily carried out indoors (with games and toys), then it may not be necessary for the cat to go outdoors.

The views of a good animal life presented so far have an important assumption in common: they both maintain that there is a standard of the good (animal) life. According to the hedonist, an animal needs to have the optimal balance of pleasure and pain to lead a good life; and according to the perfectionist, an animal can only enjoy a high quality of life if it lives in accordance with its nature, often understood in terms of its species-specific nature.

However, would we, as reflective human beings, necessarily accept that these kinds of standards would guarantee a good life for us? We might be more inclined to say that what really matters is that one gets or achieves what one considers to be important, whatever that happens to be. Some of the things that people prefer, such as engaging in extreme sports and pursuing academic careers, do seem to involve a certain amount of suffering which is not obviously compensated for by extra pleasure, and they do not appear to be (straightforwardly) 'natural'. But if that is what people really prefer, why deny that the satisfaction of the relevant preferences contributes to the quality of their lives? And if this is so for humans, why should it not be the same for other animals too?

This seems to be the reasoning underpinning the view of Peter Singer, another ethicist with a keen interest in animals. In the following passage, he explains why he claims that what matters, in a good life, is getting what one wants, that is, satisfying one's preferences:

> ... for me, a good life is one in which my own considered, informed preferences are maximally satisfied. If I hold this judgment in a form that makes no particular reference to myself – as I must, if it is to be a moral judgment as I understand the term – then I must hold that this is true for others as well, other things being equal.

> (Singer, 2002)

This view – which Singer elsewhere explicitly generalises to include animals – may be called the *preference theory*: for a good life, it is necessary to achieve what one wants or strives for, that is, to have one's preferences satisfied. If not all preferences can be satisfied, the goal is to achieve the maximum satisfaction available, which should be understood as a function of both the number of preferences satisfied and their relative strength. Typically, a requirement is added that preferences only count when they are considered and informed.

The requirement that preferences should be considered and informed is added here to avoid the objection that sometimes people (and animals) seem to prefer things that do not necessarily contribute to the quality of their lives. For example, people may prefer to do dangerous or harmful things because they do not understand the consequences; here the preference will not really be informed. Compared with humans, animals do not reflect about what they might want, so it is difficult to say that they can have 'considered and informed' preferences. Yet the reasons for including these constraints do seem relevant to animals, because they certainly could be ignorant of things that would change their preferences, and they could prefer things that are bad for them, and so would cause them, in the future, to be in states that they would not prefer.

However, it may be argued that we can make choices on behalf of animals, as well as for children, based on a concern for what would have been their considered and informed preferences had they been able to reflect and act in accordance with their long term interests. For example, it may be in the best interest of a dog not to give it the piece of chocolate that it strongly desires now, because chocolate is toxic to dogs; were the dog able to make a considered and informed choice, it would more strongly prefer not to have stomach pain and veterinary treatment that might follow.

If we return to the indoor/outdoor cat debate, the preference view may accept keeping cats indoors, as long as cats do not show signs of having strong preferences to get out (e.g. by sitting at the window, or constantly trying to slip through an open door). But if we think about what 'informed' might mean, the question is more complicated. 'Informed' in this case may mean that a cat's *actual* preference (to go outdoors) could be overridden by a *hypothetical* preference to avoid significant outdoor threats, which we might suppose the cat would have if it were fully informed about the risks to be found outdoors. On the other hand, we might equally suppose that if a cat has always been indoors, it is not fully informed about what it is missing outdoors, and that if it knew how interesting the outdoors would be, it would have a preference to go out. In the human case, preferences shaped by restricted or oppressive circumstances are sometimes described as 'deformed' or 'adaptive'; perhaps indoor cats who do prefer to stay indoors or do not prefer to go outdoors might be understood to have distorted or adaptive preferences. So, in practice, it may not always be easy to come to a clear conclusion about what constitutes good welfare if hypothetical preferences are to be counted in alongside the actual ones.

Different approaches to welfare, then, may give different answers to the question about whether a cat should be allowed to roam outdoors. It is not difficult to imagine other situations in which these approaches diverge. For example, in social animals, such as packs of dogs, fighting for a higher position in the hierarchy may be part of living a natural life, and could fit into a perfectionist vision of good welfare. But from a hedonistic view, it would be better for the animals if stressful fights were prevented, for example, by castrating the males to reduce aggression. Likewise, having preferences fulfilled may be rewarding at first, but may lead in the long run to unpleasant experiences or painful disease; for example, a dog fed according to its preferences may become obese. Thus, there may be a contradiction between what the animal desires and what will prevent it suffering in the longer term. (Of course, the comparison will be less straightforward if the preference view allows for hypothetical preferences, such as a hypothetical future preference not to suffer from diseases associated with obesity.)

However, it is not always the case that these different ideas of welfare diverge so dramatically. Positive experiences do often follow when you get what you want and you are able to express natural behaviours and potentials, and conversely, negative experiences often follow from frustrated desires and failing to fulfil natural potential or talents.

It may be possible to hold hybrid views of the good (animal) life that combine elements from different theories. Thus, one can easily imagine a view combining elements of hedonism and perfectionism, according to which it is important both to secure the best possible balance of positive and negative experiences and to express natural potentials.

So far, the discussion has concerned how to *define* the good animal life or animal welfare. But even when a definition has been adopted, there is a further question: how, in practice, should we actually assess animal welfare? It seems relevant to consider this in the context of modern discussions of animal welfare, and its links to legislation and animal welfare science.

4.3 From Farm Animal Welfare to Companion Animal Welfare

The modern idea that we should focus on 'animal welfare' and its link to so-called animal welfare science is rooted in discussions about intensive farm animal production, and dates back to the 1960s. The first clear statement appeared in a report published by the British Brambell Committee (Brambell, 1965). This committee was set up by the British government following the public outcry about intensive livestock farming prompted by Ruth Harrison's book *Animal Machines*, published in 1964. The recommendations of this committee formed the basis of subsequent British and European animal welfare legislation.

Previous legislation relating to animals had been so-called 'anti-cruelty' legislation, which only focussed on preventing people causing suffering to animals for frivolous reasons, or due to gross negligence (so-called wanton cruelty). Cruelty is still illegal, and cases involving neglect or cruelty towards dogs, cats and other companion animals make up the majority of the thousands of convictions for violations of anti-cruelty legislation made in the United Kingdom (RSPCA, 2013) and in other Western countries every year.

However, modern animal welfare legislation, in the wake of the Brambell report, also aims to protect animals from potentially adverse effects of rational attempts to make use of them, not least by increasing production efficiency (e.g. keeping laying hens confined in small cages or tethering or stalling pregnant sows). Typically, animal welfare legislation of this kind will define minimum requirements for housing and keeping animals: thus recently, in the European Union, both traditional battery cages and the confinement of pregnant sows have been banned. Some requirements to protect the welfare of companion animals have also found their way into modern, particularly European, animal welfare legislation, for example, requirements that puppies and kittens should stay with their mother for a minimum of time before being sold.

Another new development following the Brambell report was that the notion of suffering was widened to include the frustration of behavioural needs, whereas earlier, only pain was recognised as suffering. Thus, according to the Brambell report farm animals have '*behavioural urges*', often frustrated in intensive confinement systems, which they need to perform to avoid suffering (Mench, 1998). This led to the statement of a general principle of animal welfare according to which farm animals should be free '*to stand up, lie down, turn around, groom themselves and stretch their limbs*' (the so-called Brambell freedoms) (Brambell, 1965: p. 13). The committee insisted that 'suffering' should include discomfort and stress (understood to cover a wide range of mental states including frustration and fear).

Another very influential idea found in the Brambell report was that studies based on methods from physiology and ethology are necessary elements of animal welfare assessment. This was given great weight when the report's conclusions were implemented. By requiring agricultural reform to be underpinned by scientific evidence, the British Government, on the one hand, undertook to set up new research, and on the other, bought time before having to embark on controversial legislation.

The Brambell report and similar initiatives in other European countries set off significant investments in the scientific study of farm animal welfare; these investments have also benefitted other groups of animals, including companion animals. So, when researchers today study the welfare of dogs, cats and other companion animals, they typically stand on the shoulders of pioneering work done within the study of farm animal welfare.

However, the approach to the study of animal welfare following from the recommendations of the Brambell Committee also has two major limitations:

First, the focus was mainly on the *absence of suffering*; there is little mention of positive welfare. Even the central principle of the Brambell report, that animals require certain basic freedoms (later developed into the Farm Animal Welfare Council's Five Freedoms – see Box 4.1), has generally been understood to have been violated only when the infringement of a freedom led to suffering.

So, the underlying theory of animal welfare here is a very limited version of hedonism, focussing only on absence of suffering rather than on an optimal balance between pleasure and absence of suffering. Adherents of this approach may, with some justification, argue that the reduction of suffering should be considered the priority, before turning to positive welfare, which may be considered a luxury. However, it is worth noting that allowing or encouraging animals' positive states may provide an opportunity to reduce suffering, by enabling animals to better cope with any negative states they also face.

Box 4.1   The five freedoms

1. *Freedom from Hunger and Thirst* – by ready access to fresh water and a diet to maintain full health and vigour.
2. *Freedom from Discomfort* – by providing an appropriate environment including shelter and a comfortable resting area.
3. *Freedom from Pain, Injury or Disease* – by prevention or rapid diagnosis and treatment.
4. *Freedom to Express Normal Behaviour* – by providing sufficient space, proper facilities and company of the animal's own kind.
5. *Freedom from Fear and Distress* – by ensuring conditions and treatment which avoid mental suffering.

(FAWC, 2009)

This narrow hedonist view, focusing on avoiding suffering, was clearly reflected in the new field of animal welfare science that followed the Brambell report. However, measures of positive welfare have now become more prominent, although perfectionist and preference theories of animal welfare have been little recognized.

Secondly, claims regarding animal welfare could only be made on the basis of solid scientific evidence, so the burden of proof lay with those who claimed that animal welfare was threatened. This limitation strongly affects companion animal welfare, not least when taken in conjunction with the following third limitation – the lack of resources for scientific research on companion animal welfare. Substantial resources from both public and commercial sources have been spent on the study of farm animal welfare, resulting in thousands of scientific papers covering different aspects of the welfare of each of the commercially important species of farmed animals. In contrast, limited resources have been made available for the study of companion animal welfare. For example, the authors of this book searched for scientific literature published in peer review journals or books, dating back about 15 years, concerning the welfare consequences of keeping cats indoors versus allowing them out and could find very few published studies.

So, if animal welfare is taken to also include companion animals, and animal welfare science is to be used as the key source of information, we need to move beyond these limitations. It is important that a sufficient number of studies are undertaken, and that these studies consider companion animals' positive as well as negative welfare.

4.4 Assessing the Welfare of Companion Animals

Scientific studies can help to provide evidence relevant to assessing animal welfare. Staying with the example of indoor and outdoor cats, three kinds of scientific evidence are available concerning the welfare consequences of remaining indoors or going outdoors:

these concern the occurrence of behavioural problems, the occurrence of various diseases, and the involvement of cats in road traffic accidents.

The occurrences of behaviour problems in indoor and outdoor cats have been measured by means of questionnaire studies of cat owners conducted in Germany (Heidenberger, 1997) and in Spain (Amat *et al.*, 2009). One principal finding from these studies is that cats which are not, or only rarely, allowed to go outdoors show many more behaviour problems than cats which often or always have access to the outdoors. Behaviour problems are defined here as behaviours that the owners of the cats see as problematic – such as aggression or inappropriate elimination – although these may not be experienced as problems by the cat. However, such behaviours may also indicate frustration; and even if they do not, they may ultimately have bad consequences for the cat. If the owner cannot tolerate them, the cat may be euthanased (see more on behaviour problems in Chapter 9).

Buffington (2002), an epidemiologist, reviewed the veterinary literature for data on the effect of confining cats indoors on the occurrence of disease. He concluded that

> most of the epidemiologic studies of disease risk factors, conducted for more than a quarter century, have identified indoor housing as a consistent external risk factor for a variety of diseases in cats.
>
> (Buffington, 2002: p. 996)

The diseases include urinary tract disease, dental disease, obesity and endocrine disease (hyperthyroidism). The author, however, stresses that it is not possible to infer from the fact that indoor housing is a risk that the problems are *caused* by indoor housing, as there may be confounding factors. For example, most pedigree cats seem to be housed indoors and these may also be predisposed to more diseases than the mixed breed, 'domestic', cats that are more often let out to roam. Of course, outdoor cats also face risks from infectious disease; but while the risk of disease from being indoors is fairly significant, it is much less commonly noticed.

Finally, a study of cats conducted in the United Kingdom (Rochlitz, 2003a, 2003b) concluded that one in nine owned cats with outdoor access has been involved in a road traffic accident. The study discovered that a number of factors affect the risk of an outdoor cat being involved in a road traffic accident, including age (the younger the cat the greater the risk), sex (males run a greater risk), and time of day (more accidents happen at night).

Clearly, this evidence should contribute to a more balanced discussion about whether it is good for a cat's welfare to be confined indoors. The study of traffic accidents documents that there is real risk to a cat's safety (particularly if it is a young male) from being let out at night, which is perhaps not surprising. What may be much more surprising to some is that both the studies of behavioural problems and those of disease risks show that there are some real welfare concerns to be considered when it comes to keeping a cat indoors – other things being equal, it seems that cats that are confined indoors may pay a significant price for being spared the risks of traffic accidents and other outdoor hazards.

But such studies also give rise to questions and uncertainties. For example: how representative is the British study of the involvement of cats in traffic accidents worldwide? To what extent does the quality of the indoor life affect the mentioned behavioural and health problems?

Further studies would certainly help improve our understanding of the potential positive and negative effects that the way we choose to keep domestic cats has on their welfare. However, there is still no reason to believe that even a considerable investment in scientific studies would provide a definite answer about what, from the point of view of cat welfare, is the best way to keep cats. There are several reasons for this.

First, some things, for example, incidence of disease or fatality rates, are much easier to measure scientifically than others such as the pleasure that a cat can get from climbing trees or hunting. This has more general implications: it illustrates how far animal welfare science will always tend to emphasise that which is easy to measure and count.

Second, answers require that a number of very different welfare indicators are added up to create a net value or ranking. Whereas animal welfare science has a lot to contribute when it comes to assessing different aspects of what matters from the point of view of the affected animals, there is huge uncertainty and disagreement about how to aggregate across these different aspects (Veissier *et al.*, 2011).

In the case of the indoor versus outdoor cat debate, it is likely that the study of what matters will come up with an extended version of conditions and diseases that may be associated with confining a cat indoors or allowing it access to the outdoors, as seen in the following table from Rochlitz, 2007:

Cat is confined indoors	Cat has access to the outdoors
Feline urologic syndrome	Infectious diseases (e.g. viral, parasitic)
Odontoclastic resorptive lesions	Road traffic accidents
Hyperthyroidism	Other accidents (e.g. falling from a tree)
Obesity	Fights with other cats
Household hazards	Attacks by humans, dogs and other
Behavioural problems (e.g. inappropriate	animals
elimination/toileting)	Poisoning
Boredom	Theft
Inactivity	Going astray

Even with this list, which only concerns a number of possible negative effects, it is far from clear how to weigh different aspects against each other. How, for example, should an increased level of boredom be weighed against an increased risk of being poisoned?

Some of those engaged in the debate about cat welfare seem to agree that there may not be a clear-cut answer to the question about whether indoors or outdoors is best for cats. The International Cat Care (ICC) website lists the advantages and disadvantages of allowing a cat access to the outdoors, so that owners can try to make a more informed decision, for example, considering social contact, exercise, outlet for behavioural needs versus injury, disease, loss, stress (International Cat Care, 2013a). Suggestions are then offered as to how to minimise the risks to those cats allowed outdoors, including vaccination, neutering, wearing a safety collar with their owners' details, keeping the cat in at night and at peak 'risk' times, for example, morning and evening rush hour if the cat lives near a busy road. Overall, however, the ICC body suggests that while:

> Cats which have been kept indoors all their lives adapt reasonably well to their environment provided that they are given ample companionship and attention … such an enclosed environment is far from ideal and a solution which permits the cat to have access to a garden as well as the house is preferable.
>
> (International Cat Care, 2013b)

We are using the indoor/outdoor cat case as a way of making concrete a much more general problem about adding up different aspects of animal welfare, with broad implications for thinking about companion animal welfare. It is important to be aware that problem we are considering here will not necessarily go away, even if more scientific studies are forthcoming. This can be illustrated by means of an example relating to agriculture, the housing of laying hens.

In commercial egg production, laying hens are kept in a small number of different and reasonably well-defined production systems, from small cages to ranging freely. In some cases, comparisons can be made because on every indicator, such as mortality and incidence of behavioural problems of various sorts, one system is better than the other. Thus, so-called enriched cages seem in all respects to provide better welfare than the traditional cages that are smaller and more barren. However, comparisons between cage systems and outdoor systems are more difficult. These systems each have their advantages and disadvantages. This is nicely illustrated in the following quotation from a recent paper reviewing housing systems for laying hens based on nearly 200 scientific publications:

> It appears that no single housing system is ideal from a hen welfare perspective. Although environmental complexity increases behavioral opportunities, it also introduces difficulties in terms of disease and pest control. In addition, environmental complexity can create opportunities for the hens to express behaviors that may be detrimental to their welfare.
>
> (Lay *et al.*, 2011)

Thus, although scientific studies can highlight the different problems and opportunities for the animals depending on the individual system in which they are housed, science does not solve the problem of how to compare different positives and negatives in terms of animal welfare.

Most people concerned about animal welfare seem to prefer free-range systems to cage systems for laying hens despite the fact that mortality is higher in the free-range systems. Here freedom seems to matter more than safety. In the context of cats, however, many people seem to think, conversely, that safety matters more than freedom, and therefore, cats should be confined rather than free-ranging. At the end of the day, ethical assumptions, partly to do with how animal welfare is defined, will determine how we weigh different aspects of animal welfare.

Key Points

- Three theories of what constitutes a good animal life have been presented:
  - *Hedonism:* a good life is one in which there is a greater number of positive experiences relative to negative experiences.
  - *Perfectionism:* a precondition of a good life is to be able to realise significant species-specific potentials.
  - *Preference theory:* to have a good life it is necessary to achieve what one wants or strives for, that is, to have one's preferences satisfied.
- These three approaches may deliver similar conclusions about what makes a good life, but for different reasons. Equally, they may provide competing answers, such as in the question of allowing cats outdoor access. In some cases, the approaches may be combined into various kinds of hybrid views.
- The concept of animal welfare originates from the discussion of farm animals in the 1960s, when concerns developed about the negative effects of intensive production methods on animals.
- A number of limitations were found in the original concept of animal welfare – for instance, only negative welfare was emphasised, and the treatment of animals was assumed to be acceptable unless shown by scientific means to be problematic.
- We generally want cats and dogs to have 'good' and pleasurable lives, rather than simply ensuring that they have lives free of suffering.
- Although animal welfare science may enlighten us about different problems and opportunities for the animals, it is not able to give a final verdict on what is best for the animal. To come to a view on this involves an ethical judgement.

References

Amat, M., De la Torre, J.L.R., Fatjó, J., Mariotti, V.M., Van Wijk, S. & Manteca, X. (2009) Potential risk factors associated with feline behaviour problems. *Applied Animal Behaviour Science* 121 (2), 134–139.

Bentham, J. (1789/1989) A utilitarian view. In: Regan, T. & Singer, P. (eds) *Animal rights and human obligations.* Englewood Cliffs, NJ, Prentice Hall, pp. 25–26.

Brambell F.W.R. (1965) *Report of the technical committee to enquire into the welfare of animals kept under intensive livestock husbandry systems.* Command Rep. 2836. London, Her Majesty's Stationery Office.

Buffington, C. (2002) External and internal influences on disease risk in cats. *Journal of the American Veterinary Medical Association* 220 (7), 994–1002.

FAWC (2009) *Five freedoms*. Farm Animal Welfare Council. [Online] Available from: http://www.fawc.org.uk/freedoms.htm [Accessed 21 July 2014].

Heidenberger, E. (1997) Housing conditions and behavioural problems of indoor cats as assessed by their owners. *Applied Animal Behaviour Science* 52 (3–4), 345–364.

International Cat Care (2013a) *Minimising risks for the outdoor cat*. [Online] Available from: http://www.icatcare.org/advice-centre/cat-care/minimising-risks-outdoor-cat [Accessed 15 July 2014].

International Cat Care (2013b) *Fencing in your garden*. [Online] Available from: http://www.icatcare.org/advice-centre/cat-care/fencing-your-garden [Accessed 15 July 2014].

Lay, D.C., Fulton, R.M., Hester, P.Y., Karcher, D.M., Kjaer, J.B., Mench, J.A., Mullens, B.A., Newberry, R.C., Nicol, C.J., O'Sullivan, N.P. & Porter, R.E. (2011) Hen welfare in different housing systems. *Poultry Science* 90, 278–294.

Mench, J. (1998) Thirty years after Brambell: wither animal welfare science? *Journal of Applied Animal Welfare Science* 1 (2), 91–102.

Nussbaum, M. (2006). *Frontiers of Justice: Disability, Nationality, Species Membership*, Cambridge, MA, The Belknap Press, p. 392.

PETA (2013) *Why all cats should be indoor cats*. People for the Ethical Treatment of Animals. [Online] Available from: http://www.peta.org/living/companion-animals/indoor-cats.aspx [Accessed 8 May 2014].

Rochlitz, I. (2003a) Study of factors that may predispose domestic cats to road traffic accidents: part 1. *Veterinary Record* 153, 549–554.

Rochlitz, I. (2003b) Study of factors that may predispose domestic cats to road traffic accidents: part 2. *Veterinary Record* 153, 585–588.

Rochlitz, I. (2007) Housing and welfare. In: Rochlitz, I. (ed.) *The welfare of cats*. Dortrecht, Springer, pp. 177–203.

Rollin, B.E. (1993a) Animal production and the new social ethic for animals. In: Purdue Research Foundation (ed.) *Food animal well-being: conference proceedings and deliberations*. West Lafayette, IN, US Department of Agriculture & Purdue University Office of Agricultural Research Programs, pp. 3–13.

Rollin, B.E. (1993b) Animal welfare, science and value. *Journal of Agricultural and Environmental Ethics* 6 (suppl. 2), 44–50.

RSPCA (2013) *Justice for Animals*. Royal Society for Prevention of Cruelty to Animals, Prosecutions Department, Annual report 2013. [Online] Available from: http://www.rspca.org.uk/whatwedo/prosecution/report [Accessed 15 December 2014].

Singer, P. (2002) *A response to Martha Nussbaum*. [Online] Available from: http://www.utilitarianism.net/singer/by/20021113.htm [Accessed 8 May 2014].

Veissier, I., Jensen, K.K., Botreau, R. & Sandøe, P. (2011) Highlighting ethical decisions underlying the scoring of animal welfare in the Welfare Quality® scheme. *Animal Welfare* 20, 89–101.

Theories of Companion Animal Ethics

5

5.1 Introduction   73
5.2 Contractarian Approaches – Companion Animals Are
     Only Indirectly Ethically Important   75
5.3 Utilitarian Approaches – Welfare, and Only Welfare, Matters   76
5.4 Deontological and Rights Approaches – Not Only
     the Consequences Matter   79
5.5 Contextual Approaches   82
5.6 Dealing with Multiple Ethical Approaches   85

5.1 Introduction

In the previous chapter, we suggested that to ensure an animal's best possible welfare, we need to do more than simply use animal welfare science to work out what would be positive and negative from the animal's point of view. We also need to weigh these positives and negatives against one another; this weighing forms part of an *ethical judgement*. So, for example, whether it is best for a cat living in a quiet, safe neighbourhood to be allowed out to roam or to be kept indoors requires weighing the potential benefits of roaming, in terms of exercise and expression of behavioural needs, against the risks of being hit by a car or infected by disease.

By saying that *ethical judgement* is involved here, we mean that potentially conflicting values are at play. To make a decision, it is necessary to come to a view about the relative importance of these values. So far, we have only discussed values relating to the welfare

Companion Animal Ethics, First Edition. Peter Sandøe, Sandra Corr and Clare Palmer.
© Universities Federation for Animal Welfare 2016.

of the affected animals. But ethical judgements often involve much more than this. Even if two people agree about what constitutes the best welfare for a particular animal, they may still reach different *ethical* conclusions, because they disagree about whether *other* values are relevant and important and how (or whether) to factor these in. Decisions about one animal companion, for example, may have consequences for other animals, or for human welfare, or for other human values, such as aesthetic value; or they may have implications for the environment. The way people view and weigh these *other* values will affect their *all things considered* ethical decision making.

This becomes clear if we return to the indoor/outdoor cat question. Someone who thinks that overall, cat welfare would be improved by letting cats roam outdoors, may still make an 'all things considered' ethical judgement that cats should nonetheless be confined. Outdoor cats can be a significant nuisance to human neighbours and even a threat to public health. Cats also hunt wildlife, raising questions not just about the welfare of individual birds and rodents, but also about broader environmental values, such as species protection. (We will consider these questions about companion animals' negative impacts further in Chapter 14.) These concerns may outweigh those about the welfare of the cat(s) in question when deciding whether, ethically speaking, the cat(s) should be allowed to roam outdoors. When we make 'all things considered' ethical decisions, animal welfare may be only one relevant value among many. And different people may weigh these multiple values differently, leading to conflicts in ethical judgements about what we should do.

Not only are there different views as to which values matter when it comes to companion animals (many of which we will discuss in this book), there are also contrasting ways in which we apply those values. For instance, do we have an obligation to maximise what we think is valuable, such as an obligation to attempt to bring about the best possible total welfare across humans and animals? Or do our ethical commitments entail, instead, a requirement to absolutely protect what is valued – for instance, never to violate basic rights – rather than to maximise total value?

One way of enabling a structured discussion of such questions is by means of so-called *ethical theories*. These are theoretical constructs developed by philosophers to describe different approaches to understanding and weighing values, and to putting values into practice. In this chapter, we discuss four types of ethical theory, each of which outlines a distinctive approach to thinking about ethical issues involving animals. We have chosen these four approaches because we think that separately, and in combination, they provide a gateway to understanding most ethical discussions relevant to companion animal ethics.

Understanding these different theoretical approaches to ethics is important in two key ways. First, it should assist in developing, and perhaps challenging, our own ethical views about companion animals. Second, it may help in understanding why other people, who also regard themselves as behaving ethically, may support very different actions or policies from those we as individuals consider to be ethical. Such an understanding of other people's approaches to ethics is an important prerequisite for a civilised social dialogue about companion animals.

5.2 Contractarian Approaches – Companion Animals Are Only Indirectly Ethically Important

One feature that distinguishes companion animals from other domesticated animals is that most people care more about their animal companions than they do about other animals, such as those used for food production. This may seem inconsistent from a perspective from which animals with similar capacities should be similarly valued. However, this is not inconsistent in the group of views to be discussed here, according to which animals are not *directly* of ethical relevance at all. On these views, animals' values lie only in their importance to people, rather than in the good of the animal itself. As we saw in Chapter 3, many people have very close bonds with their companion animals, caring for them and seeing them as a source of affection and emotional support. From a perspective where animals matter only indirectly, harming beloved companions would be ethically problematic, not because it harms the animal, but because doing so would result in emotional or psychological harm to the animal's human owner.

From positions like this, the feelings (and perhaps the property rights) of the owner and other affected humans are not simply *a* reason, but rather the *only* reason for protecting companion animals. By implication, then, to the extent that no one cares about a particular animal, or a group of animals, they do not matter ethically. Historically, the view that animals – including companion animals – can matter ethically because, and only because, they are important to people has been widely endorsed by philosophers.

One ethical approach that (in most forms) still defends this view is *contractarianism*. Contractarians argue that morality is a kind of contract, which we join, ultimately, for our own self-interest. By adhering to certain rules of respect and decency to others, we can create a tolerable society; moral rules are conventions that serve everyone's interests. However, many forms of moral contractarianism only apply to individuals who are both able to understand and to follow the rules, and to gain from doing so. Since animals – companions or otherwise – cannot understand the rules of morality, they cannot join the contract. This means that they fall outside the sphere of beings to whom we have direct moral responsibilities. Of course, in the case of companion animals, owners care about what happens to their companions. If I steal, beat and starve your dog, I cause you considerable distress, and thereby show disrespect to you, as a member of the moral community. So I have a direct obligation to you not to do this. However, if I capture and beat a feral dog, and no one knows about it (or no one cares), then there is nothing wrong with my doing so.

However, even on contractarian views, neglect and cruelty are not normally acceptable because those who live with animal companions are usually strongly attached to them, and contractarian ethical views will provide significant protection to those particular animals. Where people extend this attachment to other members of the same species (so, someone who loves their cat may have a looser attachment to all cats), it may also provide some reason to protect all cats. However, there are important situations where this ethical approach might raise questions – as we will see in later chapters. Suppose, for instance, that an owner has a dog that is in severe pain from an incurable disease. The animal is suffering so much and has such poor welfare that we might reasonably say that it would be better off dead. But the owner, being strongly attached to her companion, wants to keep the animal alive 'no matter what', and does not take the animal to be euthanased. On this ethical theory, there is no direct reason for her to do so: only human desires matter; so what is best for the animal is ethically irrelevant.

It is for this reason that contractarianism is often regarded as inadequate in the context of animal ethics, as it implies that causing or allowing animals to suffer is morally unproblematic, so long as no human being is harmed. Indeed, this position, in a simple form, seems to take the same view of children, or people with certain mental disabilities, who are also unable to understand or keep moral rules.

However, many people consider that it is unethical *as such* to cause (or, sometimes, to allow) another to suffer for little or no reason, whether the individual concerned is a human being or an animal. An ethical theory that captures this view is *utilitarianism*.

5.3 Utilitarian Approaches – Welfare, and Only Welfare, Matters

According to utilitarianism, what we do to animals and humans alike matters ethically to the extent that we affect their welfare. On a utilitarian approach, to cause or to allow an animal to suffer always counts negatively in moral decision making, irrespective of whether humans care about it. So, one key feature of utilitarianism is that welfare matters, whoever's welfare it is. In fact, the claim is even stronger than this: according to utilitarianism, welfare is *all* that matters, and from an ethical point of view, the higher the level of welfare, the better.

In the previous chapter, we saw that there are different accounts of welfare: hedonism (focusing on the balance of pleasure and pain); a preference theory; and perfectionism, with a focus on the expression of natural abilities. Depending on which theory of welfare is adopted, there will be different varieties of utilitarianism. These are called, respectively, hedonistic or classic utilitarianism; preference utilitarianism; and ideal utilitarianism. Rather than pursuing these distinctions here, we will discuss utilitarianism more broadly, with a focus on varieties of utilitarianism on which welfare is defined either in terms of hedonism or in terms of preference satisfaction.

Utilitarianism is one family in a group of ethical theories called *consequentialist*. All consequentialist theories agree that we should bring about the best outcomes, and that only the outcomes matter. Consequentialists require us to take the *whole* outcome into account in ethical decision making, including the outcomes resulting from *omitting* to do things we could have done. Utilitarians defend a version of this view where the best outcomes are brought about by maximizing the welfare of all the beings likely to be affected by any action (whether welfare is understood in terms of pleasure versus pain, or in terms of preference satisfaction).

The calculations involved in working out what maximises welfare in practice can be complex: as we have already seen, measuring welfare is by no means straightforward; nor is trading off different aspects of welfare, even for the same animal. What is key from a utilitarian perspective, however, is that animals matter directly, and should be considered in our moral decision making. It is not only the welfare of our companion animals that matters. *Every* being that can undergo pleasure or pain or has preferences should be taken into account; there is no consistent reason for picking out companion animals and excluding other beings whose welfare may be affected.

The indoor/outdoor cat case is a good example to think about here. On a utilitarian view, we should, of course, take into account the expected pleasure and pain or preference satisfaction and frustration of the cat, comparing a life confined indoors to one that allows outdoor roaming. But we should not stop there. We should also consider the pain (and loss of the positive welfare of a future life) the cat might cause to other animals that it hunts, and the way in which being kept indoors, or allowed outside, might affect the owner(s), neighbours, and so on. Also, not all cats are the same, nor in similar circumstances; therefore, no general calculation will suffice here. The key, though, is that the expected pain and pleasure, or preferences, of every human and animal affected by any decision we make should be taken equally into account – whatever the species, and whatever relation the beings concerned have to us (Figure 5.1).

One defender of this view is the philosopher Peter Singer (1989: pp. 152–153). Singer uses the language of *interests* in outlining his position: if a being can suffer, Singer argues that it has an interest in avoiding suffering, and, he maintains, its interests should be treated equally to the similar interests of other beings, whether they are human or not.

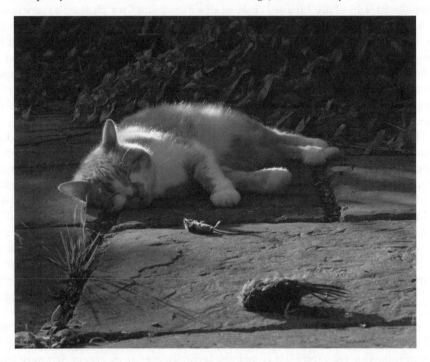

Figure 5.1 The question of whether or not cats should be allowed to outdoors is contested. Many outdoor cats predate wildlife, raising ethical concerns about the welfare of individual birds and rodents and broader environmental issues such as species protection. (*Image used courtesy of Sandra Corr.*)

Suppose we think back to the case of the owner who does not want to euthanase the incurably suffering dog. On Singer's view, the owner's interest in avoiding emotional distress should be weighed against the interests of the suffering dog. Since the dog's suffering is severe, it cannot be relieved, and it is incurable, the dog's interest in being euthanased is almost certainly stronger than the owner's interest in keeping the dog alive – especially as this is only a temporary measure. So, the action that would be expected to minimise suffering overall in this case is euthanasia.

This conclusion illustrates something else about utilitarianism: utilitarianism does not, in principle, object to killing. Killing, for utilitarians, could generate two kinds of negative outcomes: the killing process itself may cause pain, distress or frustration; and an animal's death brings an end to its possible future positive experiences, potentially reducing overall pleasure or preference satisfaction. In the case of a dog suffering intensely as a result of an incurable disease, however, no future positive experiences or satisfactions are possible, and euthanasia ends, rather than brings, suffering. For a utilitarian, in such a case, other things being equal, euthanasia is not just morally *permitted*, it is morally *required*.

However, this view has another implication that is troubling. It suggests that if animals are painlessly killed (so, no suffering is *caused*), and other animals that would not otherwise have lived are bred (so creating new possibilities for pleasant experience or preference satisfaction), then there is nothing wrong with killing them, provided the amount of new positive experience equals or exceeds whatever positive experience is lost. This seems to be the case even if the animal is healthy – and, in fact, this seems to be true of killing humans as well! So, in the case of pedigree dogs, for instance, there would be nothing wrong in principle with painlessly euthanasing a breed-imperfect but otherwise healthy litter and trying again to produce puppies that are closer to the breed ideal.

This issue has led many utilitarians to make a further distinction here, based on whether a being is thought to possess *self-consciousness* or not. What is meant by self-consciousness is difficult to define clearly, but the term is often taken to include a sense of oneself as persisting over time. In particular, some utilitarians have maintained, a self-conscious being is an individual who has a *preference* or a *desire* to go on living, and the frustration of such basic desires is morally relevant. This preference utilitarian view was adopted by Singer (1989) himself. Preference, or desire, utilitarians argue that we should minimise the *frustration of desires* in the world, especially the frustration of the most basic desire of a self-conscious creature (except in circumstances of extreme suffering) – the desire to go on living.

The first question here is what beings count as 'self-conscious'. Are adult dogs, or cats, self-conscious, in the sense of being aware of themselves as persisting over time? Are newborn kittens or puppies? There is little agreement among those who study animal cognition about who possesses this capacity – indeed, it is not clear whether even human babies are relevantly self-conscious. Secondly, even if we accept that most companion animals are relevantly self-conscious, similar problems still exist as in the earlier arguments based on pleasure and pain or preference satisfaction. As a consequentialist theory, utilitarianism must aim at best consequences. So, suppose we painlessly kill a self-conscious animal that desires to go on living. Then we breed another self-conscious animal, one that would not otherwise have existed, in its place. This new animal, after all, desires to go on living, a desire that can (for a while, at least) be satisfied. Why cannot this new desire substitute for the old desire? The philosopher Michael Lockwood considered this scenario, using a fictional case, which he called Disposapup:

> Many families, especially ones with young children, find that dogs are an asset when they are still playful puppies (capable of keeping the children amused), but become an increasing liability as they grow into middle age.... Moreover, there is always a problem of what to do with the animal when they go on holiday. It is often inconvenient or even impossible to take the dog with them, whereas friends tend to resent the imposition, and kennels are expensive and unreliable. Let us suppose that, inspired by Singer's article, people were to hit on the idea of having their pets painlessly put down at the start of each holiday (as some pet owners already do), acquiring new ones upon their return. Suppose, indeed, that a company grows up, "Disposapup Ltd", which rears the animals, house-trains them, supplies them to any willing purchaser, takes them back, exterminates them and supplies replacements, on demand. It is clear, is it not, that there can, for Singer, be absolutely nothing directly wrong with such a practice. Every puppy has, we may assume, an extremely happy, albeit brief, life – and indeed, would not have existed at all but for the practice.
>
> (Lockwood, 1979: p. 168)

Even if these puppies are self-conscious and desire to live, the obvious way of thinking about this case for a utilitarian is that the new puppies' desire to live substitutes for the frustration of the euthanased dogs' desire to live. Singer (1999) himself, in his book *Practical Ethics*, tries to argue that the creation of a new desire to live cannot be weighed against the frustration of another individual's desire to go on living – that is, that preferences are not substitutable in this way. But in maintaining this, he moves away from the aggregative, maximizing approach that defines utilitarianism, because he is suggesting that there are some goods (such as a desire to go on living) that just cannot be compensated for by the creation of more of the same goods (more desires to live). In fact, this kind of view – that some harms are just unacceptable, whatever the ensuing benefits – is much more closely associated with a cluster of different approaches to animal ethics – those that are deontological, in particular those that focus on rights.

5.4 Deontological and Rights Approaches – Not Only the Consequences Matter

An alternative set of approaches in ethical theory is often called 'deontological'. The key commitment that binds deontological views together is rejection of the fundamental premises of consequentialism – that only consequences matter, that we should aggregate values, and that, in the case of utilitarianism, we should try to maximise value. Deontologists insist that things *other* than consequences matter, that we are not always obliged to bring about the best consequences – and that sometimes we are required *not* to bring about the best consequences, if to do so means to violate an important principle or a right.

Rights theories are the most developed forms of deontology in animal ethics. There are a number of different interpretations of rights theory, but two traditions have predominated in terms of *human* rights; these two traditions persist in discussions of *animal* rights. One tradition – in the case of human rights – maintains that rights are based on something like the basic dignity of the human person; and this dignity is usually explained in terms of some high-level capacity, such as autonomy or rational thought, that humans are argued to possess. The second tradition maintains that rights are based on the protection of certain strongly important interests (Cochrane, 2012) – such as the interest in not undergoing severe suffering.

Those who argue that animals have rights maintain that – in either view – if we are to attribute rights to *all* humans, there is no valid reason to deny rights to *all* animals. After all, neither view maintains that being biologically human – a member of the species *homo sapiens* – is what gives rights; a particular configuration of DNA *in itself* is not of moral significance. Rather, it is the possession of particular capacities (such as autonomy or reason) or interests (such as not to feel pain), which being biologically human supports, that underpins humans' rights. But if it is capacities or interests rather than human DNA that is the basis for rights, it appears invalid, animal rights theorists argue, to include *all* humans and *no* animals. Aren't adult dogs, for instance, just as rational – plausibly more rational – than newborn babies? Both dogs and babies have highly significant interests in not suffering.

This argument about rights is particularly important because of the special weight rights language is usually thought to carry. Although the term 'rights' is sometimes loosely used just to mean that a being matters ethically, philosophers generally understand rights in a more restricted sense. In this restricted sense, to say that a being has rights is to make a very strong claim that those rights should be protected or promoted. Indeed, sometimes possessing a right is described as having a 'trump card' – the kind of claim that wins out over any competing claims. So, if animals have rights, they have – with respect to these rights, at least – particularly strong, overriding claims to protection.

Although a number of ethicists have argued that animals have rights, two have been of particular importance in the context of companion animals: Gary Francione and Tom Regan. Francione (2012) argues that all sentient beings – beings that are conscious and can suffer – should be regarded as having basic rights, and as being 'persons'. In light of this, he rejects the 'institution of pet-keeping' altogether. The institution of pet-keeping depends on the idea that animals can be property, which, he maintains, implicitly denies them rights – even where pets are renamed 'companion animals'. Pets, he argues, 'exist forever in a netherworld of vulnerability, dependent on us for everything and at risk of harm from an environment that they do not really understand. We have bred them to be compliant and servile, or to have characteristics that are actually harmful to them but are pleasing to us' (Francione, 2012). From this perspective, the whole idea of breeding animals to be our companions is in conflict with the idea that animals are 'persons' with rights of their own. It is an exploitative relationship that benefits people at the expense of animals. (We will return to the issue of breeding in Chapters 6 and 7.)

Francione's point is an important one for thinking about companion animal ethics. His view raises questions about what 'companionship' means, when animal companions are bred in shapes and forms pleasing to us even though they may cause the animals ill health; when animal companions are confined indoors, neutered, kept away from conspecifics, restrained with leads and crates, and so on. Is this, as Francione argues, a relationship closer to domination than companionship?

Other leading accounts of animal rights, however, do not explicitly object to companion animals. One important account here is Tom Regan's *The Case for Animal Rights* (1984). Regan (2007: p. 209) develops a view of animal rights that expands on the traditional 'dignity-capacity' based view of rights. He argues that all beings that he calls 'experiencing subjects of a life' have inherent value and rights. An experiencing subject of a life is 'a conscious creature having an individual welfare that has importance to it whatever its usefulness to others'. Such beings 'want and prefer things, believe and feel things, recall and expect things'. They can undergo pleasure and pain, experience satisfaction and frustration, and have a sense of themselves as beings that persist over time. This gives them, on his account, their own inherent value. They are not merely instruments for someone else's use and benefit. Regan argues that all mentally normal adult mammals fall into this category, and have basic rights, including the right to life and to liberty. The evidence that infant mammals and birds are experiencing subjects of a life is less clear. However, since we cannot be sure about their inner worlds, he argues that we should give them the benefit of the doubt in moral decision making, since they too may have inherent value (Regan, 1984: pp. 416–417).

On the basis of Regan's account of inherent value, the painless killing of experiencing subjects of a life is normally unacceptable. Killing an animal harms it, by deprivation of all the goods that the rest of its life would have contained (Regan, 1984: p. 99). In contrast with the utilitarian views just discussed, the creation of a new animal, even an animal that is happier, or more satisfied, cannot substitute or compensate for the painless killing of another animal. Killing an animal is rarely permissible, though it can be justified in life-or-death situations (such as in defending oneself against the attack of a dangerous and aggressive dog) or when an animal's life is of such poor quality that it is not worth living, and so loss of it is not a deprivation – as in the case of the incurably suffering dog we have already discussed. (See also Chapter 13.)

On this rights view, human practices such as keeping animals for meat are morally unacceptable – such practices violate animals' right to life; breeding new ones cannot make this loss good. But this does not necessarily mean that keeping animals as *companions* is morally unacceptable. On Regan's view, it seems at least possible in principle that one could live alongside an animal while respecting its inherent value. In his book *Animal Rights Without Liberation* (2012), Alistair Cochrane makes this argument explicit. Cochrane develops an interest-based view of animal rights in which animals' core interests – such as not to be made to suffer, and not to be killed – are protected by rights, and impose duties on others. However, he maintains, since animals do not understand what 'being property' is, unlike humans they do not have an interest in not being owned, or in not being human companions:

Some practices that are objectionable when done to humans are not objectionable when done to animals: keeping an animal as a pet is quite unlike keeping a human as a slave; using animals to undertake certain types of work is quite unlike coercing humans to labor; buying and selling animals is quite unlike trading human beings; and so on.

(Cochrane, 2012: p. 11)

Having said this, however, most animal rights views do present a number of challenges to the ways in which people generally live with their companion animals. Most companions are not free to roam, which appears to violate a right to liberty. Many companion animals are neutered, foreclosing the possibility of sexual activity or reproduction, which, if animals have rights, plausibly also constitutes a rights infringement (we will consider this in Chapter 10). And most companion animals, especially cats, are fed on food comprised from *other* animals whose rights have been violated to make it. For these reasons, even though a rights view may accept the idea of companion animals in principle, it raises serious ethical questions about many of the ways in which we actually live with companion animals, something we will consider throughout this book.

The rights view Regan defends is explicitly set up to contrast with the kinds of utilitarian view we considered in the previous section. For utilitarianism, what matters is pleasure, pain, desire satisfaction and the like – states that can be increased or decreased, maximised or minimised. Regan's focus is on *inherent value*, which belongs to individuals by virtue of their capacities, and cannot be traded off, factored into calculations about consequences, or replaced. On this view, harming or killing some beings in order to bring about good consequences for others is morally unacceptable. So, for instance, euthanasing an unadoptable feral cat in a feral cat colony that has feline immunodeficiency virus (FIV), but that still has a reasonable quality of life, in order to protect other members of the colony from FIV infection, would be unacceptable. Regan (2007) says of cases like this: 'That would be to sanction the disrespectful treatment of the individual in the name of the social good, something the rights view will not – categorically will not – ever allow.' A utilitarian, on the other hand, would likely conclude that euthanasing the infected individual would, over time, reduce overall suffering among cats in the entire colony, and so, if the cat is otherwise unadoptable or there is no prospect of adoption, would argue that we are morally required to euthanase it.

Utilitarian and rights approaches have dominated the animal ethics literature. However, several alternative approaches have recently been gaining in significance. We will deal with these approaches under the broad category of contextual approaches.

5.5 Contextual Approaches

A variety of different positions can be grouped together as advocating *contextual* approaches to animal ethics. These approaches share the view that although animal capacities – such as the capacity to feel pain – are relevant to ethical decision making, and may indeed be very important to it, we also need to take other factors into account when making ethical decisions. Advocates of contextual views argue that utilitarians and rights theorists give a limited account of what is morally relevant; that they assign no real weight to the different *relations* that humans have with different animals; that they have no substantial place for emotions such as empathy; and that they barely discuss the special obligations that humans may have towards particular animals, based on prior commitments to them or prior interactions with them.

One contextual approach with ancient roots is so-called *virtue theory*, according to which the character of the human individual is of primary ethical significance. Rather than focusing on *consequences, principles or rights*, a virtue ethicist instead asks how we should live, what it is to be a 'virtuous person', and how to make ourselves into such a person. A virtue (or a vice) is understood as a disposition or trait of character, manifested in habitual action, that it is good (or bad) for anyone to have (Rachels & Rachels, 2010: p. 161). As this definition suggests, before we can say that someone has such a disposition or a virtue, it needs to be regularly and reliably demonstrated. So, for instance, I might, in an unprecedented rage, having just crashed my new car, kick my dog out of the doorway to enter a room. But if this is the one and only time I ever kick the dog, or harm him in any way, I am not a cruel person (or even a cruel-to-dogs person). However, if I kick the dog whenever I see him, it is reasonable to think I manifest the vice of cruelty (and possibly some other vices as well!).

One striking feature of a virtue ethics view (contrasting with the theoretical approaches we have so far considered) is that it accepts the importance of what are usually called the 'moral emotions' such as *sympathy* and *compassion*, and it is concerned with our underlying emotionally influenced *attitudes* towards animals. Neither utilitarianism nor rights theory gives moral emotions a central place. Modern virtue theorists, in contrast, often argue that sympathy and compassion are virtues, and that we should endeavour to develop characters in which they are prominent. But this should not be interpreted simplistically. As the ancient Greek philosopher Aristotle argued, a virtuous person must have the practical wisdom to know how, when, to what degree, and in what way particular virtues should be expressed. This requires sufficient knowledge and understanding of a being or situation (for instance, about an animal's welfare), and the ability to make appropriate judgements. For example, Hursthouse (2011: p. 216) maintains that being so compassionate that one could not quickly kill a suffering bird mauled by one's outdoor cat would not express compassion at the right time, to the right degree and in the right way.

A virtue ethics approach to companion animals prompts us to ask different questions than utilitarianism or rights theory. Rather than asking 'What will the consequences be in terms of overall suffering if I do this?' or 'Does this violate my companion animal's rights?', we should instead ask 'What would a virtuous person do here?' or, more specifically, 'Would a compassionate and kind person do this?' or 'Would it be selfish of me to do this?' To return, for instance, to the case of the dog in intense pain from an incurable disease, a virtuous owner would ask what a compassionate and kind person would do in such circumstances, and consider whether failing to euthanase the suffering dog might be an expression of selfishness, or even cruelty, in allowing the continuance of unnecessary suffering that could be brought to an end.

Virtue provides us with a general ethical theory, but it also allows us to ask specific 'role' questions such as 'What makes a good small animal vet?' 'What makes for a good dog owner?' The most natural way of answering questions like this involves character terms, such as attentiveness, patience, sensitivity and being affectionate. Likewise, we might describe a bad dog owner or vet as callous, cruel, neglectful or impatient. So, virtue theory may be particularly useful in terms of thinking about the role responsibilities of different parties, including professional practitioners.

A closely related kind of contextual approach, sometimes called an ethics of care, emphasises the role of emotions – such as sympathy, empathy and care – in all of our transactions with others, including animals. On this view, ethics is not so much about rights and reasons, but also about our *emotional* responses to other individuals, especially those with whom we regularly interact. This approach is particularly appropriate for the kind of mutual, interactive relations people have with animal companions, relations from which emotional support is derived, and which are based on knowing the animals as particular individuals. Engaging in an ethical relationship with a particular companion animal, on this view, is not about respecting its rights, or calculating what would bring about the best consequences, but about paying attention to the animal's specific individual needs and desires, responding sensitively to it, and developing lasting emotional ties to it. Those animals that we invite into our home, care ethicists argue, have a special relationship to us; we owe them attention that we do not owe to other animals. Noddings (2003: p. 157) comments: 'When we take a creature into our home, name it, feed it, lay affectionate hands upon it, we establish a relation that induces expectations'.

If we think about the indoor/outdoor cat question from this perspective, we are likely to get quite a different answer to the one a utilitarian or a rights theorist might offer. A utilitarian is concerned with the pain and pleasure of all affected beings. A rights theorist is likely to be concerned with the cat's liberty rights and (perhaps) the rights to life of wildlife. However, an ethicist of care would emphasize the special, caring relationship the particular owner has with the particular cat; the cat's owner should adopt the policy that is most likely to develop the caring bond between himself and the cat, a policy that could not be construed as betraying or damaging the relationship.

Virtue ethics and the ethics of care, then, tend to emphasise the ethical importance of maintaining and nurturing particular special relationships, such as those we have with family members – and with companion animals. For an ethics of care, these special obligations are based on our emotional relationships with particular others. But there are other possible grounds for thinking we have special obligations to animal companions. Palmer (2010), for instance, argues that – both as individuals, and as societies in which keeping animals as companions has been institutionalised – we may have special obligations to companion animals not so much because of our emotional relationships to them, but because we have made them dependent on us. Unlike wild animals, many companion animals are not able to flourish without human support. So, we have special social responsibilities to care for domesticated dogs, for instance – responsibilities that we do not have towards wild foxes or wolves that we have not bred or brought into our homes.

All of these contextual approaches raise difficulties in practice – difficulties that may lead some people to turn back to more traditional utilitarian or rights views. For instance, it is often argued that a focus on character and 'what a compassionate person would do' is not very helpful in decision making (after all, there are occasions when, viewed in different ways, conflicting actions could all be seen as compassionate). The focus on responsive, reciprocal relationships in an ethics of care raises questions about what responsibilities we might have to those from whom we are distant. For instance, should we have no concern about the wildlife killed by outdoor cats, or about the euthanasia of millions of anonymous cats annually in animal shelters, because we do not have caring individual relations with the wild birds or with feral cats? A contextual view based on the ways in which humans have made companion animals dependent and therefore vulnerable raises other problems – in particular, who has the responsibility to assist these animals? Is everyone responsible to care for companion animals because some (other) people have been breeding them?

Contextual approaches, then, tend to be highly complex, and to present difficulties in actually working out what to do. Utilitarian and rights ethical theories both seem much more straightforward to work with, and to give much clearer ethical guidance (though this leads defenders of contextual views to argue that they are oversimplified). However, perhaps there is no need to choose between these approaches. We will consider this possibility in the final section of this chapter.

5.6 Dealing with Multiple Ethical Approaches

So far, we have outlined a number of different theoretical approaches to animal ethics. Theoretically divergent though these approaches are, in many cases, they will converge on the same action or policy. But nonetheless, there are occasions where these different ethical approaches diverge.

This may be illustrated by elaborating on an example mentioned at the beginning of Chapter 4. Suppose a cat's owner wants to go on vacation, but in order to do so has to leave the cat behind. What is it ethical for the owner to do? The answer to this question depends on which ethical approach is taken. None of the approaches we have considered is likely to accept temporary abandonment of the cat without any care. Even from a contractarian, human-centred approach, the owner's attachment to the cat is likely to mean that she will want the cat to be cared for during her absence, so that it is still alive and well on her return – although a contractarian view would permit euthanasing or abandoning the cat if the owner so wished. A utilitarian – say, a hedonistic utilitarian – would weigh the suffering and pleasures at stake. The owner would have to consider whether even the best option for the cat in her absence would outweigh the pleasure she gained by the holiday. It might be, for instance, depending on the cat's nature and circumstances, that the cat would be so distressed in a cattery that its distress would outweigh the owner's pleasure from the trip; but that if left at home and regularly fed by a neighbour, the cat would be only mildly unsettled, making the vacation permissible. From a rights perspective, it seems unlikely that temporarily leaving an animal, providing that the animal had sufficiently good care that leaving it could not be regarded as a serious harm, would be a rights violation (any more than leaving one's children to be looked after by a careful relative while making a trip would violate their rights). A virtuous owner would ask whether taking a vacation was, for instance, selfish, given the needs of her animal companion; or whether, alternatively, it would be wise to take the vacation given (for instance) her state of over-work and exhaustion, provided the companion could be well cared for. The answer here would depend on the owner, the circumstances, and the animal, and would be a matter of contextual judgement. Finally, for a care ethicist, the fundamental question is likely to be how the vacation would affect the special, caring relationship with the particular companion animal, and whether, despite the temporary separation, the relationship could resume without permanent damage.

In this example, different owners may do different things depending on their ethical conviction. However, in many cases, different people need to coordinate, or a shared policy is required. Is it necessary, in such cases, to adopt one of these approaches (or some other approach altogether) and reject all the others? Or are there ways in which people with different theoretical convictions can work together, or combine elements of different theoretical approaches to create a 'hybrid view'?

One possible approach – which might be especially useful to small animal vet practices attempting to adopt some kind of 'practice ethics' – is to draw up some 'rules of thumb', or general principles, to which most people who adopt different theoretical approaches would agree. An example of this approach – called principlism – is well known in medical ethics, and originated in biomedical research. It has now been extended to apply to many areas of ethics, including animal ethics and veterinary practice, although it is not very well developed in this field (Mullen & Main, 2001; Sokol, 2009).

The idea that biomedical research could be governed by four key principles was first proposed in the Belmont Report, a report developed to protect the use of human subjects in medical research, published in 1979 (National Commission, 1979). These four principles were later developed into a more wide-ranging approach to biomedical ethics, not confined to research situations, by Tom Beauchamp and James Childress in *Principles of Biomedical Ethics*. The four guiding principles – held by the authors to be equally important – are respect for non-maleficence (not harming), beneficence (doing good), autonomy (roughly, self-governance), and justice. Beauchamp and Childress (1994) maintain that these four principles emerge from a 'common morality' shared across many religious, cultural, ethical and philosophical traditions, and that they can, therefore, form a widely acceptable basis for moral decision making for people from many different backgrounds.

The idea that these four key principles could govern our interactions with companion animals has the appeal of simplicity. But principlism raises many difficulties. Some ethicists argue that the four principles are not sufficiently comprehensive; they fail to take account of some important moral concerns that emerge from other moral perspectives. Other critics are concerned that the indeterminate nature of all four principles – what is meant by 'non-maleficence' or 'justice', for instance – could be differently interpreted to produce *divergent* non-maleficent or just responses to the same situation, which would fail to give people sufficient guidance about how to act. Additionally, in some cases, the principles may conflict with one another: so, for instance, we may be presented with a choice between respecting autonomy and respecting beneficence. This means that a way of balancing or ranking the principles is needed, or the principles will not be useful. In the case of animals, specifically, what is meant by 'autonomy' and 'justice' needs clarification: these terms, contested enough in the human case, are particularly unclear in animal cases. After all, many companion animals are deliberately created not to be autonomous in some senses of the term; is it wrong in principle to do this, if a more autonomous being could have been created instead?

Having said this, as suggested earlier, principlism could be useful in suggesting 'rules of thumb' for how to deal with companion animals in institutions such as veterinary hospitals and animal shelters (these may vary by type of institution). Although some cases will test the meaning of the principles and their relations to one another, the principles could still provide a starting point for debate and a reference point when there is a need for quick decision making.

Other forms of hybridization between ethical theories also seem possible. For instance, it is possible to combine a rights position with certain contextual views. Most accounts of animal rights only direct us with respect to prohibited rights violations. But they do not help us to decide when, if ever, we should assist or provide for animals, or why we might have different responsibilities to care for our own cat than we do our neighbour's cat, or the equally sentient red fox that lives in the garden. Contextual ethics could help in thinking through such varied ethical responsibilities to assist and provide, while also accepting certain rights-based prohibitions. A recent account of this kind was proposed by Donaldson and Kymlicka (2012) which we discuss in Chapter 16. Likewise, there are ways of understanding virtue ethics from within other ethical theories – for instance, a virtuous utilitarian might be someone who has the disposition to act in ways that bring about the best consequences.

Some hybrid views, then, are likely to work, especially if one view is taken as 'baseline' or given priority in a situation where different approaches conflict. However, not all views hybridise with one another very easily. So, for instance, there is a deep conflict between the utilitarian idea that we should aim to bring about best expected consequences, and the claim from deontological rights theorists that certain rights should almost never be violated, however good the consequences. Yet even so, some kinds of hybridization between rights and utilitarian views may be possible. One might conclude that although there are rights that should never be violated, as long as one respects these constraints, moral reasoning should be governed by what would bring about best consequences.

Key Points

- Companion animal issues give rise to dilemmas and disagreements due to different understandings of what constitutes animal welfare, different views about which values matter, different ways of weighing or adding up the relevant values, and different ideas about how the relevant values should be put into practice.
- So-called *ethical theories* – theoretical constructs developed by philosophers to describe different approaches to understanding, weighing, and implementing values are introduced here to enable a structured discussion of such dilemmas and disagreements.

- Four groups of ethical theories are presented:

  Contractarian approaches, according to which animals only matter indirectly to the extent that humans care about them.

  Utilitarian views, according to which we should, ethically, aim at creating the best aggregate consequences in terms of welfare for *all* beings involved.

  Deontological views, according to which other things than consequences matter ethically, for example, respecting animals' rights.

  Contextual approaches, according to which human relations to the animals in question matter, for example, in the form of virtues, emotions or past commitments

- It may be possible to combine some of these approaches in the form of various hybrid approaches.

References

Beauchamp, T. & Childress, J. (1994) *Principles of biomedical ethics*. 4th edition. Oxford, Oxford University Press.

Cochrane, A. (2012) *Animal rights without liberation: applied ethics and human obligations*. New York, Columbia University Press.

Donaldson, S. & Kymlicka, W. (2012) *Zoopolis*. Oxford, Oxford University Press.

Francione, G. (2012) *"Pets": the inherent problems of domestication*. Blog entry 31 July 2012. [Online] Available from: http://www.abolitionistapproach.com/pets-the-inherent -problems-of-domestication/ [Accessed 15 July 2014].

Hursthouse, R. (2011) Virtue ethics and the treatment of animals. In: Beauchamp, T. & Frey, R. (eds) *The Oxford handbook of animal ethics*. Oxford, Oxford University Press, pp. 119–143.

Lockwood, M. (1979) Singer on Killing and the Preference for Life. *Inquiry: An Interdisciplinary Journal of Philosophy* 22, 157–170.

Mullen, S. & Main, D. (2001) Ethics: principles of ethical decision-making in veterinary practice. *Practice* 23 (7), 394–401.

National Commission for the Protection of Human Subjects of Biomedical and Behavioral Research (1979) *The Belmont report: ethical principles and guidelines for the protection of human subjects of research*. [Online] Available from: http://www.hhs.gov/ohrp/human subjects/guidance/belmont.html [Accessed 16 July 2014].

Noddings, N. (2003) *Caring: a feminine approach to ethics and moral education*. 2nd edition. Berkeley, CA, University of California Press.

Palmer, C. (2010) *Animal ethics in context*. New York, Columbia University Press.

Rachels, J. & Rachels, S. (2010) *The elements of moral philosophy*. 6th edition. New York, McGraw-Hill Higher Education.

Regan, T. (1984) *The case for animal rights*. Berkeley, CA, University of California Press.

Regan, T. (2007) The case for animal rights. In: LaFollette, H. (ed.) *Ethics in practice*. 3rd edition. Malden, MA, Blackwell, pp. 205–211.

Singer, P. (1989) All animals are equal. In: Regan, T. & Singer, P. (eds) *Animal rights and human obligations*. Englewood Cliffs, NJ, Prentice Hall, pp. 148–162.

Singer, P. (1999) *Practical ethics*. 2nd edition. Cambridge, UK, Cambridge University Press.

Sokol, D. (2009) Sweetening the scent: commentary on "What principlism misses". *Journal of Medical Ethics* 35, 232–233.

Breeding and Acquiring Companion Animals

6.1	Introduction		89
6.2	Breeding and Rearing Puppies and Kittens		90
6.3	Welfare Concerns		91
6.4	Ethical Issues		94
	6.4.1	Ethics of breeding and rearing	94
	6.4.2	Ethics and acquiring companion animals	97
	6.4.3	Possible ethical strategies and solutions	99

6.1 Introduction

When Barack Obama first moved into the White House with his family after being elected as president in 2008, he faced many difficult decisions. One of these concerned the acquisition of a dog. This decision was, of course, a very personal one, involving the whole family. However, it was also a decision with clear political implications. As a senator, Barack Obama had been involved in a campaign concerning how dogs are sourced, with a critical focus on so-called puppy mills. As a result, lobby groups campaigned for the Obamas to adopt a dog from a shelter. However, in the end, the family accepted a 6-month-old purebred pedigree dog from a breeder, to whom the dog had been returned by its previous owners. The family was criticised by some animal protection organisations for obtaining a dog from a pedigree breeder. However, the Humane

Companion Animal Ethics, First Edition. Peter Sandøe, Sandra Corr and Clare Palmer.
© Universities Federation for Animal Welfare 2016.

Society of the United States released a statement thanking the Obamas 'for taking in a second-chance dog'.

In this chapter, we review the common ways in which puppies and kittens are bred, reared, and acquired, and consider some of the ethical issues that arise at each stage. In particular, we focus on commercial breeding establishments (so-called puppy and kitten 'mills' or 'farms'), and consider ethical sources of companion animals for prospective owners. To clarify the scope of this chapter, we understand 'breeding' here as 'deliberately producing offspring, typically through intentional mating or insemination'. We consider specific questions raised by the selective breeding of purebred dogs and cats in Chapter 7, and issues raised by unwanted offspring in Chapter 13. Similar issues arise with the breeding of species other than cats and dogs; we will briefly discuss these in Chapter 15.

6.2 Breeding and Rearing Puppies and Kittens

Companion animals can be bred through natural mating, typically with selected partners, or by artificial insemination using fresh or frozen semen from a selected sire. The latter method is usually only used with purebred dog or cats, but can also be adopted in other cases where animals are not able, or willing, to be mated in the normal way.

Breeding may also take place in many different circumstances. 'Casual breeders' deliberately mate their animal companions only once or twice, while 'small scale' or

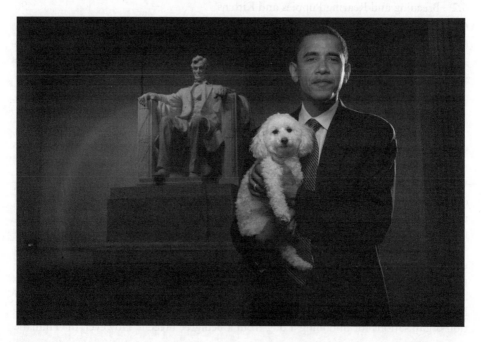

Figure 6.1 Barack Obama, while still a senator, campaigned against puppy mills by being portrayed in the Lincoln Memorial holding the three-legged former puppy mill breeding dog, Baby. (*Robert Sebree Photography, LA, USA. Reproduced with permission.*)

'backyard breeders' keep a small number of breeding dogs or cats in their homes as a side business or hobby. Pedigree breeders typically fall into the category of small-scale breeders, although they may have kennels or catteries of different sizes and quality. Commercial breeding establishments produce puppies and kittens, usually purebreds or designer breeds (see more on this in Chapter 7), on a large scale. These establishments are often called puppy or kitten 'mills' in the United States or 'farms' in the United Kingdom. However, there is no formal legal definition of these terms and some disagreement as to how they should be defined. Instead, therefore, we will use the phrase 'commercial breeding establishments', to refer specifically to those typically large-scale establishments, often with poor or questionable welfare standards, that emphasise profit over the welfare of the animals that they breed and rear (Figure 6.1).

Although there are significant welfare concerns about commercial breeding establishments (see the following section), this does not mean that they are unregulated; most countries in the industrialised West have a licensing system and require minimum standards of welfare. For instance, in the United States, dog breeders with more than three breeding bitches, who sell puppies to pet stores or puppy brokers, must be licensed and inspected by the US Department of Agriculture (USDA). Individual states often have further standards regarding the maximum number of intact animals that may be kept, the quality of housing and care that must be provided, and may require licensing and a license fee (Tushaus, 2009).

According to the American Society for the Prevention of Cruelty to Animals (ASPCA, n.d.), there are between 2000 and 3000 USDA-licensed commercial dog-breeding establishments operating in the United States. However, the ASPCA estimates that the total number of commercial breeding establishments in the United States could actually be as high as 10,000, as not all breeders need to be licensed (if they do not sell to pet stores or brokers), and many operate illegally. Some establishments are small, with only 10 breeding dogs, though others contain more than 1000. The Humane Society of the United States (HSUS, 2012a) estimates that 2 to 4 million puppies from commercial breeding establishments are sold each year in the United States.

Some European countries have stricter regulations than the United States about commercial breeding, including requirements for breeder education and a minimum weaning age. In the United Kingdom, the 1999 Breeding and Sale of Dogs Welfare Act requires annual veterinary inspections of any facility where five or more litters are produced in one year, and breeding females are restricted to one litter per year and six per lifetime. However, many breeders still operate illegally, and animals may be imported from other countries that lack such regulations: the Irish Society for the Prevention of Cruelty to Animals estimates that up to 1000 dogs are being trafficked into Britain each week from unlicensed Irish commercial breeding establishments (Forde, 2012).

6.3 Welfare Concerns

The main area of concern about the breeding of companion animals lies with commercial breeding establishments. These welfare concerns cross all areas of the animals' lives: diet, cleanliness, space, exercise, medical care and relations to both humans and conspecifics. Some commercial establishments permanently confine breeding animals without exercise, either indoors in cages, or outdoors without proper shelter. The animals may be densely packed together, and infrequently cleaned out. Females are usually bred until they are physically incapable of producing further offspring (Katz, 2009). Investigations into these commercial establishments by non-governmental organizations (NGOs) such as the ASPCA (n.d.) the HSUS (2012a, 2012b) and The Kennel Club (n.d.) report that animals often do not receive adequate veterinary care, food, water or socialization to enable them to have reasonable levels of welfare.

These welfare problems persist, despite attempts at legal regulation, for a number of reasons. First, the minimum requirements for licensing may be insufficient. For example, under the federal Animal Welfare Act in the United States, it is legal to keep a dog in a cage only six inches longer than the dog in each direction, with a wire floor, stacked on top of another cage, for the dog's entire life. Secondly, some breeders may not comply with the licensing requirements, budgets for inspections may be inadequate, inspections may not be thorough and regular enough, and fines for non-compliance may not be high enough to act as a deterrent (Tushaus, 2009). Third, many breeders may simply choose to work illegally without a license. As noted earlier, there may be an international market in puppies or kittens, where imported animals bred in poor welfare conditions are sold more cheaply than those produced in a more highly regulated domestic market. Recent legislative measures have attempted to prevent this; the import of puppies from commercial breeding establishments abroad, for instance, was banned in the United States in 2008 (United States Senate Committee, n.d.); but such imports may still happen illegally.

A recent development, also likely to have welfare implications, is the growth in selling puppies and kittens over the internet. Puppies sold online in the United States, for instance, are not subject to USDA regulation. A study by Voris et al. (2011) compared breeders selling purebred puppies online with breeders registered by the American Kennel Club (AKC). They found that breeders selling via the Internet are far less likely to carry out breed-specific health screening than breeders that are members of the AKC; they are much less likely to accept the return of puppies for any reason; and they are more likely to say they will sell puppies before they are 8 weeks old. All of these differences are likely to have welfare implications for the puppies sold online.

Demand also drives the production of puppies in large commercial establishments. Demand for purebred puppies from registered AKC breeders, for instance, significantly outstrips the number of puppies available, resulting in long waiting lists (Voris et al., 2011). Puppies and kittens bought online or from pet shops are usually much cheaper than those bought directly from AKC breeders. The Voris et al. (2011) study found that the average online price for a pedigree puppy was $736, while the average price for a pedigree puppy from an AKC breeder was $1396. Given the substantial sums involved, the flourishing of a cheaper online market is unsurprising.

Research suggests that animals born and reared, or used for breeding, in commercial establishments, often have welfare problems that persist long after they have left the establishments (McMillan et al., 2013). It is well documented in studies conducted on rodents and farm animals that factors such as avoiding stress and anxiety in the mother, providing appropriate early nutrition and opportunity to express normal behaviours, and avoiding weaning and separation from the mother when too young, are essential to the health and ability of the offspring to function well later in life. Although few studies have been conducted on cats and dogs, it seems highly likely that their health and behaviour are not simply genetic, but also significantly affected by similar environmental and early rearing factors.

Furthermore, puppies and kittens intended to live with humans as companions need to be well socialised with humans, and the right kind of handling and contact early in life are crucial (Serpell & Jagoe, 1995). Commercial establishments may try to save expensive labour costs by failing to invest in early socialization, and thereby cause severe problems for both animals and their owners later in life.

Two questionnaire studies (McMillan, Duffy & Serpell, 2011; McMillan *et al.*, 2013), both conducted in the United States, show that both puppies and breeding dogs from commercial breeding establishments suffer from reduced welfare compared to control dogs. According to the first study, former breeding dogs from commercial breeding establishments had a significantly higher rate of health problems, were more fearful, and had higher levels of other behavioural problems compared to control dogs. The other study compared dogs obtained as puppies from pet stores (which typically originate from commercial breeding establishments), with dogs obtained from non-commercial breeders. That study found that dogs from pet stores showed significantly higher aggression towards human family members, unfamiliar people and other dogs, and had greater levels of separation-related problems and house soiling than those obtained from non-commercial breeders (Figure 6.2).

These conclusions indicate that dogs originating from commercial breeding establishments have poorer welfare than dogs bred in other ways, since they have higher

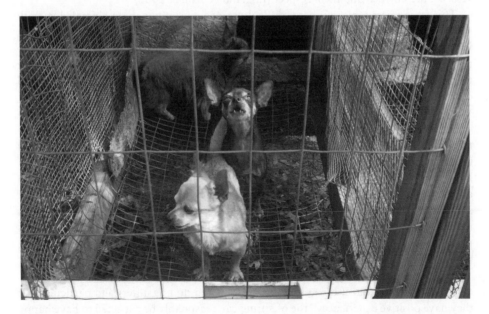

Figure 6.2 Miniature breed dogs in a puppy mill in the United States. Such animals are often in poor physical health; the dogs here have alopecia, and deformed feet with overgrown nails from standing on the mesh floors, which lack any bedding. (*By PETA (People for the Ethical Treatment of Animals), Public domain, via Wikimedia Commons.*)

levels of health and behavioural problems, which in turn are likely to increase suffering and inhibit the expression of certain species-specific behaviours. More generally, the animals produced by commercial breeding establishments are often poorly socialised to humans; Lockwood (1995), for instance, maintains that eliminating large-scale establishments that mass-produce poorly bred and unsocialised animals would reduce the level of aggression in dogs. Since aggression is one of the main reasons for relinquishment of dogs to shelters where they are likely to be euthanased (see Chapter 13), this is a further reason for concern about the welfare and the life expectancy of dogs bred in commercial breeding establishments.

6.4 Ethical Issues

The breeding and rearing of kittens and puppies raise ethical issues both in terms of supply – the ways in which companion animals are bred; and in terms of demand – the acquisition of animals by prospective companion animal owners.

6.4.1 Ethics of breeding and rearing

One very general ethical concern here relates to the idea of 'breeding animals' at all. It might be argued that making animals reproduce – in particular by forced mating or artificial insemination – inappropriately controls them, or uses them as 'reproductive vessels', thereby denying them respect (England & Millar, 2008).

This issue raises a more general difficulty: since most companion animals live with their owners, whatever happens with respect to reproduction – whether it occurs, or is prevented – is largely under the owner's control. Preventing reproduction, by neutering, raises ethical concerns from some perspectives (see Chapter 10). But deciding to permit or facilitate reproduction is equally deliberate, and may raise other ethical concerns – such as what to do with a resulting litter.

Perhaps the main concern here is whether deliberately breeding from animals – however much they appear willing to mate, and however well cared for they are – *instrumentalises* them, and whether this matters. Here, different ethical perspectives are likely to diverge. Those like Francione (2007) who regard keeping companion animals as a kind of animal slavery, might claim that breeding from companion animals treats them as reproductive vessels, and perpetuates an unethical institution in which companion animals are dependent and vulnerable. From this perspective, even if the animal is not made worse-off in terms of welfare by the reproductive process – even perhaps gains pleasure from it – there is still something unethical in principle about humans controlling animal reproduction.

But this is not the only possible ethical view. It might also be argued, from a utilitarian perspective, that if the animals that are mated do not suffer (and particularly if they have positive experiences), the offspring can reasonably be expected to have happy lives, and such breeding will not have negative impacts on other animals or humans sufficient to counterbalance the direct positive effects, then the breeding is actually ethically desirable. The animals themselves, after all, are not aware of human 'instrumentalizing attitudes', so there is no negative impact in terms of the animals' own subjective experiences.

The use of AI for breeding companion animals might be regarded as ethically problematic, even by those who do not consider there to be any general ethical difficulty with mating selected companion animals. Those who consider the performance of natural behaviours to be important, for instance, will regard AI as less satisfactory than 'natural' mating (and perhaps as denying animals the possibility of performing natural mating behaviours). Surgical intra-uterine insemination (placement of the sperm directly into the uterus through a puncture made in the uterine wall via laparotomy or laparoscopy) may cause some pain and discomfort for female animals (this practice is banned in some countries, including Norway and Sweden). Non-surgical insemination, though, probably causes little discomfort and removes the risk of catching disease from a mate. Nonetheless, even if the procedure is painless, its clinical nature and the animal's complete inability to control what is happening may seem particularly instrumentalizing if one regards 'instrumentalizing attitudes' and dominating power relationships as ethically problematic.

Of course, there are other ethical problems with commercial breeding establishments that are not *directly* due to the processes of mating and breeding, but are rather caused by the conditions in which breeding animals are kept. Suppose we take a utilitarian perspective: as noted in Chapter 5, a utilitarian would argue (roughly) that we should maximise expected pleasure, net of pain, in the world. But clearly, commercial breeding facilities that cause animals to have negative experiences including suffering, frustration, hunger and thirst, are not maximizing expected pleasure in the world. Even if the kittens and puppies produced in these establishments were to go on to have relatively happy lives, since they could have been reared in better ways, their lives could, overall, have been better.

Furthermore, it might, from a utilitarian perspective, be argued that the lives of the breeding animals confined in the worst commercial breeding establishments are often so miserable that it is reasonable to suggest that their lives are not worth living: the bad experiences they undergo outweigh any good experiences they may have. Of course, humans gain benefits from animals being bred like this – not just the breeders themselves, but also those who purchase cheap puppies and kittens. However, in some cases, the human benefits will be short lived, given the costs of dealing with the long-term health and behavioural problems of animals emerging from commercial breeding establishments (see Section 6.3). The costs to the animals are, in any case, sufficiently high that they would normally outweigh any small benefits to humans. Since alternative ways of breeding companion animals obviously exist, and are usually available to the breeder, from a utilitarian perspective, producing animals in these ways is normally ethically unacceptable.

From a rights perspective, too, breeding animals in these ways looks unacceptable. Some rights theorists – such as Francione (2007) again – would object to the idea of any commercial breeding irrespective of welfare standards, seeing the buying and selling of animals for a profit as an unethical kind of exploitation. This argument would apply to commercially bred animals, however they were treated. But even rights positions that accept that companion animals can be property – for instance, Cochrane (2012) – would reject commercial breeding establishments where both the breeding animals, and their offspring, have poor welfare. Inflicting suffering on animals, except in broadly paternalistic cases, where suffering is ultimately to the benefit of the particular animal concerned (for instance, in the course of medical treatment) violates animals' rights, on virtually all accounts of animal rights.

Contextual accounts of ethics are also unlikely to find such commercial breeding establishments ethically acceptable. One reason for this is the apparent conflict between the idea of companionship and the commercial exploitation of breeding animals that drives the breeding establishment. After all, the animals actually used for breeding are usually permanently denied the very relations of companionship for which their offspring are being bred; meaning that the existence of many much-loved companions is dependent on a 'shadow class' of the non-companion parent breeding animals used to produce them. In addition, commercial breeding establishments may produce animals less able than animals bred under better conditions to forge strong connections to their owners later in life; from a contextual perspective based on ethics of care, this may also be morally problematic.

However, there are possible objections to the idea that commercial establishments of this kind are necessarily unethical. Particularly in the United States, many commercial dog-breeding establishments developed as a profitable niche for farmers, when traditional sources of income declined. Industrial farmers usually confine their livestock and kill adults when they are no longer able to breed. If this is acceptable for livestock, why should it be unacceptable for breeding dogs or cats? It is not difficult to see why someone might object that it is ethically inconsistent for a society to accept confinement systems in pig production, yet to react with moral outrage when similar systems are used for the breeding and rearing of dogs and cats.

From the utilitarian and rights views, however, intensive rearing of *any* animal, livestock or companion – is likely to be seen as ethically problematic (Fumarola, 1998). These approaches focus on individual animals' abilities or experiences – such as sentience – irrespective of species membership. However, many people maintain that the difference between members of species that are kept as companions, and those that are not, is ethically significant, and consider it wrong to treat dogs and cats on par with pigs and cows. On this companion species-oriented view, for instance, eating dog-meat is taboo (Lien, 2004). Some justification for this view may be possible, based on the argument that since humans have created companion animal species, they have special 'companionship' or care responsibilities to companion animals that they do not have to other animals. But more commonly, this view is not defended by argument, but instead based on affective attachment to companion animal species, often derived from having lived with members of the species (see Herzog, 2011 for further discussion of this).

One further reason for objecting to commercial breeding establishments has been discussed previously: animals bred in these establishments may be less healthy, and have behavioural issues, which may create problems later on for those who buy them and which may result in a mismatch between owner and animal that results in poor animal welfare. Thus, producing puppies and kittens in such intensive ways may be problematic, since unlike piglets, they are intended to become human companions, rather than human food.

So, it seems that even those who adopt a wide range of ethical views, including views that mainly focus on human interests, are likely to agree that puppies and kittens should not be bred in commercial breeding establishments where there is poor welfare.

Alternative practices would not only produce happier, healthier and better-socialised animals, and better respect animals' rights (for those who think they have rights) but also improve relations between the animals and their subsequent owners.

Given this agreement from almost all ethical perspectives, legal restrictions on the breeding of companion animals seem justified. (We will say more about this next.) However, if this were to result in fewer animals, in total, being bred, there might be two consequences that would be problematic from some ethical views. First, fewer animals that could have fairly happy lives will come into being (a utilitarian might find this problematic), and second, people who want animals as companions may not be able to obtain them.

It is not clear how troubling these concerns should be. Currently, in most countries, more animals are euthanased in animal shelters than are bred in commercial breeding establishments, and so – in theory – restricting the latter should increase the number of shelter animals that find homes. As a result, animals that would otherwise be euthanased have the opportunity to live potentially happy lives, and breeding animals with poor welfare avoid miserable ones. However, many of the dogs that end up in shelters were bought from commercial breeding establishments in the first place, and so if this supply dries up, there may be fewer dogs available – perhaps too few to meet demand. One solution would be to increase the number of 'responsible breeders', that breed companion animals in much better welfare conditions, and for whom the breeding of animals is not primarily a commercial enterprise. Such breeders are likely to have fewer, better-cared for animals that are bred less frequently, and are kept in their homes or in enclosures with sufficient space to be comfortable. We will say more about these next.

6.4.2 Ethics and acquiring companion animals

So far, we have considered ethical questions raised by the supply of companion animals. But what about the *demand* for companion animals? What should those who want to acquire a companion animal do? Should prospective owners ever buy a puppy or kitten from a commercial breeding establishment?

There are several practical points to consider here. One is that the provenance of an animal is not always clear (Tushaus, 2009). Puppies from commercial breeding establishments are usually sold at 'neutral' locations such as pet shops, or through newspaper advertisements or Internet sites, which often use attractive websites to trick consumers into thinking that they are dealing with a small, reputable breeder (HSUS, 2012a; The Kennel Club, n.d.). In a survey by the UK Dogs Trust, dog owners were asked whether they would consider buying a dog from a 'puppy farm': although almost 95% said no, when asked from where they had got their dog, 15.1% (nearly 900,000 owners) admitted they had got them from an advert (newspaper or Internet), a pet shop or pet superstore: all outlets often supplied by commercial breeding establishments (Dogs Trust, n.d.).

It seems obvious that, if one knows or suspects that a puppy or a kitten has been bred in a commercial breeding establishment, one should not buy it. However, there are surely cases where a prospective owner has looked at such a puppy in a pet-shop, and thought that by buying it and giving it a good home, the puppy is being rescued, and that this is ethically a good thing to do. But animal welfare organizations argue strongly against this view – for instance, the Humane Society says:

Avoid the temptation to "rescue" a puppy mill puppy by buying him. Even though your intentions may be good, don't buy a puppy with the idea that you are "rescuing" him or her. Your "rescue" opens up space for another puppy mill puppy and puts money into the pockets of the puppy mill industry. Pet stores won't leave their cages empty and websites won't leave their pages blank. The money you spend on your puppy goes right back to the puppy mill operator and ensures they will continue breeding and treating dogs inhumanely. If you see someone keeping puppies in poor conditions, alert your local animal control authorities instead of buying.

(HSUS, 2013)

Although this argument seems plausible, it is not the only possible perspective. First, the HSUS 'solution' – alerting the local animal control authorities – is not necessarily helpful. The puppy may not be being kept in particularly poor conditions in the pet shop, even though it may have originated in such poor conditions. Even if the conditions in which the puppy was bred can be identified, and are poor, they may not necessarily be illegal, such that the animal control authority can act.

Second, whether or not to purchase the puppy depends on one's ethical approach. The HSUS position here looks like a form of utilitarianism. If you buy this puppy, your particular action will have specific consequences that will lead to the perpetuation of commercial breeding establishments (in general) and so cause greater suffering for breeding dogs and other puppies not yet born. This argument is not completely implausible. One individual's purchase may contribute, incrementally, to the demand that supports an industry. But (as numerous papers on other similar cases of consumer demand have argued) it is unlikely that this particular purchase is going to make much of a difference. After all, if you do not buy the puppy, someone else probably will, and that person may not know about the provenance of puppies in pet shops, and so be unprepared for the health and behavioural problems this puppy may present. In addition, there will be cases where it will make no difference at all in terms of demand whether you purchase the puppy or not – for example, if the particular pet shop is closing down, and will not be procuring any more puppies.

A stronger utilitarian argument against buying puppies in this context draws on a different version of the utilitarian view. The kind of view we have discussed so far is a form of what is called 'act-utilitarianism', which focuses on the direct consequences of particular acts – in this case, the consequences of the individual buying *this* puppy. However, strictly speaking, according to a utilitarian view, one should not only take into account the direct, short term consequences of buying a puppy from a pet shop but also the broader possible consequences in terms of, for example, setting a precedent for others. But once one starts taking these broad consequences into account, utilitarian calculations easily become very complicated. In light of this, some modern adherents of utilitarianism have argued that we should instead aim to develop simple rules that everyone can follow, rather than requiring people to calculate all the expected consequences of particular acts. This view is called 'rule-utilitarianism' (see, for instance, Brandt, 1983).

Rule utilitarians maintain that the best result is brought about not by thinking about the consequences of individual acts, but instead by following rules that, if accepted by everyone, will bring about best consequences. So, in this case, the question is 'What would the consequences be if *everyone* followed a rule that it's acceptable to buy puppies from pet shops?' rather than 'What will the consequences be if *I* buy *this* puppy?' Clearly, the demand for puppies from commercial breeding establishments would increase, and the consequences would be worse than if no one bought puppies from pet shops. So, the rule-utilitarian approach would almost certainly prescribe not buying the puppy. It is much less clear that this would be true if only a single purchase were considered.

But rule utilitarianism is *also* problematic, since there will be particular occasions where it is clear that following the rule will not bring about the best, or even good, consequences. In such cases, following a rule just seems irrational – a kind of 'rule worship', unrelated to best outcomes. So, an alternative utilitarian approach has also been developed, sometimes called a 'two-level theory', that captures elements of both act and rule utilitarianism (Hare, 1981). It recognises that while in most cases it may best to follow a simple and useful rule that generally brings about best consequences – such as 'don't buy puppies from a pet store' – there are situations where we need to stop and reflect (hence the 'two-level' theory) on whether the rule makes sense in the particular circumstances. However, these circumstances will be relatively infrequent, and generally, we should follow the rule – and in the current example, the best overall consequences will result from not acquiring puppies from pet stores.

Interestingly, it is not clear that a rights theorist would argue against buying the puppy. A puppy in a shop would, from some animal rights perspectives, be in a situation where its rights are being violated, if it is being treated solely as commercial property, something that can be bought and sold. Given this, it is likely that a rights theorist would argue that we *should* buy the puppy, if doing so would stop the violation. Buying the puppy, and treating it as an individual valuable in its own right, would mean that it was no longer being treated *solely* as commercial property (even if it is still owned). Buying the puppy would also stop other rights violations, such as not to be harmed, were it, for instance, being deprived of sufficient food and water. For most rights theorists, the violation of a right should be stopped, even if in the future, this raises the likelihood of other puppies suffering or having their rights infringed.

Some animal rights perspectives, such as Cochrane (2012), would not take the view that selling the puppy alone is sufficient to violate its rights, though depriving it of food or water would be. On views where no violation is perceived as actually occurring, a rights theorist could be neutral about purchasing the puppy, although he or she may feel compelled to buy it if a future rights violation looks likely.

In presenting these arguments, we are suggesting that the ethical conclusions here are not as straightforward as they initially might seem. Most people will probably find the rule or two-level utilitarian approach plausible – that most likely buying the puppy would contribute to a practice that generates more unhappy dogs; however, it is important to recognise that this is not the only possible ethical view here. Nonetheless, it is difficult to identify any ethical position from which commercial breeding establishments with poor animal welfare look like a good idea – this appears to be an ethical problem from almost any perspective.

6.4.3 Possible ethical strategies and solutions

Practical strategies to deal with the problem of producing puppies and kittens in commercial breeding establishments need to address both supply and demand.

In terms of *supply*, possible changes could include stricter national or state regulations at many levels. Some European countries are ahead of the United States, and some states in the United States have stricter legislation than others. For example, in the United States, there has been a move towards requiring inspection and standards not only for those dog breeders that sell puppies to pet shops and pet brokers, but also to those who sell directly to customers via the Internet (although the latter is difficult to police).

Commercial breeding and sale of dogs is regulated in many European countries. For example, a Danish ministerial order requires that a dog for sale should be kept in a room of at least 6 m^2 (Justitsministeriet, 2007). In practice, such regulations amount to a ban on the sale of puppies (and often also kittens) in pet shops. Regulations explicitly banning the sale of puppies and kittens in pet shops (unless they come from shelters or are being rehomed) have recently been passed in a number of US cities, such as San Diego (City of San Diego, 2013).

More can also be done to highlight 'consumers' rights': in the United Kingdom, The Kennel Club (2013) website advises anyone who has bought a 'poorly or problem pet' from a 'classified advert or website' to visit the Consumer Direct website: www.direct.gov.uk/en/Governmentcitizensandrights/Consumerrights/index.htm.

Regulation can also come from the business itself. Serious breeders can collaborate with third-party institutions to implement certification schemes, including better information about responsible breeders. The HSUS (2012b) characterises such breeders as aiming to improve the genetic health and well-being of the breed; screening parents for certain diseases, such as hip dysplasia; feeding nutritious food; providing veterinary care; and selling animals with a contract allowing for the puppy or kitten to be returned if the owner cannot continue care. Other practices responsible breeders may adopt include selling animals with temporary health insurance, interviewing prospective owners to determine their suitability to own the animal companion, and keeping in touch with purchasers to follow the progress of puppies and kittens. The growth in the number of responsible breeders is important for both supply of and demand for animal companions.

In terms of *demand*, possible strategies include public campaigns to educate people about the possible origin of pets purchased from pet shops or online and to encourage them to source their companions responsibly. Many animal welfare organizations already have a good deal of information about this, but government-sponsored campaigns may have greater impact. Also, vets have a role to play in educating clients about the potential consequences of acquiring dogs and cats from pet shops and online. Although most people will only visit the vet after they have acquired the animal, this may help inform decisions about acquiring further animals.

Key Points

- Puppies and kittens are bred, reared and found homes in a variety of ways – from small-scale breeders selling directly to individuals, to large commercial breeding establishments (puppy and kitten mills/farms) selling via outlets such as pet shops and internet advertisements.
- Although widely regulated, conditions within commercial breeding establishments are often poor, such that the welfare of the breeding animals may be compromised, and the offspring may be negatively affected in both the short and long term.

- People who buy such animals are often unaware of their provenance, and are subsequently faced with companions that develop health and behavioural problems as a result of their early-life conditions.
- A wide range of ethical views, including views that mainly focus on human interests, agree that the breeding of puppies and kittens should be stopped in commercial breeding establishments where there is poor animal welfare.
- When it comes to the acquisition of puppies and kittens, there may be some ethical disagreement between perspectives that emphasise the need to look after the most vulnerable individual animals, and those focusing on the effects of 'rescuing' individuals on future breeding practices.
- When looking for practical strategies and solutions, it is important both to regulate the supply of puppies and kittens, and to address the demand for them, by trying to influence the knowledge and attitudes of future dog and cat owners.

References

ASPCA (n.d.) *Puppy mills*. American Society for the Prevention of Cruelty to Animals. [Online] Available from: http://www.aspca.org/PUPPYMILLS [Accessed 16 July 2014].

Brandt, R. (1983) The Real & Alleged Problems of Utilitarianism. *The Hastings Center Report* 13, 37–43.

City of San Diego (2013) *Ordinance Number O-20280*. Available at http://docs.sandiego.gov/council_reso_ordinance/rao2013/O-20280.pdf [Accessed 17 December 2014].

Cochrane, A. (2012) *Animal rights without liberation*. New York, Columbia University Press.

Dogs Trust (n.d.) *Battery farmed dogs: battery farmed dogs campaign (puppy farming)*. [Online] Available from: http://www.dogstrust.org.uk/az/b/batteryfarmeddogs/#.UNAw12BTG1s [Accessed 16 July 2014].

England, G.C.W & Millar, K.M. (2008) The ethics and role of AI with fresh and frozen semen in dogs. *Reproduction in Domestic Animals* 43 (Suppl.2), 165–171.

Forde, E. (2012) *Dogs trafficked in 'large numbers', say animal charities*. BBC News UK 30 November 2012. [Online] Available from: http://www.bbc.co.uk/news/uk-20527281 [Accessed: 16 July 2014].

Francione, G. (2007) *Animal rights and domesticated nonhumans*. Blog entry 10 January 2007. [Online] Available from: http://www.abolitionistapproach.com/animal-rights-and-domesticated-nonhumans/#.UuaGJPZMF-U [Accessed: 16 July 2014].

Fumarola, A.J. (1998) With best friends like us who needs enemies? The phenomenon of the puppy mill, the failure of legal regimes to manage it, and the positive prospects of animal rights. *Buffalo Environmental Law Journal* 253, 253–289.

Hare, R.M. (1981) *Moral Thinking*. Oxford, Oxford University Press.

Herzog, H. (2011) *Some we love, some we hate, some we eat: why it's so hard to think straight about animals*. New York, Harper Perennial.

HSUS (2012a). *More than 2,000 pet stores take a stand against puppy mills*. The Humane Society of the United States. Press release 14 December 2012. [Online] Available from: http://www.humanesociety.org/news/press_releases/2012/12/2000-puppy-friendly-pet-stores-121412.html [Accessed 16 July 2014].

HSUS (2012b) *Three reasons responsible breeders should oppose puppy mills*. The Humane Society of the United States, 4 January 2012. [Online] Available from: http://www.

humanesociety.org/issues/puppy_mills/facts/three_reasons_oppose_puppy_mills.html [Accessed 16 July 2014].

HSUS (2013) *In the market for a puppy?* The Humane Society of the United States, 3 May 2013. [Online] Available from: http://www.humanesociety.org/issues/puppy_mills/tips /buying_puppy.html [Accessed 16 July 2014].

Justitsministeriet (2007) *Bekendtgørelse om erhvervsmæssig handel med og opdræt af hunde samt hundepensioner og hundeinternater.* Bekendtgørelse nr. 1466 af 12/12 2007.

Katz, R. (2009) *What is a puppy mill?* Animal Legal & Historical Center, College of Law, Michigan State University. [Online] Available from: http://www.animallaw.info /articles/qvuspuppymill.htm [Accessed 16 July 2014].

Lien, M.E. (2004) Dogs, Whales and Kangaroos: Transnational Activism and Food Taboos. In: Lien, E. and Nerlich, B. (eds) *The Politics of Food*, Oxford, UK, Berg Publishers, pp. 179–197

Lockwood, R. (1995) The ethology and epidemiology of canine aggression. In: Serpell, J. (ed.) *The domestic dog: its evolution, behaviour, and interactions with people.* Cambridge, UK, Cambridge University Press, pp. 131–138.

McMillan, F.D., Duffy, D.L. & Serpell, J.A. (2011) Mental health of dogs formerly used as "breeding stock" in commercial breeding establishments. *Applied Animal Behaviour Science* 135 (1–2), 86–94.

McMillan, F.D., Serpell, J.A., Duffy, D.L., Masaoude, E. & Dohoo, I.R. (2013) Differences in behavioral characteristics between dogs obtained as puppies from pet stores and those obtained from noncommercial breeders. *Journal of the American Veterinary Medical Association* 242, 1359–1363.

Serpell, J. & Jagoe, J.A. (1995) Early experience and the development of behaviour. In: Serpell, J. (ed.) *The domestic dog: its evolution, behaviour, and interactions with people.* Cambridge, UK, Cambridge University Press, pp. 79–102.

The Kennel Club (2013) *Pet advertising* [online] Available from: http://www.thekennelclub. org.uk/our-resources/media-centre/issue-statements/pet-advertising [Accessed 16 March 2015]

The Kennel Club (n.d.) *Puppy farming.* [Online] Available from: http://www.thekennel club.org.uk/stoppuppyfarming [Accessed 16 July 2014].

Tushaus, K.C. (2009) Don't buy the doggy in the window. *Drake Journal of Agricultural Law* 14 (501), 1–9.

United States Senate Committee on Agriculture, Nutrition & Forestry (n.d.) *2008 Farm Bill.* [Online] Available from: http://www.ag.senate.gov/issues/2008-farm-bill [Accessed 16 July 2014].

Voris, H.C., Wittum, T.E., Rajala-Schultz, P.J. & Lord, L.K. (2011) Characterization of advertisements for puppies sold online: determinants of cost and a comparison with parent club breeders. *Preventative Veterinary Medicine* 100, 200–209.

Selective Breeding

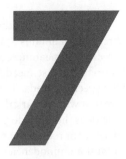

Co-author: Brenda Bonnett, BSc, DVM, PhD, Consulting Epidemiologist

B Bonnett Consulting, Wiarton, Ontario, Canada

7.1 Introduction   103
7.2 Selective Breeding of Dogs and Cats   104
7.3 Effects of Pedigree Breeding and Breed
     Standards on Welfare   105
7.4 Ethical Perspectives on Breeding   109
7.5 Possible Practical Solutions to Breeding of Healthier
     Cats and Dogs   112

7.1 Introduction

In August 2008, the British television channel BBC1 aired 'Pedigree Dogs Exposed', a documentary on the breeding of pedigree, purebred dogs. This documentary alleged that selective breeding of pedigree dogs in the United Kingdom was highly detrimental to their health and welfare. The Kennel Club, a leading British organisation in charge of dog shows, which maintains a registry for pedigree dogs (see Chapter 1), was the chief target of the criticism. The documentary gave many examples of the negative effects of current breeding practices on a wide variety of dog breeds. One of many troubling examples was a Cavalier King Charles Spaniel that showed behaviour suggestive of severe pain, due to a condition known as syringomyelia, which occurs when the skull is too small for the brain, a likely consequence of pursuing a specific flat skull shape as a breeding goal (see Figure 2.2b).

For the general public, this BBC documentary came as a shock. However, experts within the field recognised that a number of valid issues were raised: a growing body of literature had already documented the negative effects of genetic selection on the health of dogs and cats (see, e.g. CAWC, 2006; McGreevy & Nicholas, 1999).

Companion Animal Ethics, First Edition. Peter Sandøe, Sandra Corr and Clare Palmer.
© Universities Federation for Animal Welfare 2016.

The selective breeding of dogs and cats, of course, also has a positive side. Selective breeding maintains a diversity of breeds. In the case of dogs, the wide variation across breeds in appearance, temperament, function and utility is a factor in human–dog interactions. At least anecdotally, it is clear that people show intense and often lasting affinity for specific breeds. Through selective breeding, breeds and individual dogs have been created with remarkable abilities and characteristics (assistance dogs, tracking and rescue dogs, hunting dogs, etc.), and selective breeding has been used to eliminate specific diseases or reduce their prevalence (e.g. Canine Leukocyte Adhesion Deficiency (CLAD), a fatal immunodeficiency disease in Irish Setters).

However, these benefits do not eliminate the ethical issues raised by the selective breeding of purebred dogs and cats, on which we will focus in this chapter. We will begin by describing how the selective breeding of purebred dogs and cats is organised. After that, we will present what is known about the effects of breeding on animal welfare, with a focus on the negative effects on the health of purebred dogs and cats. We will then consider the issue from different ethical perspectives; finally, we will look at possible practical solutions to the problems.

7.2 Selective Breeding of Dogs and Cats

Domestication of dogs and cats goes back many thousands of years, although the precise nature and timing of the domestication of the two species is contested. Selection of dogs for specific purposes and the existence of dog 'breeds' also have a long history. However, the establishment of purebred dogs and cats based on pedigrees – that is, where breed ancestry is recorded – is relatively recent. Most of the common dog and cat 'pure breeds' have been established within the last 200 years, as has the system based on organisations that keep breeding records and organise dog and cat shows, as we saw in Chapter 1. Most modern dog and cat breeds have been established from a limited number of individuals, and only descendants of these individuals can count as belonging to a given breed – with a few exceptions, no new genes have been deliberately added after a breed has been established.

The dog population in the Western world can be divided into four groups: purebred pedigree dogs; dogs that are purebred and belong to a specific breed but that lack a pedigree; so-called designer breeds that are selectively bred crosses between one or more breeds; and random or accidental crosses between breeds. In the United States, approximately half the dogs are purebred (AVMA, 2012), whereas in European countries such as Germany and Denmark over three-quarters are reported to be purebred (Proschowsky, Rugbjerg & Ersbøll, 2003; Switzer & Nolte, 2007). Although statistics vary by country, only a minority of purebred dogs have a registered pedigree, and the proportion is falling. Designer breeds are a recent phenomenon, and anecdotal reports in both North America and Europe indicate that the numbers are rising rapidly, with many being sold for prices equal to or surpassing those of pedigree dogs.

It is generally accepted that dogs of specific breeds are relatively predictable in terms of temperament and behaviour (although because environmental factors are important too, the predictability may in specific cases be limited). Other factors, such as the level of grooming needed, are also breed specific. So, when people buy a dog or cat of a certain breed they can, to some degree, predict what kind of animal they will get, provided that they do their homework (although, unfortunately, many people do not). However, the natures of crossbred dogs and especially randomly bred dogs are less predictable, and this may have implications for the relation between the animal and the owner. There is some evidence, for instance, that crossbred dogs are more often euthanased for behavioural reasons than purebreds (Mikkelsen & Lund, 2000), although of course many other factors could be involved (e.g. the cost of the purebred dog).

In some developing countries, there are also large populations of street dogs that, although not commercially bred, share certain phenotypic, 'breed-like', characteristics. This resembles the situation of the majority of companion cats in developed countries, which are not purebred but share certain 'breed-like' phenotypic characteristics, generally being termed domestic shorthairs ('moggies' or 'country cats'). However, there are of course also pedigree purebred cats, and we discuss these in the following sections.

7.3 Effects of Pedigree Breeding and Breed Standards on Welfare

In the Western world, the breeding of pedigree show dogs and cats follows breed standards, defined and to variable degrees controlled by breed clubs. Breed clubs are often organised nationally – famous examples are the UK Kennel Club and the American Kennel Club – and may belong to larger international organisations.

Breed standards, with some local variations, currently exist for around 400 dog breeds and 40 cat breeds. Show dogs and cats are assessed by judges, appointed by the various mentioned organisations and clubs, who in turn decide how well the animals meet breed standards. Highly ranked dogs and cats will typically be used for breeding, so the opinions of show judges will have a significant effect on pedigree purebred animals, which may then trickle down to non-pedigree purebred animals.

The clubs may also set up restrictions on breeding, for example, requiring a certain outcome of a specific health test to allow an animal to be used for breeding, or making recommendations regarding norms of good breeding. However, there is often significant controversy and disagreement between breeders on the need for, and content of, breeding restrictions and recommendations.

Large numbers of apparently purebred dogs without pedigrees (recognised as specific breeds based on conformation) are also selectively bred by commercial breeders who are minimally influenced by the opinion of show judges or registry bodies. Instead, market forces drive these activities; and market forces in turn are heavily influenced by the media. An example of this is the partly celebrity-driven popularity of extra-small varieties of dog breeds such as Chihuahuas, so-called teacup or handbag dogs.

Breed standards are normally fixed, but over time their interpretation nonetheless shifts, as shown by the following three pictures of typical male German shepherds (Alsatians) spanning the period from 1910 until today. The phenotype of the 'ideal' German shepherd dog has changed gradually – but with dramatic effect – for example, in terms of a more sloping croup (hindquarters) (Figure 7.1)

Such changes in conformation (influenced by breed standards, and interpreted by show judges and breeders in the light of fashion) can have significant impacts on the

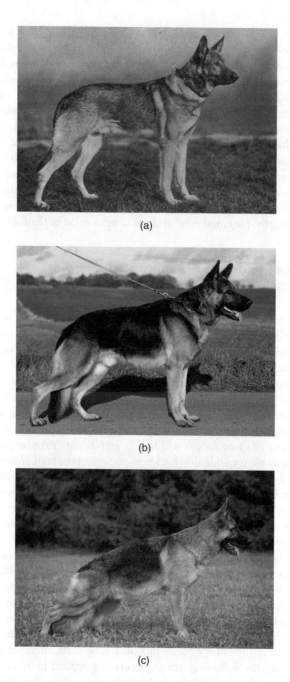

(a)

(b)

(c)

Figure 7.1 Male German Shepherds (Alsatians) at different times. (a) Tell von der Krimi-nalpolizei SZ 8770, who became a German winner in 1910. (*Rasmussen & Bertelsen*, 1980.) (b) Quax vom Aegidiendamm, a highly successful Danish show dog from the early 1970s. (*Reproduced with permission from O.B.C. Christensen.*) (c) A typical modern male show dog. (*Nikolai Tsvetkov/Shutterstock.com.*)

welfare of the animals concerned. German Shepherds, for instance, are predisposed to hip dysplasia; and they have a higher risk of dying (or being euthanased) for conditions affecting locomotion compared to all other breeds, combined (Vilson *et al.*, 2013). These effects on the health of the dogs may to a large extent be due to the heavily sloping croup (though the evidence here is not conclusive) (Wahl *et al.*, 2008).

Selective breeding of dogs and cats based on their performance in dog or cat shows is an engaging hobby for many people, and in this sense, contributes to *human* welfare. Those involved in the world of pedigrees may be intensely committed to their breed, and perceive the protection and propagation of the breed as essentially preserving a valuable cultural heritage (see more on this below).

On the other hand, producing pedigree, purebred dogs and cats also has a number of negative consequences, both on the welfare of the animals, and on the well-being, quality of life, and finances of their owners. These problems can be aggravated when purebred dogs are produced not by hobby or show breeders, but by high volume commercial or incompetent backyard breeders (see more on this in Chapter 6).

The potential negative effects of breeding of purebred dogs and cats fall into three groups: breeding extreme phenotypes, which, as a direct consequence, create health and welfare problems; increased prevalence of diseases not directly linked to the phenotypes being selected; and increased prevalence of behavioural problems.

First, then: extreme phenotypes. We have already noted that Cavalier King Charles Spaniels can suffer from syringomyelia, on account of being bred for a flat skull: a 2011 study (Parker *et al.*, 2011) found that by the age of 72 months, 70% of Cavalier King Charles Spaniels have asymptomatic syringomyelia (though it is a matter of debate to what extent the number of 'asymptomatic' carriers of a condition can serve as a predictor of the prevalence of the condition). Equally, it is suspected that the sloping croup of the German Shepherd breed will, as mentioned, predispose it to various problems. Another group of common phenotypes linked to severe health and welfare problems are the brachycephalic breeds of cats and dogs. 'Brachycephalic' means having a relatively broad, short skull, as seen in breeds such as Bulldogs, Pekingese, Pugs and Persian cats, which have been selected by humans, directly and indirectly, for their short faces and flat heads.

One prominent example of a brachycephalic breed is the English Bulldog. At the beginning of the nineteenth century, the bulldog was a working dog, used in the now universally illegal blood sport of bull baiting. When the sport was banned in the United Kingdom in 1835, bulldogs began to be bred in ways that radically changed both their character and appearance to enhance their desirability as companions. One of the most dramatic effects was a significant change in the dog's facial structure: the upper jaw and skull were reduced in length, whereas the lower jaw remained relatively unchanged (Thomson, 1996). Unfortunately, the soft tissues of the face and mouth did not shrink sufficiently to adapt to the reduced space. As a result, the redundant soft tissues can cause partial obstruction of the nose and upper airways, making it difficult for the dogs to breathe: a condition known as brachycephalic obstructive airway syndrome (BOAS).

A recent study by Packer *et al.* (2013) showed that dogs with shorter muzzles are at higher risk of suffering BOAS – so selecting for a short nose is directly linked to increased levels of this disorder. Purebred cats with short noses also suffer from much higher levels of BOAS. Dogs with BOAS may be short of breath, snore, wheeze, gag, regurgitate and vomit (Packer, Hendricks & Burn, 2012), and the symptoms may become so severe that some dogs require surgical treatment. These difficulties are not only confined to English Bulldogs. A recent Danish study (Sandøe et al., 2013) reports that 6.2 % of Pugs, 5% of French Bulldogs, and 3% of English Bulldogs among non-referred patients at the University of Copenhagen Small Animal Veterinary Hospital in 2012 had undergone surgery for BOAS. Based on Packer, Hendricks & Burn (2012), there is reason to think that this is only the tip of the iceberg. The latter study documents that 58% of owners of dogs diagnosed with BOAS by vets claimed that their dog did not have, or had not had, breathing problems. The authors of the study infer from this that owners of the dogs in question view breathing problems as normal for the breed. This is also in line with the fact that snoring or grunting sounds are often mentioned as characteristic traits of Bulldogs, Pugs and similar breeds.

However, the majority of the health problems in purebred cats and dogs are not due to breeding for an extreme phenotype, but rather due to lack of genetic diversity that leads to a predisposition to various diseases. As already mentioned, many breeds were established on the basis of few individuals, and problems are intensified when breeders use a very small number of prizewinning male dogs – 'popular sires' – to produce a large number of litters. When a young male dog is used in this way, his genes will be spread widely throughout the breed, often when he is still relatively young and his ultimate health status is unknown. In addition, as opposed to selective breeding in food animals or performance horses, little attention has been paid to progeny evaluation (in terms of health or other factors) in dogs and cats. This means that healthy carriers of inheritable diseases will not be detected.

As a consequence, predispositions for different diseases concentrate in specific breeds of purebred cats and dogs (Egenvall et al., 2005). It is estimated that each breed of dog is predisposed to between four and eight specific diseases (Brooks & Sargan, 2001). For example, Cavalier King Charles spaniels – which all descend from a very small number of individuals – not only suffer from syringomyelia, but according to the Swedish insurance company Agria, also are approximately 14 times more likely to die of heart disease compared to all breeds, combined, based on insured dogs up to 10 years of age (B. Bonnett, personal communication).

A similar pattern is found among purebred cats. For example, neoplasia (cancer) has been found to be common in Siamese cats, and Persian cats have an increased risk of eye disease (Egenvall et al., 2009, 2010), while the prevalence of polycystic kidney disease has been found to be 41.8% in Persian cats and 39.1% in Exotic Shorthair cats, whereas the disease was not detected in cats from other breeds (Barthez, River & Begon, 2003). Most of these diseases are the effect of several genes interacting with environmental factors.

The third group of problems is behavioural. As mentioned earlier, purebred dogs tend to have more predictable behaviours than crossbreds. However, if dogs or cats are bred as show animals, with a focus on their appearance rather than their temperament and performance as companions, there is a risk that breeding will result in behavioural problems. For example, some dog breeds may be prone to anxiety, or may suffer from various kinds of phobias. In spite of widespread practical experience concerning breed-specific behavioural problems, there has been little work to quantify the extent or severity of these problems. Some recent studies though have found links between breeds and specific behaviours (McGreevy *et al.*, 2013; Starling *et al.*, 2013).

7.4 Ethical Perspectives on Breeding

Humans have bred companion animals for many different reasons, for example, to have particular temperaments that make them good companions (playfulness, patience with children, lack of aggression), and in the case of dogs, to make them suitable for certain types of work. However, sometimes the breeding goals seem to serve less serious purposes.

Thus, some of the features for which dogs and cats have been bred, such as bigger eyes and flat faces, make companions more 'infant-like' and evidence suggests that these features may elicit parental-type care responses from those looking after them (Serpell, 1996: pp. 81–84). Other physical features, such as a sloping croup, or multiple skin folds, have no obvious relationship to a 'baby-like' attractiveness, but rather are features selected by breeders and show judges, and preferred by potential dog or cat owners as a result of fads and trends of the time.

However, as we have seen, some of the exaggerated features that appeal to owners do cause health problems for the animals concerned; and the preference for pure breeds, while certainly creating the advantage of predictability, means that animals may develop a greater number of diseases from inbreeding. And breeding practices that give rise to health problems do raise ethical questions.

Let us start by thinking about the case of a particular brachycephalic dog, by returning to the English Bulldog with severe breathing difficulties on account of the shape of its head. Can we say that this dog has been harmed by being bred in such a way that breathing difficulties are inevitable, and that, because (other things being equal) causing him harm is morally wrong, it was wrong to breed him? This question does capture an intuition about such cases: breeding dogs or cats that will have shortened, unhealthy lives in which they will suffer, because we like them to look a certain way, does appear morally troubling. However, it is important to be careful how this kind of worry is expressed, because of what is sometimes called the 'non-identity problem'.

This specific English Bulldog, has been bred to be brachycephalic. This is part of the genetic identity of the dog; it is part of what makes him who he is. Because of this, and other genetic problems the dog has that are typical of the breed, he suffers respiratory distress and will live (say) only 7 years. Now, it is certainly true that instead of breeding this dog, a different, healthier dog could have been bred. If one of this bulldog's parents, for example, had been mated with a mixed breed dog, the resulting dog would almost certainly not have been brachycephalic to the same degree, and would likely have had a longer, healthier life. But that healthier dog would have been a *different* dog.

The brachycephalic nature of this particular English Bulldog was decided when the dog was conceived. We cannot say '*This* dog could have been better off; in making him brachycephalic, we have harmed him'. For *this* particular English bulldog could not have been better off. It is not as though he was born non-brachycephalic and we altered him to interfere with his breathing, thereby harming him. It was in his nature to have such health problems. A healthier dog would have to be a different ('non-identical') dog.

This situation would be different if this bulldog had such a terrible life that we might say he had a 'life not worth living' – a life, let us say, where any positive experiences he might have had are completely outweighed by his pain, misery and suffering on account of his terrible breathing problems. If our bulldog's life were *that* bad, we might reasonably say that it would have been better if he had never been born, and probably that we ought to euthanase him. However, this is not the situation with our brachycephalic bulldog. He may be unhealthier, and may have a shorter life, than another dog that could have been bred instead of him. A different dog would have had a better life. But our bulldog could not have been the same dog and be any healthier – he has not been made worse off – and he has a life worth living. So, what is the problem with breeding him this way?

The non-identity problem outlined here (see Palmer, 2012 for a further discussion) may seem to be a rather academic and theoretical problem to many people, but it will be troubling from ethical perspectives that are based around what is done to particular identifiable individuals. Many rights views are like this. Suppose someone were to claim that breeding animals, such as this English Bulldog, in ways that cause health problems, violates their rights. This initially sounds plausible. But before the dog is conceived, there is no being actually in existence whose rights could be violated. Once a being is actually conceived with a particular genetic makeup, including to be brachycephalic, it is difficult to argue that the natural process of genetic development constitutes a rights infringement; the particular individual animal that comes into being, after all, could have had no other kind of life. The ethical problem about the unhealthy English Bulldog does not appear to be that his rights have been violated, even if one agrees that, as a sentient animal, he has rights.

However, even if it is difficult to argue that particular individual animals have been harmed, or have had their rights infringed, by being bred in specific ways, that does not mean that there are no ethical resources from which to judge that such breeding practices are problematic.

One way of thinking about breeding companion animals is to compare different, imaginary worlds: one world in which many companion animals suffer from diseases because of pure breeding, and another world in which breeding standards are different, and animals are healthier. The second world not only contains less animal suffering, but also more human happiness – because the emotional, social and financial costs to the owners of unhealthy companion animals can be significant. If we think about the future in this way – which is essentially a consequentialist approach – it is not only acceptable, but our duty, to breed animals in ways that enhance both human and animal welfare. If it is possible to eliminate an inheritable disease that is painful to affected dogs and has a negative impact on owners, then on this view everyone involved, opinion formers, researchers, breeding clubs, breeders and potential dog owners, have a duty to favour breeding practices aimed at reducing or eliminating that condition (though it is worth noting that in breeding to eliminate one disease, there is a risk of increasing the incidence of other diseases, or of losing related, but beneficial, traits).

Accepting this consequentialist line of argument, though, raises a further series of questions. As it seems that we should aim, through breeding, to reduce human and animal suffering by trying to eliminate breed diseases, does that also mean that we should use breeding to enhance animal health more generally? What about using biotechnological techniques such as genetic engineering to produce happier and healthier companion animals in the future?

A heated debate about enhancement in humans through applications of gene technology has been underway for some years: possibilities include 'radical extension of human health-span, eradication of disease, elimination of unnecessary suffering, and augmentation of human intellectual, physical and emotional capacities' (Bostrom, 2003). While some celebrate the possibilities that such technological changes might portend, others regard them as 'playing God' and as being 'unnatural' (and, therefore, on this view morally troubling) interventions in natural reproduction. Many of the arguments against such practices in humans stem from the view that we should not select humans for particular capabilities; that the whole process of human genetic selection is problematic. But as the principle of selective breeding is already widely accepted in animals, this argument alone would not make a successful case against 'companion animal enhancement'. For an argument against companion animal enhancement to be successful, it would have to establish a morally relevant distinction between selective breeding and biotechnological changes in the context of companion animals. To date, such an argument has not been developed.

So far, we have considered selective breeding from the perspective of rights and consequentialism. But what might someone who adopted a contextual ethic, such as an ethic of care, have to say about selective breeding? There are certainly reasons to think that selective breeding of animal companions may be important in creating strong and caring relations between owners and their animals. Selective breeding allows people to choose, as companions, animals with whom they can roughly predict that they will best bond, and therefore create the strongest relationship. There is no question that selective breeding has helped to propagate a wide diversity of breeds with specific temperaments, appearances and abilities, and there seems to be a link between such characteristics in the dogs and the level of attachment from their owners. However, if animals develop painful breed-related diseases, the very strength of the bond can be the source of great distress. In other cases, the closeness of the relationship could be undermined if an afflicted animal is no longer able to engage in long-established routines of companionship, or develops difficult behavioural problems as a result of pure breeding. So, from this perspective, we might expect that on an ethics of care view, selective breeding would continue, but in ways that reduce the likelihood of the development of stressful and distressing diseases and behavioural problems.

One further ethical issue that might be raised here concerns not so much the welfare of individual animals and their owners, but the persistence of a breed itself. Unsurprisingly, there is a range of differing views on this. Clearly, some human beings value the existence of particular breeds. This value may be aesthetic: they appreciate the appearance of animals of that kind, and would regard the world as a poorer place if there were no more individuals 'like that'. This value may also be historic and cultural: the 'form' of each breed, and how it came about, is seen as part of a cultural narrative, such as the evolution of the English Bulldog from bull-fighter to cuddly household friend that is good with children.

However, it seems difficult to sustain a further argument that a breed has ethical significance in itself – for instance, that it has some kind of independent moral status. Even though it has been argued that a breed is the kind of thing that has 'interests' and even a 'right to exist' (Hens, 2009), this is a curious claim. We may be able to make sense of the idea that something is 'in a breed's interests' (perhaps continuing in existence, as Hens (2009) proposes). But it is difficult to see why that would give us an ethical reason to protect it (as opposed to protecting individual members of the breed that can more obviously be harmed or benefited). Why would a *breed's* interests matter ethically? On the other hand, a lot of people care about protecting natural biodiversity, and it may be possible to extend that to cover culturally formed biodiversity, in the form of dog or cat breeds.

However, holding the view that breeds have some kind of independent moral significance might also imply that we have a moral responsibility to create new breeds, or to protect existing breeds even if all the living members have miserable lives and there is no way of both protecting the breed and improving the lives of its members – both troubling conclusions.

The strongest arguments for protecting breeds, then, are that people claim to love them, value them, and want to produce more members of them. However, where many of the breed's members suffer from genetic diseases, this may produce a conflict between maintaining the 'purity' of the breed and the health of its members. One way of thinking about this, though, is to note that what is meant by 'valuing' and 'loving' a breed may vary widely. For breeders and show judges, this may refer to having very precise body conformation, coat quality, or tail length, for example, but for most dog owners, what is loved and valued is often much less tangible. A dog or cat may still have a particular appearance, and similar temperament, even if some new genetic diversity has been introduced by going outside the pure, pedigreed breed. This observation leads to thinking about some more practical solutions to some of the ethical questions raised by selective breeding.

7.5 Possible Practical Solutions to Breeding of Healthier Cats and Dogs

From a number of ethical perspectives, it is problematic to selectively breed animals that tend to develop significant health or behaviour problems. So, what are the possible ways of tackling this problem? One approach here concentrates on the *supply* of animals to the companion animal market; the other focuses on *demand* for companion animals.

In terms of supply: there has already been some change in attitude on the part of key stakeholders such as kennel clubs, breeders, veterinary associations and animal protection societies, towards taking concerns about selective breeding and animal welfare seriously. The same is true of public authorities, particularly in Europe, where various boards and committees have been set up to come up with suggestions for the reform of dog breeding (see, e.g. APGAW, 2012; Bateson, 2010).

Breeding clubs in charge of individual dog and cat pedigree breeds, and to some extent kennel clubs, have the power to change breed standards and to introduce breed restrictions obliging their members to take welfare into account. A number of such initiatives have already been taken, particularly in Europe, and these mechanisms are good as far as they go. However, their effectiveness is limited by difficulties in enforcement, imports from areas or countries with less strict policies, and breeding occurring outside the influence of the leading breeding organisations.

Therefore, there is also a strong need to reduce demand for animals bred to standards that may risk ill health or behavioural problems. Potential buyers of kittens and puppies should be educated, based on the best available information, about the potential effects of breeding on the subsequent welfare of the animal. Although information resources are available, for example, http://www.ufaw.org.uk/geneticwelfareproblems.php, much more could be done to disseminate such knowledge in a more efficient and vivid way. This could, for example, include large information campaigns involving TV advertisements and other means of mass communication; but these strategies would require financial means far outstripping the capacities of the small animal welfare NGOs currently addressing the issue.

In addition, much more research is needed into the problems caused by breeding and ways to solve them, with greater collaboration between vets who treat affected animals, researchers and authorities. For example, in the United Kingdom, responsible owners of breeding animals of dog breeds where hip dysplasia is a common condition have their dogs 'hip scored' under the British Veterinary Association–Kennel Club (BVA–KC) Hip Scheme, set up in 1983 (http://www.bva.co.uk/hip_scheme.aspx). To be hip scored, the dog must be at least a year old; a specific X-ray view of the hips is taken under general anaesthetic, and nine specific features are assessed by a panel of experts, who then allocate a score for each hip. The higher the score, the worse the hip – a maximum score of 53 is possible for each hip. A *total* score of up to 10 is suggested to indicate either normal hips, or borderline changes that are unlikely to worsen with age: the recommendation is that 'ideally' only dogs with scores up to 10 be used for breeding. Similar schemes exist in other European countries, and in the United States. Prospective purchasers should, therefore, ask to see the hip scores of the parents and not buy puppies from parents where scores are high, or unavailable.

However, even though there is an indication of a positive effect in countries where the schemes have been effectively followed, these schemes have not worked as well as hoped for various reasons including that they are voluntary, and so many breeders do not have the parents screened, and some of those that do will simply not submit the radiographs for scoring if the hips look bad. Equally importantly, radiographic changes do not infallibly predict the incidence and severity of subsequent disease, which is highly influenced by environmental factors such as feeding and exercise. Thus, trying to select for healthy dogs on the basis of phenotypic indicators has had only limited success, and most experts now agree that genetic testing, which is still in its early stages, is more likely to reliably identify at-risk dogs.

A rapidly increasing number of tests are being marketed for screening for genetic diseases; however, many of them are poorly validated, especially for use in controlling disease at the population level. Even so, all breeders would still have to fully engage with the process – and given the issues previously mentioned about securing a sufficient supply of dog and cats of popular breeds – compliance by the majority of breeders, who are not members of breed clubs, may not be likely. If consumers are driving the market for dogs and cats, it may fall to them to demand documentation that the animals they buy are free of certain genetic diseases.

Economic incentives may also play an important role both in reducing supply and demand of purebred dogs and cats that are likely to be affected by inherited illnesses. First it should, in theory, be possible for owners of dogs and cats to get a significant refund from the breeder of an animal that subsequently suffers from a specific inherited illness. Although this currently happens in countries such as Denmark, it is unusual elsewhere, yet this would give breeders and suppliers an incentive to breed healthier cats and dogs. Secondly, if inherited health problems lead to increased expense for veterinary treatments, this may serve to limit demand – particularly when these costs are reflected in the price of health insurance for a cat or a dog. Some insurance companies now exclude certain inherited diseases in certain breeds from being covered, for example, treatment of BOAS in brachycephalic breeds; and this may increase the demand for dogs of these breeds which are documented to be less affected by BOAS.

In conclusion, there does not seem to be a quick fix available to solve all the problems arising from purebred pedigree breeding. However, a combination of greater awareness among potential dog and cat owners, better methods for predicting breeding-related problems, and greater pressure, including economic pressure, on breeders may serve to move things in the right direction.

Key Points

- The majority of dogs in the Western world are purebred; the rest are crosses between purebreds, either more or less at random or based on 'design'. This contrasts with cats where only a minority are purebred; the majority are 'domestic' cats.

- The selective breeding of purebred dogs and cats is influenced by breed standards, as defined by breed clubs and interpreted by judges at dog and cat shows, but consumer demand, affected by the media and other factors, also plays a role.

- Even though selective breeding of purebred dogs and cats has advantages for both human and animal welfare, there are also potential negative effects on animal welfare that fall into three groups: (a) breeding extreme phenotypes, which, as a direct consequence, have welfare problems; (b) increased prevalence of diseases not directly linked to the phenotypes being selected; and (c) increased prevalence of behavioural problems.

- From a rights view, welfare problems created by breeding may be difficult to address because of the non-identity problem.

- Viewed from a consequentialist position, it may be argued that breeding should focus on creating healthy animals likely to function well as companions.

- From an ethics of care view, it is important to breed dogs and cats that people can easily bond with, while preventing health problems for the animals that may be detrimental to the bond.
- Some people seem to care about maintaining breeds for their own sake, whereas a more defensible view seems to be that maintaining breeds has a value to the humans who care about them.
- There are a number of ways in which breeding of dogs and cats can be improved so as to avoid negative effects on health and behaviour. To make these work, it is important both to focus on the supply of, and the demand for, healthy purebred dogs and cats.

References

APGAW (2012) *A healthier future for pedigree dogs: update report.* Associate Parliamentary Group for Animal Welfare. London, The Stationary Office.

AVMA (2012) *U.S. Pet Ownership & Demographics Sourcebook.* 2012 edition. Schaumburg, IL, American Veterinary Medical Association.

Barthez, P.Y., River, P. & Begon, D. (2003) Prevalence of polycystic kidney disease in Persian and Persian-related cats in France. *Journal of Feline Medicine and Surgery* 5, 345–347.

Bateson, P. (2010) *Independent inquiry into dog breeding.* Cambridge, UK, Patrick Bateson.

Bostrom, N. (2003) Human genetic enhancements: a transhumanist perspective. *Journal of Value Inquiry* 37 (4), 493–506.

Brooks, M. & Sargan, D.R. (2001) Genetic aspects of diseases in dogs. In: Ruvinsky, A & Sampson, J. (eds) *The genetics of the dog.* Wallingford, CABI Publishing, pp. 191–266.

CAWC (2006) *Breeding and welfare in companion animals.* Sidmouth, Companion Animal Welfare Council.

Egenvall, A., Bonnett, B.N., Hedhammer, Å. & Olson, P. (2005) Mortality in over 350,000 insured Swedish dogs from 1995-2000: II. Breed-specific age and survival patterns and relative risk for causes of death. *Acta Veterinaria Scandinavica* 46 (3), 121–136.

Egenvall, A., Bonnett, B.N., Häggström, J., Ström Holst, B., Möller, L. & Nødtvedt, A. (2010) Morbidity of insured Swedish cats during 1999-2006 by age, breed, sex, and diagnosis. *Journal of Feline Medicine and Surgery* 12 (12), 948–959.

Egenvall, A., Nødtvedt, A., Häggström, J., Ström Holst, B., Möller, L. & Bonnett B.N. (2009) Mortality of life-insured Swedish cats during 1999-2006: age, breed, sex, and diagnosis. *Journal of Veterinary Internal Medicine* 23 (6), 1175–1183.

Hens, K. (2009) Ethical responsibilities towards dogs: an inquiry into the dog-human relationship. *Journal of Agricultural and Environmental Ethics* 22, 3–14.

McGreevy, P.D., Georgevsky, D., Carrasco, J., Valenzuela, M., Duffy, D.L. & Serpell, J.A. (2013) Dog behavior co-varies with height, bodyweight and skull shape. *PLoS One* 8 (12), e80529.

McGreevy, P.D. & Nicholas, F.W. (1999) Some practical solutions to welfare problems in dog breeding. *Animal Welfare* 8, 329–341.

Mikkelsen, J. & Lund, J.D. (2000) Euthanasia of dogs due to behavioural problems: an epidemiological study of euthanasia of dogs in Denmark, with a special focus on problems of aggression. *European Journal of Companion Animal Practice* 10, 143–150.

Packer, R., Hendricks, A. & Burn, C.C. (2012) Do dog owners perceive the clinical signs related to conformational inherited disorders as "normal" for the breed? A potential constraint to improving canine welfare. *Animal Welfare* 21 (Suppl. 1), 81–93.

Packer, R., Tivers, M.S., Hendricks, A. & Burn, C.C. (2013) Short muzzle; short of breath? An investigation of the effect of conformation of the risk of brachycephalic obstructive airway syndrome (BOAS) in domestic dogs. In: *Science in service of animal welfare: priorities around the world.* UFAW international animal welfare science symposium, 4–5 July 2013, Universitat Autònoma de Barcelona, Barcelona, Spain, p.26.

Palmer, C. (2012) Does breeding a bulldog harm it? Breeding, ethics and harm to animals. *Animal Welfare* 21 (2), 157–166.

Parker, J.E., Knowler, S.P., Rusbridge, C., Noorman, E. & Jefferey, N.D. (2011) Presence of asymptomatic syringomyelia in Cavalier King Charles spaniels. *Veterinary Record* 168 (25), 667.

Proschowsky, H.F., Rugbjerg, H. & Ersbøll, A.K. (2003) Mortality of purebred and mixed-breed dogs in Denmark. *Preventive Veterinary Medicine* 58 (1–2), 63–74.

Rasmussen, B. & Bertelsen, O. (1980) *Schæferhunden.* 7th edition. Copenhagen, Clausens Bøger.

Serpell, J. (1996) *In the company of animals: a study of human-animal relationships.* 2nd edition. Cambridge, UK, Cambridge University Press.

Sandøe, P., Hansen, I.K., Eriksen, T. & Fredholm, M. (2013) Hvad er der galt med min bulldog? Om mulighederne for at forebygge fremavl af hunde med brachycephalt syndrom. *Dansk Veterinærtidsskrift* 96 (12), 11–14.

Starling, M.J., Branson, N., Thomson, P.C. & McGreevy, P.D. (2013) "Boldness" in the domestic dog differs among breeds and breed groups. *Behavioural Processes* 97, 53–62.

Switzer, E. & Nolte, I. (2007) Ist der Mischling wirklich der gesündere Hund? Untersuchung zur Erkrankungsanfälligkeit bei Mischlingen in Deutschland. *Praktischer Tierarzt* 88 (1), 14–19.

Thomson, K.S. (1996) The fall and rise of the English bulldog. *American Scientist* 84 (3), 220–223.

Vilson, Å., Bonnett, B., Hansson-Hamlin, H. & Hedhammar, Å. (2013) Disease patterns in 32,486 insured German shepherd dogs in Sweden: 1995-2006. *Veterinary Record* 173, 116.

Wahl, J.M., Herbst, S.M., Clark, L.A., Tsai, K.L. & Murphy, K.E. (2008) A review of hereditary diseases of German shepherd dog. *Journal of Veterinary Behavior* 3, 255–265.

Feeding and the Problem of Obesity

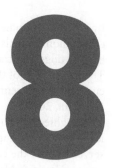

8.1 Introduction   117
8.2 How Is 'Fatness' Defined and Measured in Cats and Dogs,
    and How Many Animals Are Affected?   118
8.3 Is This a Welfare Problem?   121
8.4 Why Do Owners Allow Their Companion
    Animals to Become Fat?   123
8.5 Whether and How to Prevent and Treat Problems with
    Overweight Companion Animals   126

8.1 Introduction

One of the most basic concerns of animal care is to ensure that animals are properly fed. This is reflected in the first principle of the 'Five Freedoms' (see Chapter 4, p. 67), set up to define the basic requirements of animal welfare by the British Farm Animal Welfare Council (now Farm Animal Welfare Committee). The principle states that animals must enjoy 'Freedom from hunger and thirst – by ready access to fresh water and a diet to maintain full health and vigour' (FAWC, 2009).

Historically, underfeeding and malnutrition were major issues, although this is no longer the case for dog and cat populations in richer parts of the world. Occasionally, however – even in rich countries – individuals still keep large numbers of dogs and cats without being able to feed them a proper diet, while stray and feral cats and dogs may also suffer from thirst, starvation and malnutrition (see Chapter 13).

In general, however, companion animals are increasingly viewed as family members, clearly benefiting from the affluence of their owners. Parallel to – and partly caused by – this development, there has been a significant change in the way people feed their companion animals. Rather than feeding them scraps and leftovers, increasing numbers of dogs and cats are fed readymade feed, either in a dry or a wet (canned) form. The production of this feed is regulated to ensure a proper composition of macronutrients and a sufficient amount of vitamins, minerals and other micronutrients (Nestle & Nesheim, 2010).

Slaughter by-products not considered fit for human consumption make up a significant part of the ingredients for commercial pet food, and it may be argued that this serves to limit the environmental footprint of the growing companion animal pet food sector (Nestle & Nesheim, 2010, see also Chapter 14). Nonetheless, questions may still be raised about killing some animals to feed others, how sustainably the meat and fish in pet food have been produced, and food contamination. We will consider these questions further in Chapters 14 and 16; the rest of this chapter will focus on the consequences for companion animals of the *amount* of food they are eating.

Whatever the quality of the diet fed to companion animals, it can still be fed in too large quantities. Overfeeding, particularly in combination with too little exercise, leads to obesity and increases the risk of related diseases, including cardiovascular disease, diabetes, skeletal disease and various forms of cancer. These diseases shorten the expected lifespan of the animals, and often adversely affect their quality of life. There are also negative impacts on the owners in terms of worry and grief about their companions' health and early death, as well as the potential costs of veterinary treatment.

In this chapter, we focus on the problem of overfeeding dogs and cats, and how the problem is brought about via the animals' companionship with humans. Human lifestyles influence and affect companion dogs and cats to a significant degree, and it is not surprising that the current epidemic of human obesity in many parts of the world is increasingly mirrored in companion animals.

We begin by considering how 'fatness' is defined in dogs and cats, and then look at how their health and welfare is affected when they exceed their ideal weight. This opens up an ethical dilemma about whether maximising longevity and minimising morbidity, or avoiding the feeling of hunger, is better for animal welfare. We then review what is known about why owners of dogs and cats allow their companions to become overweight, and about the barriers that prevent dogs and cats remaining close to their ideal weight. We conclude with a discussion of various means of overcoming these barriers.

8.2 How Is 'Fatness' Defined and Measured in Cats and Dogs, and How Many Animals Are Affected?

In companion animals, as in human beings, a distinction is drawn between being overweight, and being obese. Being overweight can be defined as having a body condition where levels of body fat exceed what is considered optimal. Obesity can be defined as being overweight to the extent that serious effects on the individual's health become likely.

Various values are given in the literature for optimal % body fat, ranging from 15–20% for cats and dogs (Toll *et al.*, 2010: p. 501) to 20–30% body fat for cats

(Bjørnvad *et al.*, 2011). According to one expert, the value for optimal % body fat depends on a number of factors including the measurement technique, and age, breed and gender of the animal. He proposes the optimal % of body fat to be between 10–20% in cats, and 10–35% in dogs, depending on breed and circumstances (Alex German, personal communication).

It is possible to use relative body weight as a proxy measure of % body fat. A recent review paper defines overweight cats and dogs as being 10–20% above optimal weight, and obese animals as being more than 20% over optimal weight (Toll *et al.*, 2010: p. 501). In another review paper, obesity is defined as occurring at 30% above ideal body weight (Burkholder & Toll, 2000). However, 'these criteria have not been confirmed with rigorous epidemiologic studies, and limited data exist on the nature of an optimal body weight' (German, 2006: p. 1940).

Although most people would claim to recognise a 'fat' dog or cat when they see one, it is more difficult to distinguish between a normal versus an overweight animal and an overweight versus an obese animal. Thus, as well as agreeing on definitions of 'overweight' and 'obese', it is also necessary to develop a reasonably accurate, practical method of assessment. In the case of humans, the body mass index (BMI) has been developed: by using the BMI, an individual's body fat can be estimated based on information about the person's weight and height, and it is used to determine whether the individual is of a healthy size or not. Such a simple (albeit somewhat problematic and controversial) measure is not easily transferable particularly to dogs, as there are many diverse breeds with very different body conformations.

However, practical measures have been developed which, in a fairly easy and reliable way, enable people to score the amount of body fat of many animals, including dogs and cats. These so-called body condition scores use a number of categories, ranging from 'emaciated' to 'severely obese', based on subjective assessment of specific features. These features include the shape of the animal viewed from above, and how easily palpable the ribs are (Laflamme, 1997; McGreevy *et al.*, 2005; Toll *et al.*, 2010). Studies have shown that such measures correlate well with more advanced measurements of the amount of body fat, and, in general, there is good agreement between measurements across different users (German *et al.*, 2006) (Figure 8.1).

However, a recent Danish study (Bjørnvad *et al.*, 2011) of indoor-confined, adult neutered cats found that the body condition score tends to underestimate the level of body fat as measured using a DEXA (Dual-Energy X-ray Absorptiometry) scanner. Due to lack of exercise, these cats are in a condition that, in the human case, has been labelled 'skinny fat'. As with some physically inactive people, due to a decrease in lean body mass, these cats have a relatively high level of body fat despite what appears to be a healthy body weight; as in the human case, 'skinny fat' can lead to type 2 diabetes and other serious health problems.

A number of studies have been undertaken in North America, Europe and Australia, mainly on dogs, to determine what proportions of animals are overweight or obese: the reported prevalence was between 22% and 44% (Crane, 1991; Edney & Smith, 1986; Hand, Armstrong & Allen, 1989; Kronfeld, Donoghue & Glickman, 1991; Mason, 1970; Mcgreevy *et al.*, 2005; Robertson, 2003). Two studies (Lund *et al.*, 2005, 2006) used a cross-sectional design to measure the prevalence of overweight and obese animals

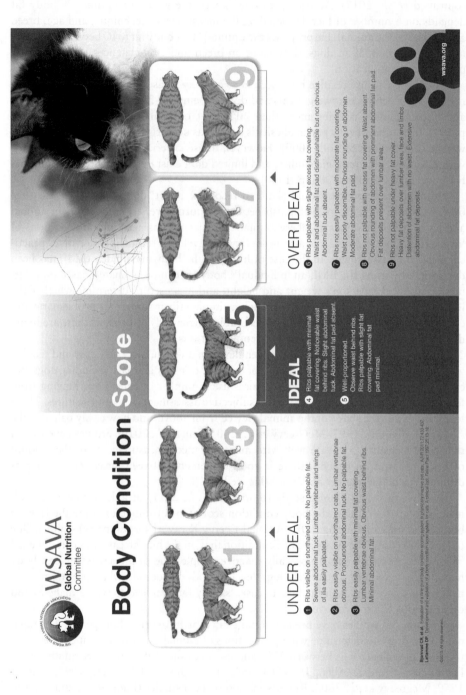

Figure 8.1 Body Condition Score chart. Many such charts are available to help owners of cats and dogs recognize whether their companion animal is in a healthy body condition. (*Image used courtesy of World Small Animal Veterinary Association Global Nutrition Committee.*)

among a large number of cats ($n = 8159$) and dogs ($n = 21,754$) seen by US veterinarians. They found that 28.7% of adult cats were overweight and a further 6.4% were obese; for adult dogs, the numbers were 29.0% and 5.1%.

The differences in the prevalence of overweight and obese animals reported in the literature may reflect differences in sampling, in who has been asked (owners or vets), or genuine local variations. Local variations are found in the levels of human obesity: in adults in the United States, it is over 30%, compared to between 8 and 25% in European countries, and less than 5% in some Asian countries, such as Japan (WHO, 2012). Nonetheless, as a rough estimate, around a third of adult cats and dogs kept as companions in the rich parts of the world are overweight, and more than 1 in 20 is obese. Experts in the field believe that the problem is increasing (German, 2006).

8.3 Is This a Welfare Problem?

There is a huge body of veterinary literature documenting that obesity in dogs and cats increases the risk of other health problems. According to one review paper, these problems include 'orthopaedic disease, diabetes mellitus, abnormalities in circulating lipid profiles, cardio-respiratory disease, urinary disorders, reproductive disorders, neoplasia (mammary tumours, transitional cell carcinoma), dermatological diseases, and anaesthetic complications' (German, 2006: p. 1940S). As these conditions shorten the expected lifespan of the affected animals, and potentially reduce their quality of life, obesity in cats and dogs has considerable potential to cause reduced welfare (Figure 8.2(a)–(c)).

Even being moderately overweight seems to have a negative effect on animal health, for example, rodents fed *ad libitum* have a shorter lifespan than those on a restricted diet (Hubert *et al.*, 2000). In a series of papers, Kealy *et al.* (2002) and Lawler *et al.* (2005, 2008) reported the results of a longitudinal study of two randomly selected groups of Labrador Retriever dogs, with 24 dogs in each group, treated identically apart from their feeding regime. One group was initially fed *ad libitum,* then fed at a level at which they stayed overweight but did not become obese (mean body condition score around 6.5 on a scale ranging from 1 – emaciated, to 9 – severely obese). The other group was fed 25% less than the first group throughout the study. Dogs in the latter group remained leaner and lived longer (median lifespan of 13.0 years compared to 11.2 years for the moderately overweight group). In addition, where the dogs in the leaner group developed the same diseases as those in the overweight group, the onset of disease came later and the symptoms of the diseases were less severe.

Thus, overweight companion animals potentially lose many years of life, despite the fact that the lifespan of dogs and cats seems to have been increasing overall (Kulick, 2009), most likely due to improvements in the quality of nutrition and better veterinary care.

On the other hand, work with rodents and pigs also indicates that a restrictive diet of the sort that secures maximum longevity and minimum morbidity causes welfare problems in the form of increased hunger, derived effects in terms of increased aggression and elevated levels of stress and the development of stereotypies (D'Eath *et al.*, 2009;

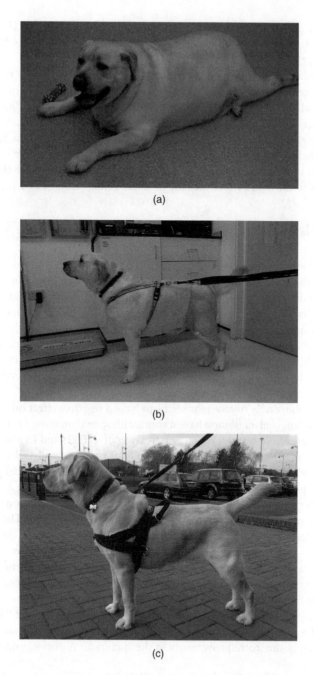

(a)

(b)

(c)

Figure 8.2 'Mighty Mike', a rescue dog. (a) Initially weighing 60 kg, Mike suffered from a rup-tured cranial cruciate ligament in the left hind leg. (b) Shortly after having surgery to stabilise his left knee, weighing 50 kg. (c) Mike required surgery for the same condition in his other knee several months later. He is shown here, fully recovered, weighing 36.6 kg. (*Courtesy of Sandra Corr.*)

Kasanen *et al.*, 2010). Assuming that the same conclusions apply to dogs and cats, there may be a real dilemma here between two of the five freedoms mentioned in Chapter 4: it may not always be possible to secure both freedom from hunger and from disease.

D'Eath *et al.* (2009) have argued that this is a significant dilemma in respect to keeping laboratory, companion and some farm animals. Kasanen *et al.* (2010: p. 40) state that: 'One could argue that the best solution is simply to proceed with feeding *ad libitum*, allowing the rats to be fat and friendly rather than lean and mean. A similar line of thought seems to apply to fattening pigs'. This solution may be appropriate for farm and laboratory animals, which are killed at a relatively young age, before they develop conditions such as osteoarthritis or heart disease later in life. However, this does not apply to cats and dogs that (barring accidents or other unexpected occurrences) normally live until they are euthanased due to a specific disease or from deteriorating health in old age.

Of course, there may be ways to make the dilemma between preventing hunger and protecting health less stark. Animals may be able to eat more without detrimental effects to their health if they also exercise more, or are fed low-calorie bulk diets that nonetheless provide a feeling of satiety. They could also be made to work for their food, thereby engaging in more feeding-related behaviours without getting too much food. However, these methods are not likely to completely solve the issue of which feeding strategy provides optimal welfare.

In fact, determining the optimal feeding strategy may depend on how welfare is defined (see Chapter 4 for more on definitions of animal welfare). If welfare is defined in terms of fitness and function, that is, as a form of perfectionism, then a very restricted feeding regime may be optimal. In contrast, if welfare is defined according to hedonism as getting the maximum amount of pleasure and the minimum amount of frustration or pain – either in total over a full life or per year lived – then a more liberal feeding regime may be preferable, as the avoidance of disease should be balanced against the potential frustration and stress relating to hunger. However, many dogs and cats end up becoming so fat that the negative health effects of obesity probably ultimately outweigh any satisfaction gained from eating.

This leads us to the obvious next question: why do owners who generally seem to love their cats and dogs allow the animals to grow fat, and, in doing so, compromise their welfare?

8.4 Why Do Owners Allow Their Companion Animals to Become Fat?

There are a number of ways in which owners can prevent cats and dogs from becoming overweight. They can feed them less in terms of volume, and/or they can feed them diets that are less dense in calories. They may be able to exercise them more (or, in the case of cats, make more opportunities for exercise available). Yet many owners find this very difficult, and a number of studies have investigated whether there is a link between particular characteristics of the owners of cats and dogs, and the risk of their companion animals becoming obese.

Firstly, these studies found a relationship between obesity in dogs and in their owners: if the owner weighs too much, it is more likely that the dog will also be overweight or obese (Colliard *et al.*, 2006; Kienzle, Bergler & Mandernach, 1998; Mason, 1970; Nijland, Stam & Seidell, 2010). However, the same relationship is not found between owners and their cats (Nijland, Stam & Seidell, 2010).

Secondly, studies seem to indicate a link with the owner's income: the poorer the owner, the more likely it is that the companion weighs too much (Courcier *et al.*, 2010; Kienzle, Bergler & Mandernach, 1998).

These first two findings reflect the well-documented but complex relationship between obesity and low social status in humans (Bove & Olson, 2006; McLaren, 2007; Paeratakul *et al.*, 2002; Robert & Reither, 2004), and it is not surprising that habits and constraints relating to people's own lives influence how they view and treat the animals in their care.

Neutering is another risk factor: even though it is possible, through careful feeding, to keep neutered cats and dogs at their ideal weight (provided that they do not scavenge), in practice, neutered dogs and cats are much more likely to be overweight or obese than intact ones (Lund *et al.*, 2006; Nguyen *et al.*, 2004). See more on neutering in Chapter 10.

So far, we have considered social, demographic and physiological factors that seem to increase the risk of an owner having an overweight companion animal. Now we will take a closer look at the possible psychological mechanisms that may be involved.

In the same way as parents of overweight children systematically underestimate their children's weight (Etelson *et al.*, 2003), a number of studies show that owners of overweight or obese dogs (Rohlf *et al.*, 2010; White *et al.*, 2011) and cats (Allan *et al.*, 2000; Kienzle & Bergler, 2006) underestimate the body condition of their animals.

Another factor seems to be linked to the dynamic of the human–animal bond, according to Shearer (2010), who suggests that owners of overweight cats and dogs use food as an acceptable form of communication and interaction with their pets. This was supported by Kienzle, Bergler & Mandernach (1998), who found that obese dogs were more often present when the owner prepared or ate their own meals, and were fed titbits then, leading the authors to suggest that 'owners of obese dogs tend to interpret their dog's every need as a request for food'. Kienzle, Bergler & Mandernach (1998) also reported that obese dogs slept more often in the owners' beds, the owners spoke more and on a greater variety of subjects to their dogs, and were less afraid of contracting diseases from their dogs, than were owners of dogs of normal weight. Owners of obese dogs also saw the animals as less important in relation to traditional dog roles such as sources of exercise, work and protection. The authors interpreted these differences as indicators of what they call 'overhumanizing' (p. 2779): 'The obese dogs were indulged as "fellow-humans" and they were no longer treated as typical companion animals.' This study also confirmed the finding that owners of obese dogs tend to be obese themselves, and found that owners of obese dogs took little interest in their own health compared to owners of normal dogs. Therefore, the authors conclude, part of the explanation of the behaviour of owners of obese dogs is a transfer of the owners' eating habits and attitude to health to their dogs (Kienzle, Bergler & Mandernach, 1998).

A follow-up study of cats by the same German group found a number of similarities between the human factors involved in dogs and in cats becoming overweight, in particular, the tendency to humanise the animals, and communicate through food. Thirty per cent of owners of overweight cats, compared with 12% of owners of normal weight cats, stated that they had not felt very happy prior to acquiring a cat, and the cat was intended to console and encourage them. The authors seem to assume that the cats fulfilled this role of consolation and encouragement, and proposed that 'the results are suggestive of (a) a closer relationship between overweight cats and their owners than between normal cats and their owners, (b) more humanization of overweight cats than of normal cats, (c) a potential role of overweight cats as a substitute for human companions' (Kienzle & Bergler, 2006: p. 1948).

Another interesting finding in the case of overweight cats had to do with the sex of the owner: the relative number of female owners was higher in the overweight (97%) than normal weight cat groups (87%). According to Kienzle & Bergler (2006), this may be linked to the results of other studies showing that women tend to have closer relationships with their cats than men do (Bergler, 1989). However, while the owners of the obese dogs studied by Kienzle, Bergler & Mandernach (1998) tended to be more obese, tended to care less about their own health, and were in general less well off than owners of normal dogs, these differences were not found in the case of cat owners.

The authors suggest that people who are not overweight or obese easily find other ways of engaging with dogs than through food, for example, by taking them on walks; however, people are less aware of alternative communication modes with cats, making feeding the main contact point between many cats and their owners. That owners of overweight cats tend to communicate with their cats via feeding is further supported by the finding that they were more likely to serve the cat homemade food and to make food available *ad libitum*, and less prone to play with their cats (Kienzle & Bergler, 2006). It should be added that all the cats in the study were indoor cats; this, of course, limited opportunities for exercise.

It has also been suggested that 'cat owners were less aware of their pet's weight problem than dog owners' (Kienzle & Bergler, 2006: p. 1949). There may be different reasons for this: cats sleep a lot, hide signs of illness more than dogs, and appear less often in public with their owners than dogs, and are, therefore, less likely to attract comments from other people. Also, outdoor cats are more likely to supplement their feeding in various ways.

Some may object to the aforementioned attempts to explain the problem of overweight companion animals by reference to a 'spill-over' of the owners' attitudes towards themselves. While a person's desire to eat may be very strong, it is less clear how such desires would cause the individual to overfeed their companion animal. After all, a person experiences her or his own food cravings, but she or he does not experience the cravings of the dog or the cat. However, this may be analogous to the situation of parents with very young children: parents do not actually feel their child's hunger pangs, but even though small children cannot open fridges they soon learn how to make their parents do it for them. Similarly, cats and dogs may manipulate their owners, if the owners are open to the signals the animals send (though we do not need to suppose that this is a conscious, worked-out strategy on the part of the animal).

Just as one would like to think that very few parents intentionally allow their children to become obese, it seems unlikely that many dog and cat owners intentionally compromise the welfare and health of their companions by overfeeding them. Rather it seems that owners of fat companions may overfeed their animals due to a number of factors, some of which they have limited control over, much in the same way as they are drawn into overfeeding themselves and their children.

So far, we have discussed work from a number of different countries linking the demographic and psychological characteristics of cat and dog owners, with the risk of the animal becoming overweight and obese. However, the total number of studies on the social and psychological mechanisms underlying the way people feed their companion animals remains small, and further factors will likely be identified as new research becomes available.

The next step, then, must be to discuss how to deal with the factors we have currently identified.

8.5 Whether and How to Prevent and Treat Problems with Overweight Companion Animals

As should be clear from the previous section, it is difficult for some cat and dog owners to prevent their companions from becoming overweight, especially if they are highly connected to their animal, have strong empathetic responses to it, and regard food as a primary means of communication with it.

One difficulty is that, for various reasons, the fact that their cat or dog is overweight or obese does not matter to the same degree to all owners. Some people simply lack the financial or personal resources to deal with their own health, or that of their family, and so the long-term health of their companion animals may not be high on their agenda.

But the issue of weight control itself is also controversial: some people and groups resist the idea that it is inevitably problematic for someone to be overweight or obese. For example, in the United States, various movements have developed in favour of so-called 'fat acceptance' (Kirkland, 2008), arguing that size is no more a reason for discrimination or prejudice than height, sex or skin colour. They resist the medicalisation of being large, arguing that fat people are normal people in large bodies, who are capable of living good lives and making a contribution work-wise and otherwise. In light of this, one might expect similar attitudes to develop in relation to companion animal obesity.

Also, there are perspectives that take a critical view of the utilitarian-like welfare maximisation approach that might be thought to permeate this chapter. Of course, from all main ethical points of view it should be granted that *other things being equal* it is a good thing that companion animals stay healthy, and if good health is maintained through regulating their weight, then this is a good thing to do. However, other things are not always equal, and therefore there may, in certain circumstances, be reasons why maintaining a normal weight may not be a priority.

For example, on some kinds of contextual view (see Chapter 5 for an overview of different ethical views and references to further literature), the key concern in our dealings with companion animals is to maintain and nurture close, caring relationships. Such a relationship may not be achievable, if the constant focus is on limiting food intake. While it will never be acceptable for someone to allow a companion dog or cat to become morbidly obese, allowing the animal to become a little overweight could be accepted as the lesser of two evils – the greater evil being the harm that constant food restriction does to the caring bond between the owner and her or his companion animal.

Assuming the need for some kind of weight control is accepted, however, there are a number of strategies that can be adopted. First, it is essential to impose a balanced feeding regime from the beginning of the animal's life, and to regularly weigh the animal and adjust feeding accordingly. It is also important to consider whether or not to neuter the animal; leaving the animal intact should reduce the likelihood of it becoming overweight (see more in Chapter 10 below). Regular exercise and other activities initiated by the owner will also help to prevent the animal becoming overweight. It is particularly important in the case of cats to find ways of engaging with them that are not linked to feeding, for example, through various forms of training and playing, especially if they are not allowed outdoors (see Chapter 9).

As many people do not recognise that their companion animals are overweight or obese, or seem unable to manage their animal's weight, vets have an important role to play in highlighting the problem when the animals are brought to the clinic for vaccination or regular health checks. A number of approaches have been developed to help owners, mainly through collaboration between pet food companies and vets.

Firstly, tools such as the body condition score (see Section 8.3) have been developed to enable owners to check whether or not their companion is a healthy size.

Secondly, a number of dietary products have been developed, some of which are low in calories and high in fibre, comparable to 'light' products for human consumption; others are high in protein. Most large commercial pet food companies now produce a range of specific diet foods for dogs and cats, some of which are prescription-only, that is, the animal must have been examined by a vet, and the product recommended. If used appropriately, these products are helpful as part of a weight loss or management plan, and, in some cases, will address the dilemma between satisfying hunger and avoiding being overweight. Feeding devices are also available that allow the animal to spend more time engaged in feeding related behaviours, without getting more food.

Thirdly, weight-loss and maintenance programs have been developed, which provide guidance for owners of overweight dogs or cats (Toll et al., 2010). There are also various books (e.g. Harvey & Taylor, 2012) and Internet-based programs, typically sponsored or run by pet food manufacturers (e.g. PetFit.com). These programs involve feeding controlled diets and regular weighing of the animal, often combined with exercise and enrichment regimes. However, persevering with such a program can be challenging, as it takes many months for noticeable weight loss to occur, and owners must remain extremely motivated. A key element of such a program therefore is regular engagement with staff at a veterinary or special weight control clinic. As in the case of human obesity, the difficulty is not only the initial weight loss, but also the long-term change of lifestyle required to maintain the weight at a healthy level.

A striking feature of many of these solutions is the size of commercial vested interests involved. In contrast to human nutrition where a significant part of the research is undertaken by independent researchers funded by government grants, and where independent institutions advise the public, nearly all research and advice on companion animal nutrition is sponsored and run by producers of pet food and pharmaceuticals. While this does not necessarily imply that the research and advice is skewed, it may give rise to lack of trust in the solutions offered. This is perhaps reflected in the large number of web pages and self-help books promoting alternative ways of feeding dogs and cats.

Another striking feature of the proposed solutions is that they all appeal to individual action, and do not consider the political, social and related human issues that seem to underlie the problem. It may be necessary for people to be able to appreciate and tackle their own unhealthy lifestyles, before they can appreciate and address the problems related to the overfeeding of their companions. Tackling these social issues will require far wider ranging solutions.

Finally, given these social issues, as well as owners' psychological states, it is important to avoid moralising, that is, condemning people for doing what they – to some degree, at least – cannot help doing. There have been cases, in Sweden and the United Kingdom (Kulick, 2009), where obese pets have been forcibly removed from their owners by the authorities. While this may be necessary if the animal's welfare is severely threatened, this cannot be a general solution to the widespread problem of canine and feline obesity. Simply condemning owners of fat companions without either helping them, or addressing the underlying social problems, may simply worsen the stigmatisation and low self-esteem that already face obese people in many societies (Puhl & Brownell, 2006). Instead, solutions must be identified to solve the underlying problem, which is to enable owners of cats and dogs to develop a healthy lifestyle for themselves and their companions.

Key Points

- In the past, insufficient feeding was a widespread problem for companion dogs and cats; however, now, in the richer parts of the world, overfeeding is the biggest problem. Approximately one in three dogs and cats kept as a companion in developed countries is overweight, and about 1 in 20 is obese.

- Simple tools have been developed to differentiate between normal, overweight and obese companion animals. Evidence suggests that being even moderately overweight results in diminished life expectancy, and obesity may lead to serious disease and related grave welfare problems.

- A restricted diet may also have a negative effect on animal welfare; however, there seems to be a real dilemma between protecting the animal against hunger and protecting its long-term health.

- Overweight and low-income owners are more likely to have an overweight dog, suggesting that the issue is indicative of broader social problems. It also seems that owners who view their animals as being like fellow humans, or, in the case of cats, have close emotional ties to them, tend to overfeed them.

- Preventing companion animals from getting fat is a good thing viewed from most ethical points of view. However, this may conflict with other concerns, such as maintaining a harmonious relation between owner and animal.
- A number of potential solutions are available to owners who want to avoid problems associated with their companion animals being overweight.

References

Allan, F.J., Pfeiffer, D.U., Jones, B.R., Esslemont, D.H. & Wiseman, M.S. (2000) A cross-sectional study of risk factors for obesity in cats in New Zealand. *Preventive Veterinary Medicine* 46 (3), 183–196.

Bergler, R. (1989) *Man and cat: the benefits of cat ownership.* London, Blackwell Scientific Publications.

Bjørnvad, C.R., Nielsen, D.H., Armstrong, J., McEvoy, F., Hølmkjær, K.M., Jensen, K.S., Pedersen, G.F. & Kristensen, A.T. (2011) Evaluation of a nine-point body condition scoring system in physically inactive pet cats. *American Journal of Veterinary Research* 72 (4), 433–437.

Bove, C.F. & Olson, C.M. (2006) Obesity in low-income rural women: qualitative insights about physical activity and eating patterns. *Women & Health* 44 (1), 57–78.

Burkholder, W.J. & Toll, P.W. (2000) Obesity. In: Hand, M.S., Thatcher, C.D., Remillard, R.L. & Roudebush P. (eds) *Small animal clinical nutrition* 4th edition. Topeka, KS, Mark Morris Institute, pp. 404–406.

Colliard, L., Ancel, J., Benet, J.J. & Paragon, B.M. (2006) Risk factors for obesity in dogs in France. *Journal of Nutrition* 136, 1951–1954.

Courcier, E.A., Thomson, R.M., Mellor, D.J. & Yam, P.S. (2010) An epidemiological study of environmental factors associated with canine obesity. *Journal of Small Animal Practice* 51 (7), 362–367.

Crane, S.W. (1991) Occurrence and management of obesity in companion animals. *Journal of Small Animal Practice* 32, 275–282.

D'Eath, R.B., Tolkamp, B.J., Kyriazakis, I. & Lawrence, A.B. (2009) "Freedom from hunger" and preventing obesity: the animal welfare implications of reducing food quantity or quality. *Animal Behaviour* 77 (2), 275–288.

Edney, A.T.B. & Smith, P.M. (1986) Study of obesity in dogs visiting veterinary practices in the United Kingdom. *Veterinary Record* 118, 391–396.

Etelson, D., Brand, D.A., Patrick, P.A. & Shirali, A. (2003) Childhood obesity: do parents recognize this health risk? *Obesity Research* 11 (11), 1362–1368.

FAWC (2009) *Five freedoms.* Farm Animal Welfare Council. [Online] Available from: http://www.fawc.org.uk/freedoms.htm [Accessed 21 July 2014].

German, A.J. (2006) The growing problem of obesity in dogs and cats. *Journal of Nutrition* 136, 1940–1946.

German, A.J., Holden, S.L., Moxham, G.L., Holmes, K.L., Hackett, R.M. & Rawlings, J.M. (2006) A simple reliable tool for owners to assess the body condition of their dog or cat. *Journal of Nutrition* 136, 2031–2033.

Hand, M.S., Armstrong, P.J. & Allen, T.A. (1989) Obesity: occurrence, treatment, and prevention. *Veterinary Clinics of North America: Small Animal Practice* 19, 447–474.

Harvey, A. & Taylor, S. (2012) *Caring for an overweight cat*. Roslin, Vet Professionals.

Hubert, M., Laroque, P., Gillet, J. & Keenan, K.P. (2000) The effects of diet, *ad libitum* feeding, and moderate and severe dietary restriction on body weight, survival, clinical pathology parameters, and cause of death in control Sprague-Dawley Rats. *Toxicological Sciences* 58 (1), 195–207.

Kasanen, I.H.E., Sørensen D.B., Forkman B. & Sandøe P. (2010) Ethics of feeding: the omnivore dilemma. *Animal Welfare* 19 (1), 37–44.

Kealy, R.D., Lawler, D.F., Ballam, J.M., Mantz, S.L., Biery, D.N., Greeley, E.H., Lust, G., Segre, M., Smith G.K. & Stowe, H.D. (2002) Effects of diet restriction on life span and age-related changes in dogs. *Journal of the American Veterinary Medical Association* 220 (9), 1315–1320.

Kienzle, E. & Bergler, R. (2006) Human-animal relationship of owners of normal and overweight cats. *Journal of Nutrition* 136, 1947–1950.

Kienzle, E., Bergler, R. & Mandernach, A. (1998) A comparison of the feeding behavior and the human–animal relationship in owners of normal and obese dogs. *Journal of Nutrition* 128, 2779–2782.

Kirkland, A. (2008) Think of the hippopotamus: rights consciousness in the fat acceptance movement. *Law & Society Review* 42 (2), 397–431.

Kronfeld, D.S., Donoghue, S. & Glickman, L.T. (1991) Body condition and energy intakes of dogs in a referral teaching hospital. *Journal of Nutrition* 121, 157–158.

Kulick, D. (2009) Fat pets. In: Tomrley, C. & Naylor A.K. (eds) *Fat studies in the UK*. York, Raw Nerve Books, pp. 35–50.

Laflamme D.P. (1997) Development and validation of a body condition score system for dogs. *Canine Practice* 22, 10–15.

Lawler, D.F., Evans, R.H., Larson, B.T. Spitznagel, E.L. Ellersieck, M.R. & Kealy, R.D. (2005) Influence of lifetime food restriction on causes, time, and predictors of death in dogs. *Journal of the American Veterinary Association* 226 (2), 225–231.

Lawler, D.F., Larson, B.T., Ballam, J.M., Smith, G.K., Biery D.N., Evans, R.H., Greely, E.H., Segre, M., Stowe, H.D. & Kealy, R.D. (2008) Diet restriction and aging in the dog: major observation over two decades. *British Journal of Nutrition* 99 (4), 793–805.

Lund, E.M., Armstrong, P.J., Kirk, C.A. & Klausner, J.S. (2005) Prevalence and risk factors for obesity in adult cats from private US veterinary practices. *International Journal of Applied Veterinary Medicine* 3 (2), 4–6.

Lund, E.M., Armstrong, P.J., Kirk, C.A. & Klausner, J.S. (2006) Prevalence and risk factors for obesity in adult dogs from private US veterinary practices. *International Journal of Applied Veterinary Medicine* 4 (2), 3–5.

Mason, E. (1970) Obesity in pet dogs. *Veterinary Record* 86, 612–616.

McGreevy, P.D., Thomson, P.C., Pride, C., Fawcett, A., Grassi, T. & Jones, B. (2005) Prevalence of obesity in dogs examined by Australian veterinary practices and the risk factors involved. *Veterinary Record* 156, 695–702.

McLaren, L. (2007) Socioeconomic status and obesity. *Epidemiologic Reviews* 29, 29–48.

Nestle, M. & Nesheim, M.C. (2010) *Feed your pet right: the authoritative guide to feeding your dog and cat*. New York, London, Toronto & Sydney, Free Press.

Nguyen, P.G., Dumon, H.J., Siliart, B.S., Martin, L.J., Sergheraert, R. & Biourge, V.C. (2004) Effects of dietary fat and energy on body weight and composition after gonadectomy in cats. *American Journal of Veterinary Research* 65, 1708–1713.

Nijland, M.L., Stam, F. & Seidell, J.C. (2010) Overweight in dogs, but not in cats, is related to overweight in their owners. *Public Health Nutrition* 13 (1), 102–106.

Paeratakul, S., Lovejoy, J.C., Ryan, D.H. & Bray, G.A. (2002) The relation of gender, race and socioeconomic status to obesity and obesity comorbidities in a sample of US adults. *International Journal of Obesity* 26, 1205–1210.

Puhl, R.M. & Brownell, K.D. (2006) Confronting and coping with weight stigma: an investigation of overweight and obese adults. *Obesity* 14, 1802–1815.

Robert, S.A. & Reither, E.N. (2004) A multilevel analysis of race, community disadvantage, and body mass index among adults in the US. *Social Science & Medicine* 59 (12), 2421–2434.

Robertson, I.D. (2003). The association of exercise, diet and other factors with owner-perceived obesity in privately owned dogs from metropolitan Perth, WA. *Preventive Veterinary Medicine* 58 (1–2), 75–83.

Rohlf, V.I., Toukhsati, S., Coleman, G.J. & Bennett, P.C. (2010) Dog obesity: can dog caregivers' (owners') feeding and exercise intentions and behaviors be predicted from attitudes? *Journal of Applied Animal Welfare Science* 13 (3), 213–236.

Shearer, P. (2010) *Literature review: canine, feline and human overweight and obesity.* Portland, OR, Banfield Applied Research & Knowledge Team (BARK).

Toll, P.W., Yamka, R.M., Schoenherr, W.D. & Hand, M.S. (2010) Obesity. In: Hand, M.S., Thatcher, C.D., Remillard, R.L., Roudebusch, P. & Novotny, B.J. (eds) *Small animal clinical nutrition.* 5th edition. Topeka, KS, Mark Morris Institute, pp. 501–542.

WHO (2012) *World health statistics 2012.* Geneva, World Health Organization.

White, G.A., Hobson-West, P., Cobb, K., Craigon, J., Hammond, R. & Millar, K.M. (2011) Canine obesity: is there a difference between veterinarian and owner perception? *Journal of Small Animal Practice* 52 (12), 622–626.

Companion Animal Training and Behavioural Problems

Co-author: Iben Meyer, DVM, PhD

Postdoctoral Fellow, Department of Large Animal Sciences, University of Copenhagen, Copenhagen, Denmark

9.1	Introduction		132
9.2	Training		133
	9.2.1	The purpose of training	134
	9.2.2	The debate about dominance	136
	9.2.3	Training methods	138
	9.2.4	Cat training	140
9.3	Behaviour Problems		140
	9.3.1	How might we prevent, solve or alleviate 'behaviour problems'?	142
	9.3.2	How might we deal with aggression and so-called dangerous dogs?	145

9.1 Introduction

Dogs and cats are domesticated animals, and their main biological niche is with the humans who take care of them. These animals have been selectively bred and have successfully adapted to fit into modern, urbanised human life, and overall their numbers have massively increased (despite a minor drop in the number of dogs recently). These animals are well fed (sometimes too well fed, as we saw in Chapter 8), they have ever more sophisticated veterinary care, and their safety is increasingly secured by various forms of control and confinement. As a result, they live much longer and safer lives than their ancestors.

However, one kind of deadly problem does not seem to be in decline. As has been eloquently claimed by Jonica Newby in *The animal attraction: humans and their animal companions:* 'The number one cause of death of dogs in the Western world is not parvovirus, it is not being hit by cars; it is bad (read: "inappropriate") behaviour' (Newby, 1999: p. 250). While this seems likely to be an exaggeration – for example, many more dogs are likely to be euthanased for 'old age' – studies have shown that euthanasia for 'behaviour problems' is common. In Denmark, for example, 'behaviour problems' were the main reason, or part of the reason, for euthanasia of about 20% of all dogs euthanased by vets (Mikkelsen & Lund, 2000). Other dogs with problematic behaviour are handed over to shelters (see Chapter 13) where they are also likely to be euthanased. Probably an even larger number of dogs with problematic behaviour have strained relations with their owners and, as a consequence of this, are more likely to suffer from reduced welfare, for example due to lack of proper care.

In the case of cats, euthanasia due to behavioural problems is also a major cause of death and reduced welfare. Often the problematic behaviour in question, as we shall see later in the chapter, is perfectly natural for both cats and dogs, but it causes inconvenience to the owner. However, particularly in the case of aggression in large dogs, behaviour problems may give rise to serious ethical dilemmas concerning human safety versus animal life and welfare.

Given the severity of the possible consequences of behavioural problems for animals' lives, and for both human and animal welfare, there are good reasons to try to prevent these problems from occurring in the first instance. The number one way to prevent behaviour problems, in the case of dogs at least, is proper education of both the dog and owner through training.

In this chapter, we review and discuss the literature on dog training from the earliest principles of dog training for military purposes. We identify three controversial assumptions on which these principles rely, and discuss them in the light of more recent literature, and in the context of different ethical views. We also consider the often-overlooked issue of cat training. Finally, the literature on behaviour problems in both dogs and cats is reviewed, and ways to deal with these behaviour problems, as well as the ethical issues to which these problems give rise, are considered. In this context, we also discuss so-called dangerous dogs.

9.2 Training

Humans have worked with dogs for thousands of years, and this has, of course, always involved some form of training. However, accounts of dog training based on psychological theory are a recent phenomenon. Konrad Most was one of the first writers to produce a systematic guide to dog training; his ideas provide a useful starting point.

Most started his career as a service dog trainer for the German police in 1906, where he developed new principles of training, published in 1910 in *Training Dogs: A Manual* (translated into English in 1954). Later, during World War I, he took charge of the organisation of canine services for the German army. He continued to work with military dogs until 1937, and was active in dog training until his death in 1954.

Most's key insight was that dogs can be trained using simple learning principles: a dog learns to do what the trainer wants it to do by being rewarded for wanted behaviour, and punished for unwanted behaviour. Most's training principles were in line with the theory of behaviourism (the major psychological school of the day), and with the work of contemporary scientists like the American psychologist Edward Thorndike, and the Russian physiologist and psychologist Ivan Pavlov. Some decades later, the famous American psychologist B.F. Skinner investigated in more detail the principles of so-called operant learning, according to which a behavioural response in the animal becomes more, or less, likely to occur, depending on its consequences. We will return to this later.

According to Most, dogs are 'beyond good or evil, living in a world without moral values, learning … solely through the faculty of memory' (Most, 1954: p. 13). So, there is no point in getting angry with a dog, or feeling disappointed about its lack of moral sense. Rather, we should give dogs the right kind of signals at the right time, allowing the dog to associate rewarding stimuli with wanted behaviour, and aversive stimuli with unwanted behaviour. Most argued that blaming or punishing the dog without creating proper associations is not only pointless, but may be damaging, by causing the dog to fear the owner.

Most maintained that the endpoint of dog training is to have a dog 'that enjoys life and is happy in his work, putting all his heart into it'; and he underlines, rather out of tune with the military ideals of the time, the need for the trainer to show the dog positive emotions. When the dog makes progress the trainer ought:

> not only to utter such words as "good boy" repeatedly in caressing tones, and fondle the dog, but also, if the exercise in hand permits it, to execute a dance of joy with the animal.

> (Most, 1954: p. 34)

These ideas are largely in line with current thinking about proper dog training. However, at least three aspects of Most's ideas are now highly controversial, concerning the purpose of training, the role of dominance in the relation between owner and dog, and the means by which dogs are trained. We now consider these ideas in more depth.

9.2.1 The purpose of training

According to Most, the purpose of dog training is 'that the dog shall only do what we find convenient and useful, and refrain from doing what is inconvenient and harmful to us' (Most, 1954: p. 24). As, on Most's view, there is a clear conflict between what is convenient and useful to us, and what is advantageous to the dog, he envisaged a significant element of compulsion involved in dog training.

Many people now reject such a human-centred view, maintaining that dogs (and cats) are worthy of respect in their own right, and so this one-sided focus on what is convenient and useful to humans is a problematic starting point. Even people who in principle favour a purely human-centred ethical view, such as adherents to a contractarian view (see Chapter 5), may love their own companion animals and disagree with the need to train them just for the sake of human convenience.

This is not to deny that human convenience is a *major* part of the reason why dogs and cats are trained. For example, housetraining is essential to allow a reasonably harmonious relation between humans and their companion dogs and cats. While it is not directly problematic to a dog or a cat to carry out what is euphemistically called 'inappropriate elimination' (e.g. urinating or defaecating indoors), this is intolerable for most owners if it occurs frequently. Since the animal is dependent on the goodwill of the owner for its life and welfare, housetraining is also indirectly beneficial for the animal. The same may apply to some other forms of basic training, for example, to not chase livestock. So, human convenience matters not only in its own right, but also because ignoring it may, indirectly, lead to harm to the animals in question.

In the case of cats, the training required to function in a normal household is usually viewed as rather minimal. The cat must learn to use its litter box, and abstain from doing certain things, such as jumping onto tables or scratching the furniture; normally no structured training procedures are applied here.

In the case of dogs, particularly larger dogs, structured training is usually thought necessary to make them well-functioning members of the household and society. In many places, dog owners attend puppy classes, where they learn to train their dog to perform basic skills including leash-walking, recall, and basic commands such as 'No!', 'Sit!' and 'Down!' Such classes have the additional benefit of socialising dogs, and may improve owners' ability to communicate with their dogs.

However, much current dog training aims to go far beyond making dogs a better fit for human lives and convenience. As we saw in Chapter 3, some dog owners engage in ongoing training with their dogs as a 'tool', as part of a sport, or as a hobby. This may be breed specific, such as tracking with hunting dogs or herding with sheepdogs. Most of the 'modern' forms of dog training – and breed specific training in particular – encourage dogs to do things they are naturally inclined to do, unlike Most's military and police dogs, which for a large part were trained *not* to do things that they were inclined to do.

Breed specific training, and other forms of hobby dog obedience training, may be intended to serve further aims. First, dogs that are being trained will be occupied and get tired, in contrast to the inactive lives of many domestic dogs. Secondly, training allows owners to build a closer, and perhaps better, relation with their dogs. Some studies, at least, have documented positive effects, including fewer behaviour problems, as a result of owners spending time training their dogs (Bennett & Rohlf, 2007; Clark & Boyer, 1993; Jagoe & Serpell, 1996), although other studies have not found such effects (Blackwell *et al.*, 2008; Casey *et al.*, 2013).

Given this, training dogs as a sport or hobby may be a positive activity (depending on the type of training), from both utilitarian and deontological views that emphasise animal welfare. Contextual ethical approaches, which focus on the building of good relations between particular humans and their companions, also understand dog training as valuable. For instance, dog trainer and philosopher Vicki Hearne claims, in *Adam's task: calling animals by name* (1982), that training dogs is not only a potential way of enriching dogs' lives, but also a human duty. If we create animals to live in the human world, then we have a responsibility to equip the animals with whom we co-exist to operate successfully in this world; so the 'proper' state for domesticated companion animals is to be trained. Using terms such as 'beauty' and 'art', Hearne claims that through training, the animals achieve a 'virtuous' character, which is unfolded and maintained in conjunction with the trainer's similarly virtuous character. Here, Hearne moves far away from Most's starting point where dogs are beyond 'good and evil'. Underlying Hearne's lofty words (it is not clear, for instance, what virtue means in the case of a dog) is the intuitively appealing idea that humans and dogs can inspire and get the best from each other through shared training activities, an idea also defended by the American philosopher Donna Haraway (2003).

Seen from this perspective, the purpose of dog training shifts from a focus largely on human convenience and benefit, to one that also promotes more fulfilling lives for dogs and their human owners. In ethical terms, this aim seems uncontroversial. However, while it may be uncontroversial that training should enable dogs to flourish, there is ongoing controversy about how far a trainer should dominate the dog.

9.2.2 The debate about dominance

According to Most, successful dog training requires that the trainer establish authority over the dog, by putting her- or himself at the top of a hierarchy:

> As in a pack of dogs, the order of hierarchy in a man and dog combination can only be established by physical force, that is by an actual struggle, in which the man is instantly victorious.... If a dog shows the slightest sign of rebellion against his trainer or leader, the physical superiority of the man as leader of the pack must be given instant expression in the most unmistakable manner.... For, each time the dog finds that he is not instantly mastered, the canine competitive instinct will increase and his submissive instinct will weaken.... We are concerned here with a struggle for authority. The object of compulsion is to obtain the permanent and unconditional surrender of the dog. The intimidated state that accompanies it soon disappears, simply because peace again reigns as soon as the man is victorious.
>
> (Most, 1954: pp. 35–37)

We can call this the Dominance Theory of dogs' natures and of their relation to humans.

The most popular way to support the Dominance Theory is as follows: dogs originated from wolves, and their behaviour derives from that of wolves. Wolves naturally live in packs with a clear hierarchy, and an alpha-male and a dominant female at the top, a view supported by studies of groups of wolves kept in captivity (Zimen, 1975). To maintain the hierarchy, the alpha-male must dominate the subordinate members of the group, who regularly try to challenge the dominant members, and prevent them from becoming dominant by showing aggression. When we live with dogs, they view us as pack members and will naturally strive to rise above us in the hierarchy. To avoid this ongoing competition, we must confront and dominate dogs effectively, so that they accept their place below us in the hierarchy.

The Dominance Theory was widely accepted for most of the twentieth century, and following its premise, many dog owners adopted a training style where they would, for example, confront a dog protecting a bone, and forcibly remove the bone, to show the dog 'who was boss'. When dogs showed signs of dominance, owners would engage in somewhat violent confrontations, such as doing an 'alpha-roll' on the dog (forcing it to lie on its back, and holding it there while staring into its eyes).

However, this theory has recently been the subject of intense controversy among experts in the field of animal behaviour. In 1999, the wildlife biologist David Mech published a study based on observations of wolves in the wild, rather than in captivity. He found that these wolves lived in family groups led by two parents. According to Mech:

> The typical wolf pack, then, should be viewed as a family with the adult parents guiding the activities of the group and sharing group leadership in a division-of-labor system, in which the female predominates primarily in such activities as pup care and defense and the male primarily during foraging and food-provisioning and the travels associated with them.... Dominance displays are uncommon except during competition for food.... Active submission appears to be primarily a food-begging gesture or a foodgathering motivator.
>
> (Mech, 1999: p. 1202)

So, on this view, the natural life of a wolf is not a constant fight for dominance. Rather, wolves live in family structures where hierarchies are defined by family role; where young animals will naturally become leaders by leaving their parents and establishing their own families.

Following Mech's study, influential dog trainers and experts in dog behaviour published further papers aiming to debunk the Dominance Theory. Wendy van Kerkhove (2004) argued that a number of earlier studies on feral dogs showed that they live in loosely organised groups rather than packs, which speaks against making assumptions about the social behaviour of dogs based on wolf behaviour. Further, she argued that aggression between dogs is better addressed by rewarding non-aggressive behaviour than by trying to punish signs of dominant behaviour.

A subsequent review paper by the ethologist John Bradshaw and colleagues from Bristol University, expanded van Kerkhove's arguments, and questioned the usefulness of the Dominance Theory, concluding that:

> ... where a dog is anxious about the approach of an owner in a particular context (perhaps because the owner has previously forced the dog into an "alpha roll"), it may show appeasement, avoidance, or aggression to avoid the perceived threat. Since the first two are unsuccessful when owners persist in approaching and pulling their pet out from its hiding place, and the latter is successful, even if only momentarily, it is the aggressive response that is reinforced. Over subsequent encounters, if this response is consistently successful, the dog will become more confident in showing this behavior in that specific context. Similar associations can be used to explain how behavior that originates as defensive can metamorphose into the type of offensive behavior that is commonly categorized as "dominant".
>
> (Bradshaw, Blackwell & Casey, 2009: p. 143)

So, it is suggested here that the Dominance Theory, when applied in dog training, may serve as a self-reinforcing hypothesis: by using physical force, the owner elicits an aggressive response from the dog, which in turn is interpreted as a sign of dominance; alpha-rolls and other forms of physical confrontation may actually increase the risk of aggressive responses from the dog (Herron, Shofer & Reisner, 2009). Bradshaw and colleagues conclude that it is

> doubtful whether the concept of "dominance" can make any useful contribution to explaining dog–dog aggression, and it is therefore even less likely to be applicable to aggression directed at humans, given the added complexities of interspecies communication.
>
> (Bradshaw, Blackwell & Casey, 2009: p. 143)

However, recently researchers have argued that it is premature to claim that dominance plays *no* role in dog–dog and human–dog relations (Schilder *et al.*, 2014; Trisko, 2011). They argue that dominance can be used to explain the relation between individuals, that stable relations of dominance are observed for some (but not all) dyads of dogs, but also that, in contrast to the Dominance Theory, dominance relationships are maintained primarily by the low-ranking dogs voluntarily showing submissive signals to high-ranking dogs. The high-ranking dogs on the other hand mainly demonstrate their rank by posture and threats, and almost never by overt aggression (Trisko, 2011: p. 40).

These researchers agree with critics of the Dominance Theory that forceful behaviour is not a good way of ensuring that dogs are submissive to their owners. Instead, 'adequate socialization of the dog and a clear and consistent behaviour by the owner' is needed (Schilder *et al.*, 2014: p. 7). So, even though the role of dominance is highly contested, there seems to be agreement among academics studying dog behaviour that Most's idea of forcefully dominating dogs should be rejected. In fact, forceful dominance may increase the risk of aggression and other behaviour problems. This debate about dominance leads us directly into a more general debate about training methods.

9.2.3 Training methods

Most's ideas about animal training were later, independently, given a scientific basis by Skinner, based primarily on his studies of rats. Some of Skinner's students then applied his ideas to dog training. Skinner's simple idea was that an individual's behaviour is modified by its consequences: consequences that increase the likelihood of the behaviour are called 'reinforcers', while those that decrease the likelihood of the behaviour are called 'punishers' (Chance, 1999: pp. 135–140, 188–190).

Both reinforcement and punishment can in principle come in two forms; a positive form where the trainer adds something to the situation, and a negative form where the trainer removes something from the situation. For example, in training a dog not to jump on people, there are four ways to condition the dog's behaviour using operant learning:

• Positive reinforcement: treats for staying on the ground (reinforcing relaxation and staying on the ground)

- Negative reinforcement: holding on to the dog's collar to keep it on the ground, then releasing this lightly aversive stimulus when the dog relaxes (reinforcing relaxation and staying on the ground)
- Positive punishment: hitting the dog when it jumps (punishing jumping behaviour)
- Negative punishment: turning your back to the dog when it jumps, thereby removing the possibility of pleasant social contact with the human (punishing jumping behaviour).

In this context, there need not be anything positive, in the usual sense of the word, about positive punishment – it just refers to adding something to, rather than removing something from the situation – and punishment as defined here need not involve any violence: saying 'NO' to a dog in a deep voice can be just as much a positive punishment as hitting it.

Positive reinforcement methods are widely accepted, and techniques for employing it have been much improved in recent decades. One example is the use of so-called clicker training, which became popular following the publication of Karen Pryor's book *Don't shoot the dog* (1984). Here a dog is trained to connect the positive reinforcer, for example, a piece of food, with a 'click', a short, distinct sound made by a mechanical device operated by the trainer. This enables the trainer to reinforce behaviour in a more precise way than would otherwise be possible.

Most, and some of his followers, notably the American William Koehler, on the other hand, used rather harsh methods of punishment in dog training. Koehler's immensely popular book *The Koehler method of dog training* (1962) recommended throw chains and electric shocks for 'emphatic corrections' in addition to a spiked collar and beatings with a switch, as had previously been used by Most. Koehler presented his views very passionately, ridiculing 'the prattle of "dog psychologists"' (Koehler, 1962: p. 6). This contributed to a heated debate, which also involved several court cases against Koehler, and resulted in his books being banned in Arizona for a while (Hearne, 1982: p. 10).

Even today deep divisions still exist about the use of positive punishment in training. One approach is championed by the television personality and trainer Cesar Millan, who uses different forms of positive punishment in his television shows, as well as physical handling that aims at making the dog submit to the trainer (e.g. alpha rolls). A rather different approach is defended by Victoria Stilwell, who in her books and television shows favours what she calls 'positive training', which features the principle of 'avoiding the use of intimidation, physical punishment or fear' (Stilwell, n.d.).

This debate about physical punishment clearly has an ethical component. Adherents of animal rights and similar views maintain that the use of pain and other negative states to motivate an animal is wrong on principle. Utilitarians, on the other hand, will decide based on the apparent empirical consequences of using positive punishment, and if the alternative to positive punishment is worse – for example, confinement of dogs chasing livestock – some argue that it could warrant the use of, for example, shock collars to train such dogs. Still, the use of shock collars can have negative consequences for dog welfare, and studies show that dogs trained with shock collars are more stressed than dogs trained without them, not only in the training context, but in general. This is at least part of the reason why the use of such devices is legally banned in a number of European countries. However, if the dogs can predict and control the shock, that is, they know that they can avoid it by not performing a particular behaviour, then they are much less stressed than if they cannot predict the shock, that is, if the shock is administered unpredictably (Schalke *et al.*, 2007; Schilder & van der Borg, 2004), as might occur with incompetent trainers.

As mentioned before, a number of studies show that people who use more forceful forms of positive punishment in dog training run a greater risk of the dogs having severe behaviour problems, particularly in the form of aggression (Blackwell *et al.*, 2008; Herron, Shofer & Reisner, 2009; Hiby, Rooney & Bradshaw, 2004; Rooney & Cowan, 2011). So, returning to a utilitarian perspective, evidence suggests that even if positive punishment may be an effective and (perhaps) a better alternative to euthanasia, harsh and forceful forms of positive punishment subject dogs to negative experiences without much in the way of behavioural benefits, either to their owners, or indirectly to the dogs themselves. Given these results, and the widespread sense that dogs are friends and family members (see Chapter 3), it is more common today to emphasise positive reinforcement in dog training and to reject harsh or forceful forms of positive punishment.

9.2.4 Cat training

Until recently, there has been little formalised cat training. Other than basic training to use a litter tray (largely done by the mother cat), behaviours such as climbing onto kitchen surfaces, eating their owners' food and scratching furniture are dealt with on an *ad hoc* basis.

However, basic skills that can improve most cat–owner relationships, such as socialisation, acceptance of handling, and willingness to use a carrier can quite easily be taught, and many cats will also happily engage in more fun-based training. There is a growing and very committed community of people who engage in clicker training of cats (see e.g. http://www.clickertraining.com/cat-training). As with dogs and other animals, clicker training of cats is based on positive reinforcement of desirable behaviour, rather than punishing unwanted behaviour (Figure 9.1).

Cat training plausibly serves three main purposes (similar to dog training): first, it is good for cat welfare, as it engages cats in activities that both provide exercise and prevent boredom, especially important for indoor cats (see Chapters 4 and 8). Second, it allows owners to interact more with their cats, which may develop human attachment to the cat and the bonding of the cat to the owner. Third, training may make it easier for owners to deal with issues such as nail clipping, tooth cleaning, brushing and administration of medicine. However, so far there are no scholarly studies looking at the effects of cat training, so while it seems likely to have benefits, they have not yet been empirically substantiated.

9.3 Behaviour Problems

Some people do not bother to try to train their dog; and as we have seen, formal cat training is very rare. However, even when people engage in training activities with their dog or cat, the animal may still manifest a 'behaviour problem'. What makes a behaviour problem a 'problem' is that it is viewed as such by the owner, or other people with whom the animal is in contact. This is, of course, a very human-centred definition,

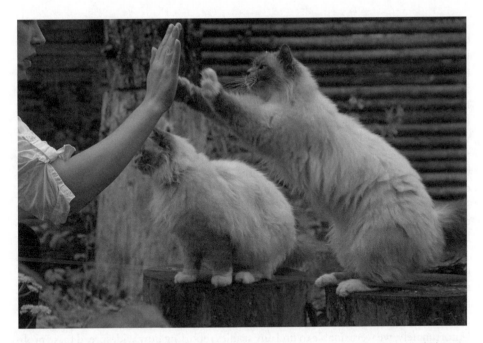

Figure 9.1 Clicker training of cats. In this instance, the training was to address a behaviour problem where one cat felt intimidated by the other. Through the training, the intimidated cat gained more confidence and was able to tolerate the company of the other cat. (*Reproduced with permission from* Pressefolden.dk.)

but it reflects the social reality that humans decide what behaviours are acceptable in companion animals.

Statistics about the different kinds of behavioural problems and their prevalence mainly come from two sources: records from veterinary and behaviour clinics, and questionnaires aimed at owners. The former gives an insight into problems that are so severe and difficult to live with that people seek professional help, whereas the latter includes a wider range of problems, some of which are perceived as less severe.

Two papers by Michelle Bamberger and Katherine Houpt provide statistics for the prevalence of behaviour problems seen at the Animal Behavior Clinic at Cornell University Hospital for Animals, for dogs and cats respectively, during the period 1991–2001.

By far the most frequent problem in dogs seen at the clinic was aggression, mostly directed at humans. Over 60% of all the cases seen belonged to this group, and in most of the cases, the owner was the target. The second most common group of problems consisted of so-called anxieties, and affected nearly 20% of the dogs seen in the clinic. Of these, around three-quarters suffered from separation anxiety, meaning that the animals 'display destructive behaviour, vocalization, salivation or elimination when being separated from their owners'. Other prevalent behaviour problems were 'unruly behaviour' ('behaviours resulting from control and obedience problems'), affecting about 12% of the dogs, and house soiling, affecting around 8% of the dogs (Bamberger & Houpt, 2006b).

In contrast, a study based on information given by a randomly selected population of suburban dog owners in Australia found the most frequently reported problems to be 'overexcitement' (63%) and 'jumping up on people' (56%), 'rushing at people/dogs' (38%), 'excessive barking' (32%), 'constant running around' (29%), 'digging' (28%) and 'chewing' (25%) (Kobelt *et al.*, 2003). These could all be loosely classified as 'unruly behaviour' (mentioned in the preceding paragraph), making it the most widespread behaviour problem in the general population of dogs. 'Nervousness', on the other hand, which seems similar to what the clinic called 'anxieties', at 20%, is at a similar level to the Cornell behaviour clinic. The most significant difference concerns problems relating to aggression towards humans, which in the Australian study occurred at a frequency of less than 10%, but was the most widespread problem found in the clinic. This is not surprising, however, as people are more likely to seek professional help for a problem they consider more serious, such as aggression, than one perhaps less so, such as 'unruly behaviour'.

The Cornell data on cats gives a very different picture from that concerning dogs: the majority of cats, nearly 60%, were presented for house soiling. The second most widespread problem, in about a quarter of cats, was aggression towards other cats, typically other cats in the household. Finally, the third most common problem was aggression towards humans, typically the owner (13%) (Bamberger & Houpt, 2006a). Unfortunately, we were unable to find any studies reporting how widespread these problems are in the general cat population.

Behaviour problems in dogs and cats are costly in terms of animal welfare, human well-being and animal lives. Some behaviour problems have a clear, direct effect on animal welfare in terms of increased levels of anxiety and fear. Others, such as excessive barking or digging, may in the short term be conducive to the animal's welfare but may indirectly affect the animal negatively via a strained relation with the owner, which may in turn have negative welfare impacts for the animal, for instance, by making the owner less willing to invest in good veterinary care (Todd, Pantenburg & Crawford, 2008). For the owner, behaviour problems are directly linked to frustration and often also distress, and they may also be costly, both because of harm done by the animal and through the need to spend time dealing with the problem and paying for professional assistance. Finally, the sad end point of many behaviour problems is that the animal is likely to be euthanased or in other ways relinquished (Patronek *et al.*, 1996).

Viewed from almost every ethical perspective, there are good reasons to seek ways to prevent, solve or alleviate behaviour problems in dogs and cats. In the rest of this chapter, we first try to give a brief overview of possible ways of achieving this, and then deal specifically with ethical dilemmas relating to aggression in dogs, since this appears to be the most serious problem.

9.3.1 How might we prevent, solve or alleviate 'behaviour problems'?

So far, we have talked of behaviour problems as being linked to insufficient, or inappropriate, training. However, this is far too simplistic a picture. Behaviour problems are multifactorial, that is, they have many causes as illustrated by Figure 9.2.

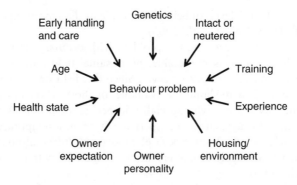

Figure 9.2 Causal factors affecting the level of behaviour problems in dogs and cats.

As we saw in Chapter 6, the early care of puppies and kittens – their socialisation with humans and how stressful their early environment is – may affect behaviour later in life. Furthermore, as we saw in Chapter 7, the genetic makeup of an animal, affected by selective breeding, may also have a significant effect on behaviour. For example, some lines of dog breeds carry a higher risk of compulsive disorders (Luescher, 2004). Similarly, dogs of certain breeds bark more than others: it will be no surprise to those familiar with the breed that Cairn Terriers, for instance, 'vocalise' much more than most dogs in the general population (Bamberger & Houpt, 2006b).

As we will see in Chapter 10, whether or not a dog or a cat is neutered may also affect behavioural problems. For example, neutering male dogs may prevent roaming, and neutering male cats may prevent urine spraying. Bad past experiences, for example, with other animals, children or environments, may also result in the development of fearfulness, phobias or fear-related aggression, whereas positive experiences, much like good early handling, can prevent or alleviate such problems. As we saw in Chapter 4, some behavioural problems in cats, for example, inappropriate elimination, may be affected by whether or not they are allowed outdoor access.

We noted in Chapter 3 that owner expectations affect attachment to companions and probably what owners see as being a behavioural problem. The availability of so-called convenience surgery such as debarking and declawing, which we will discuss in Chapter 11, to prevent normal but inconvenient forms of behaviour, may also affect owner expectations. Finally, health problems may cause behavioural problems; for example, inappropriate urination may be caused by urinary tract infections and aggression may be caused by pain (e.g. Neilson, 2003; Reisner, Shofer & Nance, 2007). Conditions such as senility or limited motor control, more frequent with increasing age, may also give rise to behaviour problems. Thus, proper training from an early age is just one of many factors that may prevent behaviour problems, although it is an important one.

Behaviour problems, then, can be dealt with in several ways. First, the owner could consider whether illness or age may be causing the problem, or whether neutering may resolve it, and seek advice from a vet. Second, he or she could consider living with the problem, as in many cases, the 'problem' may be a natural behaviour, and the real issue is the owner's expectations. That some people do change their expectations of companion animals through living with them may explain the finding in some studies that first-time dog owners perceive higher levels of behaviour problems than more experienced owners (Jagoe & Serpell, 1996; Kobelt *et al.*, 2003).

Owners may also try addressing the problem with ordinary training. If this does not work, and the problem is intolerable, professional help may be sought from a dog trainer, a behavioural therapist or a vet. Since this field has grown substantially, as we saw in Chapter 2, help should be available for those who can pay for it. Apart from training and advice, vets who specialise in behaviour problems will sometimes prescribe psychoactive drugs, either on a permanent or on a temporary basis (Bowen & Heath, 2005; King *et al.*, 2000; Seksel & Lindeman, 2008), although it is usually recommended that pharmacological intervention is combined with behavioural therapy (Bowen & Heath, 2005).

Finally, owners may part with their companion, for instance, by relinquishing it to a shelter or having it euthanased; the ethical issues arising from this will be discussed in Chapter 13. Here we will consider ethical perspectives on whether and how to respond to behavioural problems in a companion animal.

On some ethical views – such as contractarian approaches (see Chapter 5), only human interests matter directly. The interests of the problematic animal companion matter only inasmuch as they matter to the owner (or others, for instance, other people affected by a dog's intrusive barking). If the owner, or other members of the family (for instance children) are very attached to the animal, then trying to resolve the problem looks like the best solution. However, if the problem is difficult or impossible to resolve, and the loss of the animal would not be devastating to those who live with it, it may be rational to get rid of the animal – for instance, a cat that persists in house soiling.

However, most people do think that the animal's interests should factor into decision making here. Those with broadly utilitarian perspectives, for instance, will argue that the affected animal's welfare, in terms of pleasure and pain, or desire satisfaction, should be considered. If the 'problem' behaviour arises from pain, fear or frustration, it is a problem both for the owner and the animal; resolving it would improve the state of affairs for everyone affected. Even if the gains to the owner from, say, behavioural therapy do not, from the owner's perspective, outweigh the cost of paying for it, benefits to the animal may justify the expense overall. However, a utilitarian would not necessarily argue that an animal should be kept at all costs. If an animal and/or an owner is highly distressed, and no solution can be found, euthanasia may be the solution that minimises pain and distress overall.

Three other kinds of ethical views should be mentioned here. First, a view on which animals have rights would require the owner to avoid violating the rights of the animal to life (either directly by euthanasia, or by exposing animals to the risk of euthanasia in a shelter). We discuss this further in Chapter 13. Second, as we saw in Chapter 4, there are also some views on which naturalness is an important value, and should be protected or promoted. Since some 'problem' behaviours (e.g. barking and scratching) are natural behaviours, these behaviours should be permitted as valuable expressions of what is natural to the species or breed, even if it is inconvenient to the owner. (It is less clear on this view what to think about highly anxious behaviours that may seem less 'natural'.)

Finally, contextual ethical views may take different approaches here. Those that emphasise the importance of specific past commitments – in this case, the commitment that comes from acquiring a companion – are likely to argue that individuals who take

on animals have very strong responsibilities to care for their welfare and not to abandon or kill them – that was part of the 'moral deal' when the animal was acquired.
Other contextual views, though, that focus on care and emotional attachments, may
take a different view. If the problem behaviour causes the relationship to break down,
or if one or both parties are made miserable by the relationship, then parting from the
animal may be the best outcome.

However, there is one kind of behaviour problem that gives rise to special ethical
issues: aggression that affects not only the welfare of the aggressive animal, but also
the safety of the owner, other humans and other dogs/animals nearby. To this and the
related ethical issues we will now turn.

9.3.2 How might we deal with aggression and so-called dangerous dogs?

Aggression is, as previously described, the behaviour problem in dogs that is most likely
to lead people to seek professional help. Whereas other behaviour problems may be
highly inconvenient to the owner, the aggressive dog often poses *a serious danger* to the
object of its aggression, be it the owner, children in the family, strangers or other dogs.
When it comes to human-directed aggression in dogs, bite statistics show a distressing
picture of children, who already know the dog, being the prime victims (Rosado *et al.*,
2009; Weiss, Friedman & Coben, 1998).

Aggression in dogs, like other behavioural problems, is typically multifactorial and
there seems to be different kinds of motivation behind aggression in dogs (Bowen &
Heath, 2005). In some cases, aggression may be related to dominance or territorial
defence. However, in several studies, a link has been found between fear-related
problems and aggression in dogs (Bamberger & Houpt, 2006b; Haverbeke *et al.*, 2009;
Hsu & Serpell, 2003).

Unfortunately, in popular debate, aggression is often viewed as a trait-like feature
that follows the dog irrespective of the object of aggression, the context of aggression
and prior learning. Typically, this trait has been linked to certain breeds of dogs, for
example, Pit Bulls, which are then viewed as 'dangerous dogs'. In some countries, for
example, Denmark and the United Kingdom, official lists of banned dog breeds exist.
These bans can be very difficult to administer, partly because, pedigree dogs apart, it
can be almost impossible to prove that a dog belongs to or is genetically related to a
certain breed.

Of course, there are differences between breeds as regards aggression; however, these
differences do not match public prejudice. Studies have found that some of the small
breeds, such as Chihuahuas and Dachshunds, are among the most aggressive breeds of
dogs; here there seems to be a clear link between fearfulness and aggression (Duffy, Hsu
& Serpell, 2008). However, since these are very small dogs, the risk of injury to the
object of their aggression is much less than from a larger dog. Other dog breeds, such
as Greyhounds, have a high level of fear, but a low level of aggression, whereas some
guard-dog breeds, such as Rottweilers, tend to be aggressive towards, but not fearful
of, strangers. There also seems to be a marked difference in the propensity of breeds
to show aggression, and also in whether the aggression is directed towards humans or
other dogs (Duffy, Hsu & Serpell, 2008).

In scientific studies, some of the dog breeds that are typically perceived as dangerous, such as Pit Bulls and American Staffordshire terriers, have not been found to be

particularly aggressive on tests constructed to evaluate dog aggression towards humans and inanimate objects (Ott *et al.*, 2008; Schalke *et al.*, 2007). This should speak against banning these breeds. However, it has been argued that breeds with a history of being used for dog fighting are more dangerous to other dogs, which does seem to be supported by a study showing an over-representation of dogs of the pit bull type in situations where guide dogs were attacked by other dogs (Brooks & Moxon, 2010). Unfortunately, literature on dog–dog aggression is scarce.

It is possible that dogs of the pit bull type have a reputation for being dangerous because they are often acquired by socially marginalised young men who have little idea of responsible dog ownership, resulting in the development of problematic behaviour in the dog. In fact, ownership of breeds perceived as dangerous has been linked to higher levels of violent criminal behaviour in the owner (Barnes *et al.*, 2006; Harding, 2013; Ragatz *et al.*, 2009). To conclude that dogs of these breeds are always aggressive and dangerous, even when being brought up by responsible dog owners, may be an unjustified attitude that does not take into account the multifactorial nature of aggression in dogs.

Aggression towards both humans and other dogs can sometimes be successfully treated. However, in many cases, such treatments are not tried because of the danger these dogs may pose to people, and particularly to children. This is an understandable reaction to a very real ethical dilemma: while it may be possible to treat the dog, there is always a risk that the intervention will fail, or that someone will be seriously bitten before it works. For the same reasons, aggressive dogs are difficult to re-home.

There are several different ethical approaches to this dilemma. From a human-centred view such as contractarianism, human interests are of primary importance. Unless strong emotions are invested in the aggressive dog, the most obvious strategy would be to put human safety first and to have the dog euthanased without trying other options. A utilitarian will favour looking for a solution that maximises well-being across individuals, human and canine. This may allow for attempts to treat the dog while implementing safety precautions with children and other vulnerable individuals.

On a rights view, the issue may be complicated by the fact that rights are ascribed both to the affected dogs and to the vulnerable humans. So, the dog has a right to life, and it may be argued that the child has the right to be protected by adults from foreseeable dangers. Some adherents of animal rights, such as Tom Regan, claim that all humans have a right to self-defence in the face of dangerous animals. So, in principle, these views will not completely exclude the option of euthanasing a dangerous dog. However, since euthanasia involves taking a life, on a rights view it should be viewed as the last and not the first option.

Key Points

- Systematic accounts of dog training principles based on psychological theory originate in the early twentieth century with the pioneering work of Konrad Most.
- Most's key idea, later independently given a scientific underpinning by B.F. Skinner and his pupils, is that dogs and cats learn through conditioning by means of reward and punishment.
- Most and other early trainers had a purely human-centred view on the purpose of dog training; more recently, training is also seen as enriching dogs' lives.

- Most understood violent domination and harsh punishment to be a necessary precondition for successful dog training, but recent ethological studies reject this approach, although the role of dominance in dog–dog and dog–human relations is still disputed.
- There is no tradition of cat training, but there are reasons to believe that cat training may have positive effects, particularly on indoor cats.
- Problematic behaviour is one of the prime causes for relinquishment and euthanasia of dogs and cats; the problems are multifactorial, with links to most of the issues discussed in this book.
- Depending on the ethical perspective, there will be differences regarding the best way to deal with a dog or a cat with a behaviour problem.
- Aggression in dogs is a complex problem, and the widespread tendency to stigmatise certain so-called 'dangerous' dog breeds as particularly aggressive is so far scientifically unfounded.
- Dog aggression gives rise to a special dilemma, between, on the one hand, saving a dog's life, and on the other protecting human safety.

References

Bamberger, M. & Houpt, K.A. (2006a) Signalment factors, comorbidity, and trends in behavior diagnoses in cats: 736 cases (1991-2001). *Journal of American Veterinary Medical Association* 229 (10), 1602–1606.

Bamberger, M. & Houpt, K.A. (2006b). Signalment factors, comorbidity, and trends in behavior diagnoses in dogs: 1,644 cases (1991-2001). *Journal of American Veterinary Medical Association* 229 (10), 1591–1601.

Barnes, J.E., Boat, B.W., Putnam, F.W., Dates, H.F. & Mahlman, A.R. (2006) Ownership of high-risk ("vicious") dogs as a marker for deviant behaviors: implications for risk assessment. *Journal of Interpersonal Violence* 21, 1616–1634.

Bennett, P.C. & Rohlf, V.I. (2007) Owner-companion dog interactions: relationships between demographic variables, potentially problematic behaviours, training engagement and shared activities. *Applied Animal Behaviour Science* 102, 65–84.

Blackwell, E.J., Twells, C., Seawright, A. & Casey, R.A. (2008) The relationship between training methods and the occurrence of behavior problems, as reported by owners, in a population of domestic dogs. *Journal of Veterinary Behavior: Clinical Applications and Research* 3, 207–217.

Bowen, J. & Heath, S. (2005) *Behaviour problems in small animals: practical advice for the veterinary team*. Edinburgh, Elsevier Saunders.

Bradshaw, J.W.S., Blackwell, E.J. & Casey, R.A. (2009) Dominance in domestic dogs: useful construct or bad habit? *Journal of Veterinary Behavior: Clinical Applications and Research* 4, 135–144.

Brooks, A. & Moxon, R. (2010) Incidence and impact of dog attacks on guide dogs in the UK. *Veterinary Record* 166 (22), 778–781.

Casey, R.A., Loftus, B., Bolster, C., Richards, G.J. & Blackwell, E.J. (2013) Inter-dog aggression in a UK owner survey: prevalence, co-occurrence in different contexts and risk factors. *The Veterinary Record* 172 (5), 127.

Chance, P. (1999) *Learning and behavior*. 4th edition. Pacific Grove, CA, Brooks/Cole Publishing Company.

Clark, G.I. & Boyer, W.N. (1993) The effects of dog obedience training and behavioural counselling upon the human-canine relationship. *Applied Animal Behaviour Science* 37, 147–159.

Duffy, D., Hsu, Y. & Serpell, J. (2008) Breed differences in canine aggression. *Applied Animal Behaviour Science* 114 (3–4), 441–460.

Haraway, D. (2003) *The companion species manifesto: dogs, people, and significant otherness*. Chicago, Prickly Paradigm Press.

Harding, S. (2013) 'Bling with bite': the rise of status and weapon dogs. *Veterinary Record* 173 (11), 261–263.

Haverbeke, A., Smet, A., Depiereux, E., Giffroy, J. & Diederich, C. (2009) Assessing undesired aggression in military working dogs. *Applied Animal Behaviour Science* 117 (1–2), 55–62.

Hearne, V. (1982) *Adam's task: calling animals by name*. New York, Vintage books.

Herron, M.E., Shofer, F.S. & Reisner, I.R. (2009) Survey of the use and outcome of confrontational and non-confrontational training methods in client-owned dogs showing undesired behaviors. *Applied Animal Behaviour Science* 117, 47–54.

Hiby, E.F., Rooney, N.J. & Bradshaw, J.W.S. (2004) Dog training methods: their use, effectiveness and interaction with behaviour and welfare. *Animal Welfare* 13, 63–69.

Hsu, Y. & Serpell, J. (2003) Development and validation of a questionnaire for measuring behavior and temperament traits in pet dogs. *Journal of the American Veterinary Medical Association* 223 (9), 1293–1300.

Jagoe, A. & Serpell, J. (1996) Owner characteristics and interactions and the prevalence of canine behaviour problems. *Applied Animal Behaviour Science* 47, 31–42.

King, J.N., Simpson, B.S., Overall, K.L., Appleby, D., Pageat, P., Ross, C., Chaurand, J.P., Heath, S., Beata, C., Weiss, A.B., Muller, G., Paris, T., Bataille, B.G., Parker, J., Petit, S., Wren, J. & The CLOCSA (Clomipramine in Canine Separation Anxiety) Study Group (2000) Treatment of separation anxiety in dogs with clomipramine: double-blind, placebo-controlled, parallel-group, multicenter clinical trial. *Applied Animal Behaviour Science* 67 (4), 255–275.

Kobelt, A.J., Hemsworth, P.H., Barnett, J.L. & Coleman, G.J. (2003) A survey of dog ownership in suburban Australia: conditions and behaviour problems. *Applied Animal Behaviour Science* 82, 137–148.

Koehler, W. (1962) *The Koehler method of dog training*. New York: Howell Book House.

Luescher, A. (2004) Diagnosis and management of compulsive disorders in dogs and cats. *Clinical Techniques in Small Animal Practice* 19 (4), 233–239.

Mech, D. (1999) Alpha status, dominance, and division of labor in wolf packs. *Canadian Journal of Zoology* 77, 1196–1203.

Mikkelsen, J. & Lund, J.D. (2000) Euthanasia of dogs due to behavioural problems: an epidemiological study of euthanasia of dogs in Denmark, with a special focus on problems of aggression. *European Journal of Companion Animal Practice* 10, 143–150.

Most, K. (1954) *Training dogs: a manual*. London, Popular Dogs Publishing Co. Ltd.; reprinted 2001 by Dogwise Publishing (Wenatchee, WA).

Neilson, J.C. (2003) Feline house soiling: elimination and marking behaviors. *The Veterinary Clinics of North America, Small Animal Practice* 33 (2), 287–301.

Newby, J. (1999) *The animal attraction: humans and their animal companions.* Sydney, ABC Books.

Ott, S.A., Schalke, E., von Gaertner, A.M. & Hackbarth, H. (2008) Is there a difference? Comparison of golden retrievers and dogs affected by breed-specific legislation regarding aggressive behavior. *Journal of Veterinary Behavior: Clinical Applications and Research* 3(3), 34–140.

Patronek, G.J., Lawrence, T., Glickman, L.T., Beck, A.M., McCabe, G.P. & Ecker, C. (1996) Risk factors for relinquishment of dogs to an animal shelter. *Journal of the American Veterinary Medical Association* 209, 572–581.

Pryor, K. (1984) *Don't shoot the dog!: the new art of teaching and training.* New York & Toronto, Bantam Books.

Ragatz, L., Fremouw, W., Thomas, T. & McCoy, K. (2009) Vicious dogs: the antisocial behaviours and psychological characteristics of owners. *Journal of Forensic Sciences* 54, 699–703.

Reisner, I.R., Shofer, F.S. & Nance, M.L. (2007) Behavioral assessment of child-directed canine aggression. *Injury Prevention* 13, 348–351.

Rooney, N.J. & Cowan, S. (2011) Training methods and owner-dog interactions: links with dog behaviour and learning ability. *Applied Animal Behaviour Science* 132, 169–177.

Rosado, B., Garcia-Belenguer, S., Leon, M. & Palacio, J. (2009) A comprehensive study of dog bites in Spain, 1995-2004. *The Veterinary Journal* 179, 383–391.

Schalke, E., Stichnoth, J., Ott, S. & Jones-Baade, R. (2007) Clinical signs caused by the use of electric training collars on dogs in everyday life situations. *Applied Animal Behaviour Science* 105, 369–380.

Schilder, M.B.H. & van der Borg, J.A.M. (2004) Training dogs with the help of the schock collar: short and long term behavioural effects. *Applied Animal Behaviour Science* 85, 319–334.

Schilder, M.B.H., Vinke, C.M. & van der Borg, J.A.M. (2014) Dominance in domestic dogs revisited: Useful habit and useful construct? *Journal of Veterinary Behavior: Clinical Applications and Research* 9 (4), 184–191.

Seksel, K. & Lindeman, M.J. (2008) Use of clomipramine in the treatment of anxiety-related and obsessive-compulsive disorders in cats. *Australian Veterinary Journal* 76 (5), 317–321.

Stilwell, V. (n.d.) *What is positive training?* Positively®. [Online] Available from: http://positively.com/dog-training/positive-training/what-is-positive-training/ [Accessed 19 August 2014].

Todd, W.L., Pantenburg, D.P. & Crawford, P.M. (2008) Impact of the owner-pet and client-veterinarian bond on the care that pets receive. *Journal of the American Veterinary Medical Association* 232, 531–540.

Trisko, R. (2011) *Dominance, egalitarianism and friendship at a dog daycare facility.* A dissertation submitted in partial fulfillment of the requirements for the degree of Doctor of Philosophy (Psychology) in the University of Michigan.

van Kerkhove, W. (2004) A fresh look at the wolf-pack theory of companion-animal dog social behavior. *Journal of Applied Animal Welfare Science* 7(4), 279–285.

Weiss, H., Friedman, D. & Coben, J. (1998) Incidence of dog bite injuries treated in emergency departments. *The Journal of the American Medical Association* 279 (1), 51–53.

Zimen, E. (1975) Social dynamics of the wolf pack. In: Fox, M.W. (ed.) *The wild canids, their systematics, behavioral ecology and evolution.* New York, Cincinnati, OH, Toronto, London & Melbourne, Van Nostrand Reinhold Company, pp. 336–362.

Routine Neutering of Companion Animals

10

10.1 Introduction   150

10.2 Chemical Sterilisation   152

10.3 Surgical Neutering and Its Impacts on Animal Welfare   152

    10.3.1 The question of whether to neuter in light of potential effects on health-related welfare   153

    10.3.2 The question of when to neuter   156

    10.3.3 Conclusions (based on medical evidence)   157

10.4 Neutering and Positive Welfare   158

10.5 Neutering and Ethical Theories   158

    10.5.1 Utilitarian approaches   158

    10.5.2 Deontological and rights approaches   161

    10.5.3 Contextual approaches   163

10.1 Introduction

The American Veterinary Medical Association (AVMA), among others, strongly encourages owners of dogs and cats to have their companion neutered.

Companion Animal Ethics, First Edition. Peter Sandøe, Sandra Corr and Clare Palmer.
© Universities Federation for Animal Welfare 2016.

By having your dog or cat sterilized, you will do your part to prevent the birth of unwanted puppies and kittens. Spaying and neutering prevent unwanted litters and may reduce many of the behavioral problems associated with the mating instinct … Early spaying of female dogs and cats can help protect them from some serious health problems later in life such as uterine infections and breast cancer. Neutering your male pet can also lessen its risk of developing benign prostatic hyperplasia (enlarged prostate gland) and testicular cancer … Most pets tend to be better behaved following surgical removal of their ovaries or testes, making them more desirable companions.

(AVMA, n.d.)

However, not all vets take this view. Across continental Europe, vets have traditionally been more reluctant to neuter companion animals, especially dogs. (We will use 'neuter' to refer to sterilisation of both sexes.) In Sweden, for example, it was illegal to castrate a male dog until 1988, unless there was a specific medical reason for doing so. The official view of Swedish vets is still much more restrictive than that of the AMVA. The section of the Swedish Veterinary Association dealing with companion animals issued a statement (SVS, 2011) in which routine surgical neutering of dogs is rejected as sound policy. However, the idea of routine neutering of companion animals seems to be spreading. (By *routine* neutering, we mean neutering of healthy animals becoming the norm or 'default setting'.)

Neutering may be of ethical significance in several ways. It plays an important role in discussions about unwanted and unowned cat and dog populations, which raises ethical issues; we will explore these issues about populations in Chapter 13, and put them on one side here. In this chapter, we are interested in a narrower set of concerns: the routine neutering of companion animals kept indoors and not permitted to roam, or always kept under restraint when outdoors – that is, animals living in situations where it is impossible, or extremely unlikely, that mating will occur. This applies to cats kept wholly indoors, and to many dogs living in urban or suburban environments in Western industrialised countries.

Neutering is not the only form of reproductive control in companion animals, although it is by far the most popular. So we will begin this chapter with a brief discussion of other forms of reproductive control, and why they are not widely used. Then we will move on to the substance of the chapter: surgical neutering. We will consider the short- and long-term impacts of neutering in terms of animals' welfare, and the relations between humans and their animal companions. Then we will explore broader ethical issues that neutering may raise from different ethical perspectives, including the ideas that neutering may deprive animals of certain aspects of positive welfare, that it may infringe on their rights, and that it might be either an expression of care, or alternatively of domination, within a human–animal relationship.

10.2 Chemical Sterilisation

While surgical neutering is by far the most popular form of reproductive control in companion animals, temporary/reversible control of reproduction and behaviours related to reproduction ('chemical sterilisation') is also possible for cats and dogs of both sexes, and can be achieved pharmacologically, using hormonal products. Many hormonal products cause similar side effects to those seen following neutering, for example, increased body weight, hair coat changes, or predisposition to diabetes mellitus (see below); but most side effects resolve when the treatment is stopped. Some hormonal products have additional side effects, for example, progestogens may predispose bitches to pyometra (a uterine infection) and oestrogens may cause dose-related bone marrow suppression, which can result in a severe and possibly fatal blood disorders, although side effects are less common with more modern preparations (Romagnoli & Sontas, 2010).

Although chemical sterilisation is sometimes used as a temporary measure in breeding animals, or to test whether loss of hormones would alter unwanted behaviour (particularly in male dogs) prior to surgical neutering, it is not routinely used for long-term reproductive control of companion animals. This may be due to concerns about potential adverse effects with prolonged or repeated use of hormonal products, but equally, there are concerns about convenience and confidence. Neutering is a one-off procedure guaranteed to permanently prevent reproduction and associated behaviours. Chemical sterilisation is temporary, and to remain effective, may require daily administration of oral tablets, or repeated injections (although implants lasting 6–12 months are available, and vaccines are being developed). Chemical sterilisation, as a means of reproductive control, therefore involves some inconvenience to the owner, and in some cases stress to the animal of repeated visits to the vet, and these 'costs' – as well as economic ones – over the lifetime of the animal may therefore compare unfavourably with neutering. Since neutering is far more common than chemical sterilisation, we will, in the rest of this chapter, focus on neutering as the principal means of controlling reproduction in companion animals.

10.3 Surgical Neutering and Its Impacts on Animal Welfare

Neutering involves removal of the animal's reproductive organs, and is, therefore, permanent. Cats can become pregnant from 4 months onwards, although most reach puberty between 8 and 10 months (Joyce & Yates, 2011). Puberty in dogs is more variable, from 6 months onwards in smaller breeds, but often much later in large breeds. Routine neutering has traditionally been performed at around 6 months in cats and bitches, with male dogs castrated a few months later. However in some parts of the world, notably the United States, it has recently become common to neuter much earlier (6–16 weeks); we consider special questions raised by early neutering in Section 10.3.2.

Welfare impacts of neutering include the direct effects of the surgery itself, which involves an animal being left in unfamiliar surroundings with strangers, undergoing general anaesthesia and surgical trauma, and enduring some degree of pain; the risk of negative short-term side effects (e.g. inflammation at the site of the incision), and longer term costs and benefits, relating to incidence of disease, suffering, and length of life. However, research suggests that these impacts vary depending on the sex and species of the neutered animal. So, we will consider welfare within four categories here: female dogs (bitches), male dogs, female cats (queens) and male cats (toms).

10.3.1 The question of whether to neuter in light of potential effects on health-related welfare

10.3.1.1 Female dogs

Neutering female animals involves removal of the ovaries; in bitches, it is normal also to remove the uterus. Studies have shown, however, that there are no clear advantages from removing the uterus too; and just removing the ovaries is a more straightforward and less invasive surgery (Van Goethem *et al.*, 2006). So, there seems in most cases to be a welfare justification here for changing the *normal method* of neutering bitches (in addition, laparoscopic – or 'keyhole' – procedures are becoming increasingly available). But what about the health and welfare issues raised by neutering itself, independent of the method?

Neutering bitches prevents complications from pregnancy and potential diseases in the ovaries and uterus, such as developing the uterine infection, pyometra, which occurs in 15.2% of entire bitches by 4 years of age (Fukuda, 2001), and thereafter becomes increasingly common. It also significantly reduces the risk of mammary tumours, the most common tumour of female dogs, of which 50% are malignant (Robbins, 2003). Reducing the risk of mammary tumours is frequently quoted as a major reason for early neutering; neutering before the first season reportedly reduces the risk of developing mammary tumours to less than 0.5% (Schneider, Dorn & Taylor, 1969). However, a recent systematic review of the evidence by Beauvais, Cardwell & Brodbelt (2013) concluded that due to limited evidence and potential bias in studies, the evidence that neutering reduces the risk of mammary tumours is weak and not a sound basis for firm recommendations. Nonetheless, it is widely accepted that neutered bitches on average live longer than intact ones, perhaps because of the decreased incidence of reproductive disease.

There are, though, also negative impacts of neutering: complication rates of up to 20.6% have been reported (Burrow, Batchelor & Cripps, 2005), and occasionally, bitches die from peri-operative bleeding. One of the main complications is the development of urinary incontinence, particularly in large breeds: neutering increases the risk 7.8-fold (Thrusfield, Holt & Muirhead, 1998). In most cases, the incontinence is treatable, although half of the bitches may require surgery. Furthermore, as we saw in Chapter 8, neutering increases the risk of obesity. There are also impacts that may make neutered bitches more difficult to live with: some studies suggest that neutered bitches are more aggressive than entire bitches, though the reasons for this are unclear.

Two recent studies, concerning both male and female dogs, investigated the risk of neutered dogs of specific breeds developing hip dysplasia (HD) or cranial cruciate ligament disease (CCL), or three kinds of cancer – lymphosarcoma (LSA), hemangiosarcoma (HSA), and mast cell tumour (MCT) – compared to entire animals. In the first, Torres de la Riva *et al.* (2013) found that the incidence of all five diseases increased in Golden Retrievers of both sexes – to some extent depending on whether neutering was performed 'early' (before 1 year of age) or 'late' (after 1 year of age). Late neutered bitches had four times the incidence of HSA (8%) of intact and early neutered females, and 6% had MCT, compared to none in intact females.

In a follow-up paper, Hart *et al.* (2014) compared the effects of neutering Golden Retrievers and Labrador Retrievers on the occurrence of three joint disorders (HD, CCL and elbow dysplasia) and four types of cancers (LSA, HSA, MCT and mammary cancer). The study found that breeds respond very differently to the effects of neutering. The incidence of joint disease in intact males and females of both breeds is around 5%, but this was nearly doubled in Labrador Retrievers, and increased four- to fivefold in Golden Retrievers, neutered before 6 months of age. The occurrence of one or more cancers in intact dogs ranged from 3% to 5%, except in Golden Retriever males where incidence was 11%. While neutering Labrador Retrievers of either sex at any stage had little effect on increasing cancers, and the same was found for male Golden Retrievers (except for LSA which increased significantly if they were neutered before 6 months old), neutering a female Golden Retriever at any period beyond 6 months increased the risk of one or more cancers to three to four times that of intact females.

Despite these findings, on balance, in welfare terms, it appears that the long-term health related welfare of bitches – that is, with respect to longevity and risk of suffering from disease in later life – is likely to be improved, or at least not reduced, by neutering.

10.3.1.2 Male dogs

Male dogs are typically castrated by surgical removal of the testicles. This surgery itself rarely causes immediate complications. However, unlike the case of female dogs, overall there are probably increased risks of significant negative long-term consequences for health-related welfare. Castration of male dogs removes the risk of testicular disease (e.g. testicular cancer), and reduces the risk of androgen-dependent diseases such as perineal hernias. However, as well as increasing the risk of obesity, neutering also significantly increases the risk of prostate and bladder cancer: although prostate cancer is rare in male dogs (0.2–0.6% incidence), it is almost always malignant (Bryan *et al.*, 2007). Castration also slightly increases the risk of other cancers such as bone and cardiac cancer; for example, osteosarcoma (OSA), a highly aggressive bone tumour, occurs twice as frequently in neutered dogs compared to intact dogs (Ru, Terracini & Glickman, 1998). Breed also appears to be significant: Rottweilers neutered before 1 year of age have a 1 in 4 lifetime risk of developing OSA, which is significantly higher than entire dogs (Cooley *et al.*, 2002). A similar increase in certain serious diseases in neutered males of specific breeds was found by Torres de la Riva *et al.* (2013) and Hart *et al.* (2014) (see previous section). Torres de la Riva *et al.* (2013) also found that 'early' neutered male Golden Retrievers had double (10%) the incidence of HSA of intact males, and 10% had LSA (three times the number seen in intact males).

Sometimes, male dogs are castrated to limit aggression and other behavioural problems (which can cause injury to the dogs themselves, as well as being problematic for their owners; see Chapter 9). However, the effect of neutering on male dog behaviour seems to be variable. One study suggests that neutered male dogs over 1 year old were most likely to have bitten someone (Guy *et al.*, 2001) – though the biting behaviour may have been the reason these dogs were neutered, and not all studies support this finding. Neutering does seem to reduce roaming and urine marking in male dogs, and there is some evidence that neutering males of certain breeds makes them more trainable (e.g. Rottweilers and Shetland Sheepdogs) (Serpell & Hsu, 2005).

Bringing all these findings together, with respect to the animals' own welfare, the costs of routinely neutering male dogs, in terms of the increased risk of very serious diseases, probably outweigh the benefits. So, justification for routine neutering of confined male dogs, then, does not seem to follow from claims about the dogs' own welfare.

10.3.1.3 Female cats

Female cats, like female dogs, are usually neutered by removing the uterus and the ovaries, and the surgery itself can cause complications (Figure 10.1). However, there are longer-term benefits to the surgery. Health risks from pregnancy are avoided (and since confined cats may escape, this is a more significant possibility than with bitches).

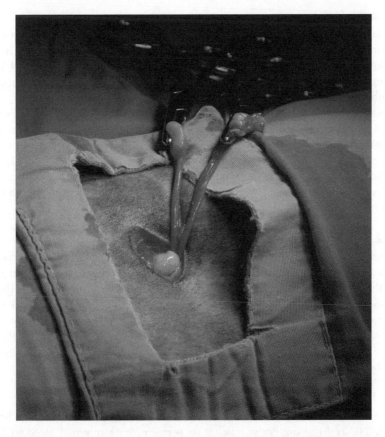

Figure 10.1 Cat spay. The procedure is often performed through a small flank incision, and both the ovaries and uterine horns are exteriorised and removed. (*Image used courtesy of Sandra Corr.*)

Neutering female cats significantly reduces the risk of mammary tumours, which in cats have an 80–90% chance of being malignant, although they occur at a much lower frequency than in bitches. Neutering before 6 months results in a 91% reduction in the risk of developing mammary carcinomas (Overley *et al.*, 2005), and prevents other mammary diseases. Neutered female cats do not have more urinary tract problems, and appear to show less aggression than intact female cats (Finkler & Terkel, 2010). The main health-related welfare problem for neutered cats (of both sexes) is a substantially increased risk of obesity, which can lead to diabetes and other problems (see more about this in Chapter 8). Neutered cats of both sexes are significantly more likely to become obese than entire cats (Nguyen *et al.*, 2004) and are at significantly greater risk of becoming diabetic (Panciera *et al.*, 1990).

On balance, then, there are some welfare benefits to female cats from being neutered, although in terms of avoiding serious disease, these seem weaker than the welfare reasons to neuter bitches. The welfare costs, at least in terms of obesity, are to some degree avoidable. So, on this basis at least, neutering looks as though it will improve, or at least not reduce, welfare.

10.3.1.4 Male cats

In male cats (toms), as in male dogs, castration is the only practiced form of surgical neutering. Unlike in dogs, both testicular and prostate disease are very rare in toms (Reichler, 2009), so neutering has little positive *or* negative direct impact on these aspects of welfare. The main welfare issue for the tomcat itself is, as with female cats, a significantly increased risk of obesity and of diseases that follow obesity, such as diabetes.

Tomcats are frequently neutered, however, to make them easier to live with – in particular to reduce urine spraying, aggression and roaming. Castration does seem effective in eliminating or significantly reducing urine spraying, and somewhat effective in reducing aggression and risky behaviour. So, neutering may reduce the likelihood of tomcats experiencing negative welfare impacts (by reducing risks from fighting and roaming), and it could indirectly benefit welfare, through creating better relations with owners than entire male cats could have; we will consider this further below.

10.3.2 The question of when to neuter

Many associations, such as the AVMA and Association of Shelter Veterinarians, are increasingly recommending early neutering (pre-pubertal gonadectomy) primarily to reduce the unwanted pet population. In this context, 'early' typically means between 6 and 16 weeks of age (Kustritz, 2002; Looney *et al.*, 2008) not just under 1 year, as in the studies reported in the previous section. Early neutering has been slow to gain widespread acceptance amongst European vets however, due to concerns over the safety of general anaesthesia and surgery in young animals, and the effects of removing reproductive hormones before sexual maturity. But what does the evidence show?

10.3.2.1 Peri-operative concerns

No increased anaesthetic risks have been associated with early neutering, (Brodbelt *et al.*, 2008), and the surgery is quicker to perform, with minimal bleeding (Howe, 1997; Kustritz, 2002) and fewer post-operative complications (Aronsohn & Faggella, 1993; Howe, 1997).

10.3.2.2 Long-term effects

Studies comparing early neutering to traditional neutering have produced conflicting results. Some studies have failed to identify differences in potential long-term effects, either generally (Kustritz, 2002), associated with the occurrence of hip dysplasia, urinary incontinence or vaginitis in puppies (Howe *et al.*, 2001), obstructive urinary tract disease (Howe *et al.*, 2000), or urethral diameter (Root *et al.*, 1996; Stubbs *et al.*, 1996) in male cats, or obesity levels (Howe *et al.*, 2000; Root, 1995; Stubbs *et al.*, 1996). However, other studies have found effects: Thrusfield, Holt & Muirhead (1998) and Spain, Scarlett and Houpt (2004b) reported an increased risk of urinary incontinence in dogs and cats neutered at a younger age, as well as an increased risk of hip dysplasia in dogs. Spain *et al.* (2004a) also found that early neutering was associated with a lower incidence of asthma, gingivitis and hyperactivity in both sexes, and a significantly lower incidence of abscesses, sexual behaviours, urine spraying and aggression towards vets in male kittens. As discussed earlier, increased rates of certain diseases were reported by Torres de la Riva *et al.* (2013), who consequently recommend delaying neutering of Golden Retriever males to well beyond puberty; advice on females is more problematic, as early neutering significantly increased the incidence rate of CCL rupture (from near 0% to almost 8%), but late neutering increased the rates of certain tumours.

The effect of early neutering on behaviour is not clear. Dunbar (1975) and Leiberman (1987) reported that early neutered puppies were at least three times less likely to show behaviour problems. However, Spain, Scarlett & Houpt (2004b) reported in both male and female dogs, early neutering was associated with increased incidence of sexual behaviours and noise phobias, but a decreased risk of separation anxiety, escaping behaviours, and consequent relinquishment. Early neutering of kittens is reported to increase their shyness and tendency to hide (Spain, Scarlett & Houpt, 2004a).

A final area of controversy is the effect of early neutering on skeletal growth (growth plate closure): some studies report no difference (Root, Johnston & Olson, 1997; Stubbs *et al.*, 1996), others delayed closure (Salmeri *et al.*, 1991), but none have identified a clinical problem as a result.

10.3.3 Conclusions (based on medical evidence)

Current best evidence suggests that bitches may benefit from neutering, while the evidence weighs against routine neutering of male dogs. The case of cats is less clear either way; there are no significant welfare benefits or costs to neutering, but it may improve welfare inasmuch as it makes the animals into better companions and therefore leads to more satisfactory relationships with owners. In general, the evidence suggests that neutered animals have a longer life span than intact animals, perhaps due to a combination of less risky behaviour, fewer reproductive diseases and possibly the increased level of care given by owners who neuter their animals (Kustritz, 2007).

Early neutering appears to be a quick and safe procedure with no increase in short-term complications compared to traditional age neutering; evidence for a significant difference in long-term complication rates and effects on long-term health is currently uncertain; so, at the moment, there is no clear health-related welfare grounds for a recommendation.

However, so far, we have only really considered the potential for neutering to avoid or generate *negative* welfare, in particular in terms of disease and suffering. We have not discussed whether animals might lose some *positive* welfare when they are neutered – and whether this matters.

10.4 Neutering and Positive Welfare

Neutering an animal removes a number of possibilities from its life: the possibility of sexual behaviours including (in males) roaming, fighting, seeking mates and mating; in females, mating, pregnancy and tending to offspring. What carrying out these behaviours means to cats and dogs and whether the animals in some sense may, in their absence, miss them, we have little idea. However, these behaviours do seem relevant to welfare, on some interpretations of welfare at least.

Suppose we adopt a hedonist idea of welfare (see Chapter 4), one that focuses on positive and negative experiences. It is likely that male cats and dogs gain some pleasurable experiences from mating, and that it is certainly possible that female cats and dogs gain pleasurable experience from tending to their offspring. On this view, neutering may deprive animals of positive experiences they might otherwise have had (even if they do not miss them), and this might matter ethically, as we will suggest below.

There seems to be less ambiguity concerning what to think about neutering from a preference-oriented view of welfare. Neutering changes what animals prefer; a male cat no longer desires to roam and mate, for instance, so neutering avoids preference frustration. However, in Chapter 4, we considered the possibility of hypothetical preferences. If a cat were to understand what neutering entailed, it is at least possible that he or she would prefer not to undergo it because of the loss of future positive experiences or desire–satisfactions it would entail. So, we cannot be quite sure what to conclude from a preference-oriented view. If welfare is understood as concerning the fulfilment of cats' natures or what counts as flourishing for a cat, it is also not at all clear what to think about neutering. It might be argued that engaging in reproductive behaviours and producing offspring is part of what is good for a cat. On this view, there is something ethically problematic about neutering cats; they are being prevented from fulfilling their natures. On the other hand, one might argue that neutering actually *changes* cats' natures. On this view, reproductive behaviours would no longer be part of the *nature* of an animal that lacks the ability or desire to engage in them.

Neutering, then, raises a number of difficult questions about animal welfare. To explore these issues further, we will consider how such concerns about neutering relate to the different ethical theories we outlined in Chapter 5.

10.5 Neutering and Ethical Theories

10.5.1 Utilitarian approaches

On a utilitarian approach to ethics, only the consequences of our actions/practices – here, neutering – matter directly. The aim is to maximise what is good and minimise what is bad. We will take *maximum net positive welfare* as what is optimal, though this will have different forms, depending on what welfare is understood to be.

Let us start by thinking about neutering in a utilitarian context with a *hedonist view* of welfare. First, surgery likely causes negative experiences such as pain and stress, though these are unlikely to be long lasting or serious provided that anaesthesia and painkillers are used. But if maximising net positive welfare is the goal, then positive experiences or the prevention of other negative experiences would have to arise from the surgery to outweigh the certain negative experiences it causes (though these positive experiences need not be to the neutered animal itself).

As we have seen, in the case of bitches, this does seem to be the case: the expected benefit from gaining extra life in better health is likely sufficient to outweigh the certain negative experiences associated with neutering now. This is not the case for male dogs; in fact, since neutering actually increases health risks for male dogs, the likelihood of suffering later adds to the negative experiences of surgery now.

For cats of either sex that are kept indoors, it is debatable how pleasure and pain add up, as we have noted. But if neutering makes cats easier to live with, and less likely to express 'inappropriate' behaviour, then their owners' and their own experiential welfare is likely to improve. This may be generally true where neutered animals make better companions – although neutered bitches may not make better companions, if their aggression increases and they suffer from urinary incontinence. Of course, a utilitarian might argue that an even better outcome is possible: where humans treat their entire companions well *despite* any 'inappropriate' behaviour, and the animals remain entire. But this is an unlikely expected consequence, particularly when it comes to male cats.

There are other, additional, factors to consider here, in particular the loss of neutered animals' *positive* welfare because the animals cannot undergo sexual and reproductive experiences that may (for instance) be positively stimulating and exciting. The concern here is not that neutered animals have *negative* experiences of frustration or longing (since it is very implausible that neutered animals could feel these in relation to their missing sexual opportunities) but rather that they do not have relevant positive experiences, even if they do not know what they are missing, or indeed that they are missing anything. If there is less positive experience in the world, on this view, the world is, overall, less good.

But we could counter this worry by considering what the alternatives actually are for most companion animals. After all, *not* neutering an animal raises similar concerns, if the animal is not allowed to mate or breed. In fact, the concerns here will be stronger, if the animal additionally actually has feelings of frustration. So, an unneutered tom may undergo negative experiences if consistently prevented from accessing female cats; if a bitch on heat is kept indoors and not walked while she is in heat, then even if she has no sexual desires, she has negative experiences from having to miss her walks. If animals are not to be allowed to breed, nor to behave sexually, then leaving them entire may mean not only that they do not have *pleasurable* experiences, but that they actually have *frustrating* ones. From a utilitarian point of view, a frustrated entire animal is worse off than an unfrustrated, neutered one.

In contrast, a utilitarian view that takes welfare to concern satisfaction and frustration of animals' preferences – in brief, about animals getting what they want – would understand neutering rather differently. As noted earlier, a question is raised here about hypothetical preferences – whether, if an animal knew what neutering meant, he or she would prefer not to undergo it (we know, of course, that most humans who do understand what neutering means prefer otherwise!). However, we will leave this complex issue on one side, and focus here instead on the *actual* preferences animals are likely to have. During the stressful period surrounding surgery, it is reasonable to say that animals would prefer not to be in the negative states of fear, pain, or discomfort that may ensue. But beyond this, neutering does not seem to involve frustrated actual preferences. Animals do not prefer not to be neutered (since animals cannot comprehend what this could mean); nor does a neutered animal have frustrated sexual preferences. Nor do such animals have second-order preferences to *have* such preferences (as one might imagine in the case of a human being who had been castrated at a young age, longing to have, or to understand, sexual or parental feelings). On this view, then, the only relevant animal preferences are those involving the surgery, and any subsequent preference not to undergo the pain from diseases related the neutering (which is primarily relevant to male dogs). So – if we leave aside hypothetical animal preferences – if a human prefers an animal to be neutered, the only relevant animal preferences/frustrations concern the surgery, the neutering has the effect of directly causing human satisfaction, and the animal indirectly has more preferences fulfilled by having a better-disposed companion human, then routine neutering looks ethically unproblematic or desirable, with the possible exception of male dogs.

On a third view of welfare, where welfare is based around animals' flourishing in accordance with their *natures* – perfectionism – it is rather unclear what we should think about neutering, as noted earlier. What constitutes a 'good life' for an animal is contested (as it is for human beings). It is at least plausible to argue that the expression of sexual behaviour and/or producing offspring is part of what it is to flourish for a cat or a dog, even if the animal itself does not miss such experiences when neutered. But an alternative view is also plausible: that whatever makes for an excellent cat or dog life, given the kinds of beings that they are, it need not include sexual activity or reproduction. It might also be argued that neutering *changes* an animal's nature, so that what it is to flourish for a neutered animal differs from what it is to flourish for an unneutered animal. But the plausibility of the view that sexual activity and reproduction means that animals flourish according to their natures should at least give pause for thought. Routine neutering, on this view, denies animals the possibility of living the best lives possible for them (even if the animals themselves are unaware of this) and thereby reduces the amount of flourishing in the world.

There's one other, rather different, issue worth noting here in the context of utilitarianism: the long-term potential consequences of routinely neutering young animals. Take dogs as an example. Though modern dogs represent an extraordinary variability in phenotypic traits, the majority of the breeds emerged from a limited gene pool, and breeding practices have led to the loss of genetic diversity (see Chapter 7). Yet for populations to maintain good health, and certain useful functions, they need genetic diversity, which requires adequate population sizes and breeding from dogs with diverse genetic material. Routine neutering, especially of very young animals, makes this difficult; by the time it is discovered that an animal has particularly useful genetic traits (e.g. in terms of disease resistance), it has been neutered, and so cannot be bred from. Interestingly, here the welfare of particular individual dogs may be in tension with the welfare of dog populations. As we have seen, in terms of welfare related to an individual's health, bitches are better off neutered before they are able to reproduce, since this reduces their chance of disease. But from the perspective of genetic diversity, there are reasons to wait in order to leave breeding options open. A more diverse genetic population matters on some forms of utilitarianism. It is likely to make for a healthier population (which is likely to improve dogs' experiences over time).

In summary, then: from a utilitarian view on which satisfied preferences are what matters, neutering looks relatively untroubling, unless we are concerned about hypothetical preferences. However, where mental states are concerned, *routine* neutering is problematic, although neutering will be permissible, or even required, in many cases. It is unclear what we should think ethically on a view where welfare is understood as flourishing according to one's nature; at the least, on this view, routine neutering raises an ethical question.

10.5.2 Deontological and rights approaches

Suppose we thought that animals have some basic rights, such as the right not to be killed. Would neutering infringe on an animal's rights? What rights could be at stake? Possible candidate rights would be a right to reproduce (it is sometimes argued that humans have this right); a right not to be harmed; and a right to bodily integrity. Let us consider these in turn.

There is some dispute about whether even people have a 'right to reproduce' – or, indeed, what this right amounts to. Where rights to reproduction are claimed (e.g. UN, 1994), they are usually understood as rights to *autonomy* in reproductive matters – rights to be able to decide whether to have children, when to have them, and how far apart to space them. These kinds of autonomy rights to reproduction could not apply in the animal case, since animals are obviously not able to make these kinds of reflective decisions. *Coercive sterilisation* has, though, historically, been viewed as an infringement of human rights to reproduction. It is possible that neutering could be conceived of as a rights violation in this way, although non-coercive sterilisation is not possible in an animal's case.

Francione (2007) – one of the most vehement defenders of animal rights – explicitly denies that domesticated animals have a right not to be coercively sterilised. This flows from his argument that animal domestication, including companion animal domestication, is wrong, creating dependent and servile animals to be 'truly animal slaves' (Francione, 2007). On this view, allowing domesticated animals to breed is to perpetuate a cycle of vulnerability and dependence; neutering stops the cycle.

There is something problematic in this argument, though, even if one accepts Francione's premises. His argument seems to be that individuals born into an institution (the institution of being a companion animal) that on his view ethically should not exist, do not have the same rights as similar individuals born outside this institution. So, while Francione would probably find it wrong coercively to sterilise *wild* animals, according to his view, this would not apply to domesticated companion animals. This attaches the rights animals have partly to their contexts rather than their capacities. Such a view may be defensible; it would require an argument that the right not to be coercively sterilised is not a universal right, or that there are some circumstances in which infringing on this right can be justified (see Donaldson & Kymlicka, 2012 for a discussion of this).

Neutering, however, may fall under a more general right: a right not to be harmed, or a right to respectful treatment. That animals have the latter right is defended by Regan (1984), though not in the context of neutering; Boonin (2003) however, does apply this right to neutering. Boonin argues that neutering an animal imposes non-trivial harms on it. Neutering is not (usually) carried out for the benefit of the particular animal being neutered, unlike, say, surgery to remove a tumour. In the tumour case, we might say either that the animal would voluntarily relinquish its rights, were it to be able to understand what was happening, or that surgery to cure an animal is not harmful or disrespectful in the first place. But most neutering is justified by reference to benefit for the owners or to improve population welfare levels (though this may not apply to neutering bitches, who as we have seen are likely to benefit as individuals from being neutered). Rights theorists normally insist that an individual's rights may not be violated to benefit populations or other individuals. So, it looks as though, on this view, neutering would not be permissible unless it would clearly benefit the individual concerned.

However, Boonin (2003: p. 7) – who thinks that an animal rights view that cannot endorse companion animal neutering is indefensible – proposes an amendment to this kind of rights view. He argues that 'it's permissible to impose relatively minor harms on animals (and relevantly analogous humans) in at least some cases, where this produces great benefits for others, and that is not only consistent with the attribution of rights to animals, but is motivated by the same sorts of considerations that justify such attribution'. On this view, neutering is a relatively minor harm in comparison with avoiding the production of potentially miserable offspring. However, while this might be applicable to the cases we will consider in Chapter 13 – cats in trap-neuter-return programmes, for instance – this argument does not apply to the cases we are considering here, where companion animals are not free-ranging, and thus would not be producing miserable offspring anyway. So, given that this qualification does not seem to work here, this kind of rights argument raises very serious questions about the routine neutering of companion animals.

A third right that might be at stake is a right to bodily integrity – a right that it is sometimes argued that humans have, and that has played a significant role in recent debates in Germany about the practice of circumcision. Here it is argued, in the human case, that humans have a right not to be physically interfered with in ways that affect their bodily integrity, in particular by submitting to unchosen surgeries to alter parts of the body. (This claim may depend on a perfectionist idea of welfare.) This could translate in the animal case as follows: individual animals were born in particular ways, with specific bodily features: tails, ears, claws – and gonads. These features are all part of an animal's bodily integrity – part of what it is to be *that* physical individual. Surgically to remove or alter any of these parts is to infringe on this bodily integrity, and can be seen as a rights violation. (See Chapter 11 on other animal surgeries performed for non-medical reasons.)

In the human case, the right to bodily integrity can, presumably, be voluntarily relinquished where there are significant welfare benefits from doing so. Even though animals are not able to understand or to choose to relinquish rights voluntarily, it seems reasonable to say that if a dog has testicular cancer, for instance, it would be permissible to remove the testes, even though this would affect his bodily integrity. However, the welfare benefits from neutering are not in all cases so clear-cut that we could say that if *healthy* animals were able, they would choose voluntarily to relinquish their right to bodily integrity in order to allow routine neutering, as some women choose prophylactic mastectomies to prevent serious disease. Given the evidence we have reviewed, the 'prophylactic' argument seems only to be applicable to bitches.

Overall, then, *routine* neutering appears problematic on all of these rights arguments. Benefits to others do not usually justify rights infringements; so it is only in cases where neutering benefits the animals being neutered that we can make a more straightforward argument that rights could be waived. An amendment such as Boonin's might work for free-ranging animals, but does not obviously apply to animals that will not be allowed to reproduce anyway. So, arguments flowing from animal rights perspectives are very unlikely to support the practice of *routinely* neutering companion animals, at least.

10.5.3 Contextual approaches

A third group of theoretical approaches focuses on the contexts in which animals are located and the *relationships* between companion animals and their owners. Prominent among these approaches is the ethics of care (outlined in Chapter 5). Key features of this approach include the importance of responsive attention to others, the value of caring emotional bonds, and paying attention to a particular animal's specific needs and desires (Donovan & Adams, 2007; Gilligan, 1982).

How might neutering be regarded here? Could it be part of a caring relationship? This has not, to our knowledge, been explicitly discussed by ethicists of care; and there are different possible ways of thinking about it. One approach might be to see neutering as *enhancing* the relationship between humans and companion animals. Companion animals have been bred in ways that make them well-suited to live alongside humans, and ill-suited to other lives. What is best for them is to fit well into domestic households and to bond well with their owners. If neutering helps to develop a responsive, caring relationship which it plausibly does, then it seems to be ethically desirable. Still, given that an ethics of care focuses on knowing animals as particular individuals (see Chapter 5) general principles – such as are implied by *routine* neutering of companion animals might be questioned. On this view, each owner should ask themselves whether neutering their companion animal actually does fit into an emotionally attentive relationship that takes care of the needs, interests, and desires of the other. It is certainly possible to imagine situations where this question is answered positively – where, for instance, an animal companion is driving an owner to desperation through unmanageable behaviour that is undermining the caring relationship. But on the other hand, we can imagine a different story being told (even about a similar case). For companion animals are, almost always, ultimately vulnerable to their owners, and neutering can be seen as one (of many) ways that humans control 'badly behaved' animals. It has been suggested that neutering is a form of – or promotes – human *domination* over companion animals (Palmer, 2001); that its purpose is not so much to strengthen human–animal relationships, as to make animals more docile, less habitually offensive, or, more generally, into better companions for people. On this view, routinely neutering animals is a way of shaping them to fit better into human households, in a way they cannot resist. After all, this caring relationship (like many caring relationships) is not an equal one; companion animals are completely vulnerable to being neutered (Palmer, 2001). Seen like this, it is difficult to defend the idea that neutering could be part of a relationship that is supposed to be built on care, responsive attention, and taking account of the others' needs and desires. The language of companionship, it might be argued, serves to conceal the ways in which such animals are actually being coercively manipulated to meet human preferences.

Clearly, neutering can be seen in different ways from a contextual perspective of an ethics of care. It may be seen as a caring way of deepening a bond between animal and owner, or alternatively as a dominating, manipulative practice to be rejected. In fact, a thoroughgoing contextual approach is likely to see some instances of neutering as caring, and others as dominating, depending on the particular factors at stake in any particular case. But what does seem clear here is that neutering should not, at least, be *routine* from the perspective of a contextual approach, because there are likely to be ethically relevant relational factors present in one context that are absent from another.

These considerations suggest that the neutering of companion animals is a complex and largely unexplored ethical issue. What to think about it, ethically, depends partly on how animal welfare is understood, and on what approach to ethical theory is adopted. On any ethical view, though, the routine neutering of all companion animals, of both sexes, where uncontrolled reproduction is not an issue, looks ethically questionable. Nonetheless, on almost all views, there are many, or at least some, particular occasions where neutering of companion animals that will not otherwise reproduce, will be permissible or ethically required.

Key Points

- The claim that neutering should become routine is becoming increasingly popular, although different cultures have different attitudes towards the practice.
- The health and welfare effects of neutering vary by gender, breed, species, and the stage in an animal's life at which it is carried out.
- Evidence suggests that bitches may benefit from neutering, in terms of reducing their risk of serious diseases, but that the same is not true of male dogs, who are exposed to some increased long-term health risks from neutering.
- There is less evidence of impact either way on the health and welfare of cats from neutering. However, neutering cats, especially male cats, makes them better companions and therefore may indirectly improve welfare; in the case of cats, escape from confinement and accidental pregnancies may be more likely.
- In terms of positive welfare, neutering might deprive animals of the positive experiences associated with sexual and reproductive behaviour. Furthermore, sexual and reproductive behaviour might be part of a flourishing life for a cat or dog, irrespective of animals' experiences or desires.

- Where welfare is interpreted in terms of preferences, the question is raised whether animals might have a hypothetical preference not to be neutered. If this possibility is laid aside, from a preference-oriented perspective, neutering seems largely unproblematic; unneutered but frustrated animals might be better off if they are neutered.
- Where welfare is interpreted in terms of what promotes animals' natural flourishing, it is unclear what to think about routine neutering, since neutering may change their natures; but it is at least plausible that neutering is ethically problematic.
- On almost all accounts on which animals have rights, neutering is ethically problematic.
- On contextual accounts of ethics, in particular an ethics of care, it is unlikely that *routine* neutering would be permissible, since what to do depends on particular caring relationships. Neutering *may* strengthen the emotional bonds between companion animals and their owners but conversely, neutering *may* be a dominating practice.

References

Aronsohn, M.G. & Faggella, A.M. (1993) Surgical techniques for neutering 6- to 14-week-old kittens. *Journal of the American Veterinary Medical Association* 202 (1), 53–57.

AVMA (n.d.) *Spaying and neutering*. American Veterinary Medical Association. [Online] Available from: https://www.avma.org/public/PetCare/Pages/spay-neuter.aspx [Accessed 17 July 2014].

Beauvais, W., Cardwell, J.M. & Brodbelt, D.C. (2013) The effect of neutering on the risk of mammary tumours in dogs: a systematic review. *Journal of Small Animal Practice* 53, 314–322.

Boonin, D. (2003) Robbing PETA to spay Paul: do animal rights include reproductive rights? *Between the Species*, III, 1–8.

Brodbelt, D.C., Pfeiffer, D.U., Young, L.E. & Wood, J.L. (2008) Results of the confidential enquiry into perioperative small animal fatalities regarding risk factors for anesthetic-related death in dogs. *Journal of the American Veterinary Medical Association* 233 (7), 1096–1104.

Bryan, J.N., Keeler, M.R., Henry, C.J., Bryan, M.E., Hahn, A.W. & Caldwell, C.W. (2007) A population study of neutering status as a risk factor for canine prostate cancer. *The Prostate* 67 (11), 1174–1181.

Burrow, R., Batchelor, D. & Cripps, P. (2005) Complications observed during and after ovariohysterectomy of 142 bitches at a veterinary teaching hospital. *Veterinary Record* 157, 829–833.

Cooley, D.M., Beranek, B.C., Schlittler, D.L., Glickman, N.W., Glickman, L.T. & Waters, D.J. (2002) Endogenous gonadal hormone exposure and bone sarcoma risk. *Cancer Epidemiology, Biomarkers & Prevention* 11, 1434–1440.

Donaldson, S. & Kymlicka, W. 2012. *Zoopolis: towards a political theory of rights for animals*. Oxford: Oxford University Press.

Donovan, J. & Adams, C. (2007) *The feminist care tradition in animal ethics: a reader*. New York, Columbia University Press.

Dunbar, I.F. (1975) Behaviour of castrated animals. *Veterinary Record* 96, 92.

Finkler, H. & Terkel, J. (2010) Cortisol levels and aggression in neutered and intact free-roaming cats living in urban social groups. *Physiology and Behavior* 99, 343–347.

Francione, G. (2007) *Animal rights and domesticated nonhumans.* Blog entry 10 January 2007. [Online] Available from: http://www.abolitionistapproach.com/animal-rights-and -domesticated-nonhumans/#.UuaGJPZMF-U [Accessed: 16 July 2014].

Fukuda, S. (2001) Incidence of pyometra in colony-raised Beagle dogs. *Experimental Animals* 50, 325–329.

Gilligan, C. (1982) *In a different voice.* Cambridge, MA, Harvard University Press.

Guy, N.C., Luescher, U.A., Dohoo, S.E., Spangler, E., Miller, J.B., Dohoo, I.R. & Bate, L.A. (2001) Demographic and aggressive characteristics of dogs in a general veterinary caseload. *Applied Animal Behaviour Science* 74 (1), 15–28.

Hart, B.L., Hart, L.A., Thigpen, A.P. & Willits, N.H. (2014) Long-term health effects of neutering dogs: comparison of labrador retrievers with golden retrievers. *PLoS ONE* 9(7): e102241. doi:10.1371/journal.pone.0102241

Howe, L.M. (1997) Short term results and complications of prepubertal gonadectomy in cats and dogs. *Journal of the American Veterinary Medical Association* 211 (1), 57–62.

Howe, L.M., Slater, M.R., Boothe, H.W., Hobson, H.P., Fossum, T.W., Spann, A.C. & Wilkie, W.S. (2000) Long-term outcome of gonadectomy performed at an early age or traditional age in cats. *Journal of the American Veterinary Medical Association* 217 (11), 1661–1665.

Howe, L.M., Slater, M.R., Boothe, H.W., Hobson, H.P., Holcom, J.L. & Spann, A.C. (2001) Long-term outcome of gonadectomy performed at an early age or traditional age in dogs. *Journal of the American Veterinary Medical Association* 218 (2), 217–221.

Joyce, A. & Yates, D. (2011) Help stop teenage pregnancy! Early age neutering in cats. *Journal of Feline Medicine and Surgery* 13, 3–10.

Kustritz, M.V.R. (2002) Early spay–neuter: clinical considerations. *Clinical Techniques in Small Animal Practice* 17 (3), 124–128.

Kustritz, M.V.R. (2007) Determining the optimal age for gonadectomy of dogs and cats. *Journal of the American Veterinary Medical Association* 231 (11), 1665–1675.

Leiberman, L.L. (1987) A case for neutering pups and kittens at two months of age. *Journal of the American Veterinary Medical Association* 191 (5), 518.

Looney, A.L., Bohling, M.W., Bushby, P.A., Howe, L.M., Griffin, B., Levy, J.K., Eddlestone, S.M., Weedon, J.R., Appel, L.D., Rigdon-Brestle, Y.K., Ferguson, N.J., Sweeney, D.J., Tyson, K.A., Voors, A.H., White, S.C., Wilford, C.L., Farrell, K.A., Jefferson, E.P., Moyer, M.R., Newbury, S.P., Saxton, M.A. & Scarlett, J.M. (2008) The Association of Shelter Veterinarians veterinary medical care guidelines for spay-neuter programs. *Journal of the American Veterinary Medical Association* 233 (1), 74–86.

Nguyen, P. G., Dumon, H.J., Siliart, B.S., Martin, L.J., Sergheraert, R. & Biourge, V.C. (2004) Effects of dietary fat and energy on body weight and composition after gonadectomy in cats. *American Journal of Veterinary Research* 65 (12), 1708–1713.

Overley, B., Shofer, F.S., Goldschmidt, M.H., Sherer, D. & Sorenmo, K.U. (2005) Association between ovarihysterectomy and feline mammary carcinoma. *Journal of Veterinary Internal Medicine* 19 (4), 560–563.

Palmer, C. (2001) "Taming the wild profusion of existing things"? A study of Foucault, power and human/animal relationships. *Environmental Ethics* 23, 339–358.

Panciera, D.L., Thomas, C.B., Eicker, S.W. & Atkins, C.E. (1990) Epizootiologic patterns of diabetes mellitus in cats: 333 cases (1980-1986). *Journal of the American Veterinary Medical Association* 197 (11), 1504–1508.

Regan, T. (1984) *The case for animal rights.* Berkeley, CA, University of California Press.

Reichler, I.M. (2009) Gonadectomy in cats and dogs: a review of risks and benefits. *Reproduction in Domestic Animals* 44 (Suppl. 2), 29–35.

Robbins, M. (2003) Reproductive oncology. In: Slatter, D. (ed.) *Textbook of small animal surgery.* 3rd edition. Philadelphia, PA, Saunders, vol. 2, pp. 2437–2444.

Romagnoli, S. & Sontas, H. (2010) Prevention of breeding in the female. In: England, G. & von Heimendahl, A. (eds) *BSAVA manual of small animal reproduction and neonatology.* 2nd edition. Gloucester, UK, British Small Animal Veterinary Association.

Root, M.V. (1995) Early spay-neuter in the cat: Effect on development of obesity and metabolic rate. *Veterinary Clinical Nutrition* 2, 132–134.

Root, M.V., Johnston, S.D., Johnston, G.R. & Olson, P.N. (1996) The effect of prepuberal and postpuberal gonadectomy on penile extrusion and urethral diameter in the domestic cat. *Veterinary Radiology and Ultrasound* 37, 363–366.

Root, M.V., Johnston, S.D. & Olson, P.N. (1997) The effect of prepuberal and postpuberal gonadectomy on radial physeal closure in male and female domestic cats. *Veterinary Radiology and Ultrasound* 38 (1), 42–47.

Ru, G., Terracini, B. & Glickman, L.T. (1998) Host related risk factors for canine osteosarcoma. *Veterinary Journal* 156, 31–39.

Salmeri, K.R., Bloomberg, M.S., Scruggs, S.L & Shille, V. (1991) Gonadectomy in immature dogs: Effects on skeletal, physical, and behavioral. *Journal of the American Veterinary Medical Association* 1998 (7), 1193–1203.

Schneider, R., Dorn, C.R. & Taylor, D.O.N. (1969) Factors influencing canine mammary cancer development and postsurgical survival. *Journal of the National Cancer Institute* 43, 1249–1261.

Serpell, J. & Hsu, Y. (2005) Effects of breed, sex and neuter status on trainability in dogs. *Anthrozoös* 18 (3), 196–207.

Spain, C.V., Scarlett, J.M. & Houpt, K.A. (2004a) Long-term risks and benefits of early-age gonadectomy in cats. *Journal of the American Veterinary Medical Association* 224 (3), 372–379.

Spain, C.V., Scarlett, J.M. & Houpt, K.A. (2004b) Long-term risks and benefits of early-age gonadectomy in dogs. *Journal of the American Veterinary Medical Association* 224 (3), 380–387.

Stubbs, W.P., Bloomberg, M.S., Scruggs, S.L., Shille, V.M. & Lane, T.J. (1996) Effects of prepubertal gonadectomy on physical and behavioral development in cats. *Journal of the American Veterinary Medical Association* 209 (11), 1864–1871.

SVS (2011) *Norm angående kirurgisk kastration av friska hundar [Norm regarding the surgical neutering of healthy dogs]* Sveriges Veterinärförbund. [Online] Available from: http://svf.se/sv/Sallskapet/Smadjurssektionen/Normgruppen/Normer-av-medicinsk-karaktar/Norm-angaende-kirurgisk-kastration-av-friska-hundar/ [Accessed 17 July 2014].

Thrusfield, M.V., Holt, P.E. & Muirhead, R.H. (1998) Acquired urinary incontinence in bitches: its incidence and relationship to neutering practices. *Journal of Small Animal Practice* 39 (12), 559–566.

Torres de la Riva, G., Hart, B.L., Farver, T.B., Oberbauer, A.M., Messam, L.L.M., Willits, N. & Hart, L.A. (2013) Neutering dogs: effects on joint disorders and cancers in Golden Retrievers. *PLoS ONE* 8 (2), e55937.

UN (1994) *Human rights: supporting the constellation of reproductive rights.* United Nations. [Online] Available from: http://www.unfpa.org/rights/rights.htm [Accessed 21 July 2014].

Van Goethem, B., Schaefers-Okkens, A. & Kirpensteijn, J. (2006) Making a rational choice between ovariectomy and ovariohysterectomy in the dog: a discussion of the benefits of either technique. *Veterinary Surgery* 35, 136–143.

Performing Convenience Surgery: Tail Docking, Ear Cropping, Debarking and Declawing

11

11.1 Introduction   170
11.2 Convenience Surgeries   170
    11.2.1 Tail docking (dogs)   170
    11.2.2 Ear cropping   171
    11.2.3 Debarking   172
    11.2.4 Declawing (and tendonectomy)   172
11.3 Ethical Perspectives on Convenience Surgeries   172
    11.3.1 Possible health benefits   173

Companion Animal Ethics, First Edition. Peter Sandøe, Sandra Corr and Clare Palmer.
© Universities Federation for Animal Welfare 2016.

11.3.2 Possible indirect benefits, and effects on
        human attachment   174
11.3.3 Possible harms: pain, suffering and other negative
        effects on animal welfare   176
11.3.4 Weighing costs and benefits   178
11.3.5 Violating animals' bodily integrity   178
11.3.6 The preservation of dog breeds   180
11.3.7 Professional veterinary ethics   181

11.1 Introduction

Surgery is not always performed on companion animals to prevent, alleviate or cure disease. Some surgical procedures are performed for non-medical reasons, such as to make the animals more aesthetically appealing to their owners, to meet a breed standard, or to create 'better' companions with whom to co-habit. Such procedures can be termed 'cosmetic' procedures, 'convenience' procedures (Jefferson, 2011) or 'utility' surgeries (Rutgers & Heeger, 1999). We will use the terms 'convenience surgeries' or 'procedures' here. These surgical procedures are distinctive in that they are not normally performed for the direct benefit of the animal concerned. However, the boundary between procedures performed for medical reasons, and convenience surgeries, may be unclear – for example, routine neutering of an animal, as discussed in Chapter 10, may to some extent be considered a 'convenience' procedure. Here we build on some of our earlier ethical discussion relating to neutering. We focus on the four most common convenience surgeries: tail docking, ear cropping and debarking dogs, and declawing cats. We briefly review these procedures from a veterinary and legal perspective, and then consider different ethical perspectives on them.

11.2 Convenience Surgeries

11.2.1 Tail docking (dogs)

Tail docking is defined as the removal of part of a healthy tail from a healthy dog. Traditionally, this procedure was routinely performed in a number of specific breeds including Boxers, Rottweilers and Dobermans, as well as in many Spaniel and Terrier breeds. Puppies are usually tail docked at less than 5 days of age, and a varying amount of the tip of the tail is removed, depending on the breed, normally by using a scalpel blade or nail cutters. In some countries, tail docking is carried out by breeders or other lay persons rather than by vets; in others, only vets are legally permitted to perform this surgery. When performed by vets, a general anaesthetic or analgesic may be administered.

So why are dogs' tails docked? The Council of Docked Breeds, a UK-based organisation set-up 'to protect the freedom to choose the tail docking option', says that docking is performed 'to avoid damage to the tail in heavy vegetation and thick brambles, or down holes; for hygiene (avoiding faecal fouling with potential for maggot infestation), and to maintain breed standards (and the genetic pool, otherwise some breeds could be lost forever)' (Council of Docked Breeds, 2010a). Some, but not all, of these reasons sound as if they may be of benefit to the animal concerned; we will return to this issue when discussing ethics in a later section.

Laws on tail docking vary between countries: while legal in the United States, tail docking is illegal in most European countries, unless medically indicated (Neumann, 2008). Although the procedure is legal in Canada (with the exception of Newfoundland), veterinary medical associations in a number of provinces do not permit their members to perform it. Exceptions to legal bans are made for working dogs in some countries, such as England and Wales but not Scotland (British Veterinary Association, n.d.), Denmark (Justitsministeriet, 1991) and Germany (Council of Docked Breeds, 2010b). The definition of a 'working dog' in England and Wales is tightly controlled, and veterinary certification is required; the dog must be docked before it is 5 days old and must also be microchipped. However, this exception for working dogs is difficult to police, as there is no guarantee that dogs once docked will ultimately be used as working dogs.

11.2.2 Ear cropping

Ear cropping is the procedure by which the ears of certain breeds of dog such as Great Danes, Dobermans and Boxers, are surgically re-shaped (cut), to give the dogs a more alert or aggressive appearance. It is usually performed under general anaesthesia at 8–12 weeks of age, and the ears are then 'posted' or 'racked' (wrapped or taped up) for several weeks or months, to train them to stay erect (Figure 11.1).

Ear cropping is illegal in Australia, New Zealand, and many European countries including the United Kingdom (Gumbrell, 1984). It is legal in the United States, although several states have repeatedly tried to outlaw ear cropping (and tail docking). In 2008, the American Veterinary Medical Association adopted a policy opposing both

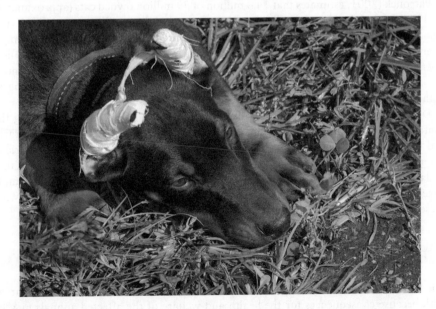

Figure 11.1   A Doberman puppy with cropped ears. The ears are bandaged after the surgery to encourage them to stay erect. (*Budimir Jevtic/Shutterstock.com.*)

ear cropping and tail docking for cosmetic purposes, and 'encouraged its elimination from all breed standards' (AVMA, n.d.a). However, the American Kennel Club has fought such initiatives, arguing that, as prescribed in certain breed standards, ear cropping and tail docking 'are acceptable practices integral to defining and preserving breed character, and/or enhancing good health' (American Kennel Club, 2012).

11.2.3 Debarking

Debarking (devocalising) is a surgical procedure that involves removing a dog's vocal cords under general anaesthetic. It is performed mainly to prevent nuisance noise, but sometimes also to create silent attack dogs.

Debarking is banned in the United Kingdom and other European countries, but is permitted in most states of the United States other than New Jersey, while Ohio restricts the surgery to dogs not considered 'vicious'. The American Veterinary Medical Association (AVMA, 2013) recommends that the surgery only be done 'as a final alternative to euthanasia after behavioural modification to correct excessive vocalization has failed and after discussion of potential complications from the procedure with the owner'.

11.2.4 Declawing (and tendonectomy)

Declawing (onychectomy) involves amputation of a cat's distal phalanges (the last bone in the toe) of the front paws, usually simultaneously, to prevent the cat scratching (furniture or people). The amputations may be performed by using a scalpel, guillotine or laser. An alternative technique involves cutting or removing part of the deep digital flexor tendon of each toe (tendonectomy or tenectomy). This is a less invasive procedure that results in the claws remaining retracted (limiting the cats ability to scratch), but the claws become thick and brittle, and must be trimmed regularly.

Patronek (2001) estimates that 14.4 million of 59 million owned cats (approximately 24.4%) in the United States are declawed, and quotes other studies reporting between 19.6% (Morgan & Houpt, 1989) and 45.1% (Pollari & Bonnett, 1996). Declawing is often performed along with neutering, when the animal is 6–8 months old. It requires a general anaesthetic, application of a tourniquet (a constricting device used to control blood supply to an extremity for a period of time), and post-operative bandaging of both front paws.

Declawing and tendonectomy are illegal in more than 25 countries (including the United Kingdom and other European countries, Australia and New Zealand, Brazil, and Israel), but are legal, and widely performed, in the United States. The American Veterinary Medical Association does not recommend tendonectomy, but maintains that declawing should remain an option, but that it should be considered 'only after attempts have been made to prevent the cat from using its claws destructively or when its clawing presents an above normal health risk for its owner(s)' (AVMA, n.d.b).

11.3 Ethical Perspectives on Convenience Surgeries

The four procedures described raise ethical issues, but how these are interpreted varies, both because consequences for the health and welfare of the affected animals may be evaluated differently, and because different theoretical approaches to ethics disagree about what is actually at stake.

The only ethical perspectives from which convenience surgeries seem largely unproblematic are human-centred approaches such as contractarianism, in which animals do not count in their own right, and where the potential positive effects on human welfare are all that matter. From other ethical perspectives, significant concerns are raised about convenience surgeries.

We will begin by considering convenience surgeries from a utilitarian perspective, focusing on direct and indirect benefits and costs to animal and human welfare, and on the impacts of surgery on animals' natural behaviours. Then we will outline objections based on non-utilitarian claims that such surgeries affect the 'integrity' of animals' bodies; we will also consider concerns that relate not so much to the individual animal, but to the breed to which it belongs. Finally, we will discuss some ethical implications for vets, as at least three of the convenience surgeries require the involvement of a vet.

11.3.1 Possible health benefits

The surgery that seems most likely potentially to offer direct health benefits to individual animals is tail docking. The argument, made largely in the case of working dogs (i.e. dogs that are not only, or not primarily, kept as companions), is that pre-emptive tail docking can prevent or limit the risk of painful injuries to dogs' tails. However, evidence to support this argument is mixed.

Houlton (2008), for instance, looked specifically at *gundogs*, and found that for Springer Spaniels and Cocker Spaniels, there was a highly significant association between tail injuries and undocked dogs. A subsequent large study by Diesel *et al.* (2010) reported 281 tail injuries in a *general population* of 138,212 dogs. Within specific breed groups, Spaniels, Greyhounds, Lurchers and Whippets were at significantly higher risk of tail injury compared to Labradors and other Retrievers, yet of these, only Spaniels are traditionally docked. Most tail injuries occurred in the home, usually due to trapping the tail in a door, rather than when the dogs were working (as the legislation in the United Kingdom, for instance, is designed to address). The results also indicated that while dogs with docked tails were significantly less likely to sustain a tail injury, approximately 500 dogs would need to be docked in order to prevent one tail injury.

More recently, two linked studies, funded by the Scottish Government, investigated the prevalence of tail injuries in dogs in Scotland. In the first study, Lederer, Bennett & Parkin (2014) collected data by Internet questionnaire from owners of working dogs used during the 2010/2011 shooting season. They found that 13.5% of 2860 working dogs sustained at least one tail injury (nearly 42% of these dogs sustained two or more tail injuries, and 13.2% sustained four or more tail injuries). Spaniels and Hunt Point Retrievers (HPRs) with undocked tails were at greatest risk: 56.6% and 38.5% of undocked dogs of each breed, respectively, suffered at least one tail injury. The degree of docking (one-third, one-half or shorter) made no statistically significant difference to the likelihood of injury. The authors noted that while any benefit from docking would be likely to be sustained for the number of years that the dog was worked, docking as a puppy does not entirely remove the risk of subsequent tail injury. The authors also acknowledged potential bias in the study, which was publicised through country sports associations, known for their opposition to the complete tail-docking ban in Scotland.

In the second study, records from 16 veterinary practices in Scotland were retrospectively searched to identify the prevalence of more 'severe' tail injuries in working and non-working dog breeds between 2002 and 2012 (Cameron *et al.*, 2014). Severe injuries were defined as those deemed by owners to require veterinary treatment; the overall prevalence was 0.59%, with significantly more injuries in working breeds (0.9%) compared to non-working breeds (0.53%). Within working breeds, Pointers and Setters were most likely to sustain a tail injury requiring veterinary attention (1.69%). Tail injuries severe enough to require amputation (0.12%) were significantly more common in working breeds (0.19%) than in non-working breeds (0.09%). Data was also available from eight practices for tail injuries in Spaniels before (April 29, 2007) and after the introduction of the tail-docking ban. Tail injuries were seen in 14/2607 Spaniels (0.54%) before the ban, and 36/2942 spaniels (1.22%) after January 2009: the odds of suffering a tail injury were 2.3 times greater after the ban.

However, the number of dogs that must be docked to prevent a tail injury seems high, even though both Scottish studies estimate lower numbers than the 500 proposed by Diesel *et al.* (2010). To prevent a tail injury in working breeds, Lederer *et al.* (2014) suggest that between 5 and 54 puppies across all working breeds – or in the case of Spaniels or HPRs, between 2 and 18 puppies – would have to be docked. To prevent a 'severe' tail injury, Cameron *et al.* (2014) calculated that approximately 232 puppies across the working breeds – or between 81 and 135 Pointer/Setter, HPR or Spaniel puppies – would need to be docked. To prevent one tail amputation in Spaniels, 320 Spaniel puppies would need to be docked.

The authors of both Scottish studies propose that it may be appropriate to consider changes to the current legislation for specific breeds of working dogs, suggesting that the difference in risk is most likely due to the different tail conformation, and the fact that the breed groups work in very different terrains (most 'worst tail injuries' occurred during 'rough' or 'driven shoots' while dogs were in 'cover' or 'woodland'). However, with the exception of Spaniels, most of the breeds identified in the aforementioned studies as being most at risk of tail injuries (Greyhounds, Lurchers, Whippets, Pointers, Setters and Retrievers) have historically not been docked.

While there may be some benefits to some dogs of being tail docked, potential benefits seem to be much less clear in the case of the other three surgeries. Although there are anecdotal claims that ear cropping reduces ear infections and makes dogs' ears less vulnerable to tearing, no systematic evidence of health benefits from ear cropping has been uncovered. There do not appear to be any direct health benefits to the animals concerned from debarking and declawing either. But do these practices provide *indirect* benefits?

11.3.2 Possible indirect benefits, and effects on human attachment

Convenience surgeries raise interesting questions about the attachment between humans and their animal companions. For example, preventing barking and scratching – perceived as problems by some owners – by devocalisation and declawing, although offering no direct health benefits for the animals, may result in a better relationship between the owner and the animal. Consequently, the animal may have a better life; for instance, fewer punishments for anti-social behaviour, and a reduction in the likelihood of the animal being abandoned, rehomed or euthanased.

The American Kennel Club (2010) states that:

> debarking is a viable veterinary procedure that may allow a dog owner to keep a dog that barks excessively in its loving home rather than to be forced to surrender it to a shelter.

Similar claims could be made for scratching behaviour undermining the attachment of owners to their cats; declawing could end the disruptive behaviour and allow for the continuance of the relation. However, evidence that declawing is a protective factor against relinquishment is weak. One study reported that considered in isolation, declawing made relinquishment less likely; but when all other related factors were taken into consideration, declawed cats were at an increased risk of relinquishment (Patronek, 2001), perhaps because declawing may trigger other unwanted behaviours such as biting or inappropriate urination (Jefferson, 2011). However, the evidence here remains contested.

In considering the indirect benefits argument, a number of further issues are raised. First, the acceptance of convenience procedures, especially in the United States, may result from an unrealistic expectation about what is involved in owning and caring for an animal. As discussed by Sandøe et al. (2008a), if owners are unfamiliar with normal animal behaviour, they will be unable to make the distinction between normal behaviours that they just do not want (scratching, barking) and abnormal behaviours created by a bored or frustrated animal (e.g. destroying the carpet). While in many cases abnormal behaviour can be changed by training, behavioural guidance, or environmental alterations (see Chapter 9), normal behaviours are likely to persist, and should be expected when living with a dog or a cat.

In a similar vein, some critics of such surgeries raise questions about the nature of a human/companion animal bond in which such surgeries are seen as acceptable:

> Does one really foster a healthy human–animal bond while condemning and forcibly altering part of the animal, with no benefit to the animal? And, is it unreasonable to think that if one views an integral part of the animal as disposable that he/she may be more likely to view the whole animal as disposable?

> (Jefferson, 2011)

Jefferson's argument seems to be almost the reverse of the main argument in favour of convenience surgeries. The implication here is that rather than convenience surgeries making animals easier to live with and so strengthening the bond, performing such surgeries instead stems from, or fosters, an attitude of disposability, reflecting a willingness to dispose of the animal itself, for instance, by relinquishing it to a shelter. Jefferson may be right in making this claim, but as we have already noted in the case of declawing, evidence about the relationship between relinquishment and convenience surgery remains unclear.

11.3.3 Possible harms: pain, suffering and other negative effects on animal welfare

All four surgical procedures raise concerns, to different degrees, about both short- and longer-term pain and discomfort for the animals concerned.

To begin with tail docking: little research has been carried out concerning the effects of tail docking on individual dogs, but there has been debate over whether young puppies can feel pain from the docking process itself (Bennett & Perini, 2003). A single study exists that made behavioural observations of 50 puppies undergoing tail docking, and reported that all the puppies vocalised intensely at the time of amputation and for 138 seconds afterwards (range of 5 to 840 seconds) (Noonan *et al.*, 1996). The authors suggested that the animals did experience pain, but reported that most puppies settled to sleep a mean of 3 minutes later (range of 35 seconds to 14 minutes). Tail docking may also have longer-term effects, although these are uncertain. Studies on dogs and rats have shown that the first post-natal week is a critical period, when infliction of surgical pain may affect changes in sensory processing resulting in hyperalgesia (increased sensitivity to pain) in response to subsequent surgical pain (Walker, Tochiki & Fitzgerald, 2009). It is also possible that chronic pain could arise from neuromas in tail stumps (Bennett & Perini, 2003), and the neuromas may become permanent; one study describes this happening in six dogs (Gross & Carr, 1990).

Similar concerns over potential suffering also exist with the other convenience surgeries. Ear cropping likely causes acute peri-operative discomfort, and medium-term discomfort when ears are held in an abnormal position during healing. Debarking carries the risk of complications, including chronic coughing, aspiration pneumonia, and nerve damage (and the surgery is not always successful, as scar tissue regrowth may allow vocalisation again (Jefferson, 2011)).

Declawing, in particular, can result in significant pain and complications (Figure 11.2). Tobias (1994) reported that of 163 cats undergoing declawing, 50% had one or more complications immediately after surgery, including pain (38.1%), bleeding (31.9%), lameness (26.9%), and swelling (6.3%), or were non-weight-bearing (5.6%). Follow-up was available for 121 cats; 19.8% developed complications after discharge. Late postoperative complications included infection (11.6%), regrowth of claws (7.4%), bone protrusion (1.7%), abnormal stance (1.7%), and prolonged, intermittent lameness persisting up to 45 days (0.8%). Other late complications include chronic infection, radial nerve paralysis, and tissue death from improper bandage placement (Jankowski *et al.*, 1998; Landsberg, 1991; Martinez, Hauptmann & Walshaw, 1993), and almost 1% of cats, according to one study, suffer persistent lameness after declaw surgery (Pickett, 2012). Cats undergoing tendonectomy suffer similar, though fewer, complications.

Other negative experiences following these surgeries are also possible, although again there are few studies to draw on here. Convenience surgeries could make animals more vulnerable to future painful experiences – for instance, declawed cats are much less able to defend themselves, and debarked dogs may suffer due to their inability to communicate vocally with other dogs or human beings. Ears and tails also appear to play important roles in canine communication, potentially leading to negative

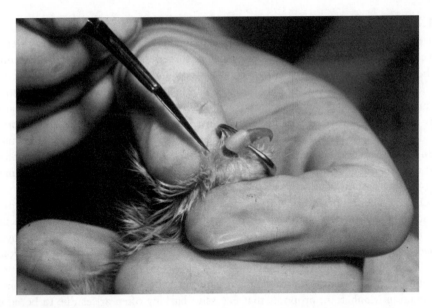

Figure 11.2 Cat being declawed: the nail and last bone of each digit are surgically removed. (*Reproduced with permission.*)

experiences for those dogs physically altered through cropping or docking (Jefferson, 2011; Leaver & Reimchen, 2008; Neumann, 2008).

Some of these surgeries may also cause experiences of frustration, as dogs may still try to bark after devocalisation and cats may try to scratch after declawing, which can also lead to chronic stress (Patronek, 2001). This is in contrast to neutering, where sexual desires are likely to disappear after the procedure. As well as producing negative experiences, some forms of convenience surgeries may also deny animals *positive* experiences they otherwise would have had (for instance, tree climbing for a cat).

So far, in this section, we have worked with a *hedonist* conception of welfare. However, as described in Chapter 4, there are also other ideas of welfare. Many people focus more on animals' *capacities*, arguing that we should not inhibit the ability of animals to engage in 'natural behaviours'. On this view – described in Chapter 4 as perfectionism – something important is lost when companion animals are deprived of the capacity to carry out natural behaviours such as barking, scratching or communicating with their tails (Leaver & Reimchen, 2008). To be clear, the concern here is not so much that animals' desires to carry out particular actions are frustrated (though they might be). According to the perfectionist view, there is something independently problematic about preventing animals from realising significant natural or species-specific potentials. Something important is lost in the life of a dog that cannot bark and a cat that cannot scratch, even if the animal does not itself miss those capabilities. All the forms of convenience surgery considered here, perhaps with the exception of ear cropping, will lead to a reduction in welfare if it is defined in perfectionist terms.

11.3.4 Weighing costs and benefits

On utilitarian ethical views (see Chapter 5), decision making should be guided by weighing costs and benefits. In the case of convenience surgeries, there appear to be a number of benefits to owners (in particular, reduced stress and annoyance with animal companions, at least in the case of debarking and declawing) and indirect benefits to some animals, who experience better relations with their owners, and, in more extreme cases, may avoid the negative experiences that follow from being relinquished. On the other hand, surgery may be associated with significant negative experiences for the animals, both in the short and long term. Furthermore, with a wider, perfectionist, notion of animal welfare, there are additional negative consequences in terms of preventing animals carrying out natural behaviours.

One consideration here is that some of the benefits of convenience surgery could be achieved by other means (though not without considerable human commitment). For instance, regularly cutting cats' claws, or applying soft claws (soft rubber covers glued over the nails) can prevent furniture being scratched; some barking behaviours can be reduced by environmental alteration, appropriate training, or medication. Dr. Louise Murray, director of medicine at the ASPCA's Bergh Memorial Animal Hospital in Manhattan, proposes that excessive barking often arises due to boredom or underlying frustration, and suggests that this should be addressed instead (Dolnick, 2010). However, such measures are unlikely to be universally effective.

Although there may be disagreement about how to weigh these human and companion animal experiences, it is likely that in many cases – from a broadly utilitarian perspective – the costs to the animals concerned (in terms of pain, frustration, loss of positive experiences and inability to exercise natural forms of behaviour) will outweigh the benefits to all parties. However, in certain cases, where an animal's behaviour seriously threatens the human–companion animal bond, convenience surgery may be considered the least bad option for both humans and animals. This is much more likely to apply in the case of preventing barking and scratching, than to removing ears and tails. Overall, though, utilitarian logic would suggest that even though some individuals could benefit from some forms of convenience surgery, the negative effects of generally allowing these forms of surgery very likely far outweigh these benefits. Utilitarian approaches, then, would probably support legal bans on convenience surgeries.

11.3.5 Violating animals' bodily integrity

So far, we have considered utilitarian views that judge the moral acceptability of conducting convenience surgeries on animals in terms of weighing the effects that these surgeries will have on animal and human welfare. Other ethical theories, though, construe this issue in terms of rights or principles that should be very seriously respected or protected, and should only ever be overruled if they conflict with a principle that is even more important, for instance, an animal's right to life. A key concern of these non-utilitarian approaches is the idea of bodily integrity (although utilitarians and other consequentialists *could* be concerned about this, in practice, most discussions of animals' bodily integrity have been non-utilitarian).

In Chapter 10, we considered the argument that bodily integrity should be respected, and therefore an animal should not have to undergo surgery without a clear medical benefit to the animal from doing so. With the possible exception of some cases of tail docking, therefore, convenience surgeries also raise significant ethical concerns for views on which animals' bodily integrity is to be respected. A similar ethical concern could be raised over neutering; in particular, castrating confined male dogs, which is difficult to justify on the basis of it being medically beneficial to the animal (see Chapter 10).

An argument might be made here that humans undergo cosmetic surgeries to alter noses, eyelids, breasts, and so on that do not have medical benefits. Does this differ from surgeries such as ear cropping? On some versions of this view, it does not: humans should not normally interfere with their own bodily integrity, unless there is some medical need to do so (Wilkinson & Garrard, 1996). However, a more widely accepted argument is that humans are able to reflect on and to choose such surgeries, whereas animals are not. People may believe (rightly or wrongly) that they will benefit psychologically and/or socially from having cosmetic surgery, and can decide that the benefits are worth the financial cost, risk and discomfort of the surgery itself. Companion animals are unable to make such choices; they will not gain psychological benefits from having surgery, and while there may be some post-surgical changes as to how they are regarded by human beings, these are not changes that we can reasonably think would overrule a principle as serious as respect for an animal's bodily integrity.

There is room for discussion, however, about the principle of respect for bodily integrity. A concern here is that the idea of 'bodily integrity' is itself rather difficult to define. Its boundaries are unclear: is a cat's bodily integrity affected by trimming its claws (as opposed to declawing it)? Would removing an ugly, but harmless, growth on a dog's face that appeared to be causing it no difficulties impinge on its integrity? These issues raise questions such as whether 'bodily integrity' must concern actions that *irreversibly* impact on a physical body (this is not normally thought necessary in the human case, where, for instance, sexual assault is usually thought of as infringing on bodily integrity) and whether, in the animal case, 'integrity' concerns the norm for a particular individual, or for a breed or species.

Having said this, convenience surgeries do impact on bodily integrity on most plausible definitions; from value perspectives on which integrity should be respected, or on which animals have a right not to have their bodily integrity interfered with, such surgeries are ethically troubling.

Of course, not all ethical views accept that bodily integrity matters. For instance, according to utilitarian views that adopt a hedonist view of welfare, bodily integrity *in itself* does not matter. If convenience surgery does not change human or animal experiential welfare, it is ethically irrelevant. So, while pain, discomfort, frustration, happiness and so on matter, integrity violations in themselves do not. A rights view, also, may be primarily concerned with pain and other forms of suffering, rather than bodily integrity. For instance, it might be argued that an animal has a right not to be subjected to pain and suffering unless it is for the sake of the animal's own health, even if inflicting such suffering would bring about overall benefits to all affected, and that violating this right is what is wrong with convenience surgery, not a loss of bodily integrity. Certain contextual approaches to ethics, such as an ethics of care, also focus on issues other than bodily integrity. For instance, it might be maintained that a companion animal bond that enforces the pain and discomfort of surgery on one party for the convenience of the other party, cannot be based on the affection, respect and the 'willingness to compromise' that should characterise a caring relationship (Neumann, 2008). Nonetheless, the argument that convenience surgeries fail to respect bodily integrity does play an important role in this debate.

11.3.6 The preservation of dog breeds

So far, we have considered ethical arguments that focus on the affected individuals – be they human beings or animals. However, two forms of convenience surgery, tail docking and ear cropping of dogs, are also discussed in the literature in the context of their effects on dog *breeds*. While debarking may be carried out on any breed of dog, tail docking and ear cropping have been important in the breed standards for certain dogs. It has been argued that banning these procedures will cause breeders to slow down or stop breeding these dogs, and so the genetic pool will diminish, perhaps ultimately leading to the end of the breed. And the loss of breeds, it is sometimes argued, matters ethically. This concern has two different but related aspects: an empirical one (will genetic pools shrink/breeds become extinct if tail docking and ear cropping are banned?) and a value-oriented one (would it matter if this happened?)

Why might fewer dogs of the traditionally docked breeds be bred after a docking ban, especially if revised breed standards permit undocked dogs to be shown? One possibility is that the docked (and cropped) appearance pleases people aesthetically, and that, without this, enthusiasm for the breed might decline. Another possibility is that show dogs of these breeds have not so far been selected for their tails, and dogs that may otherwise be good show dogs may not have good tails. If the requirement to have a good tail is added to existing breed standards, a smaller number of dogs will be bred from, potentially further reducing the genetic pool of the breed and threatening its continuance. A third possibility is that owners of working dogs may feel that the dogs' ability to work is compromised, if they are made more susceptible to injury.

Very few statistics have been published on the effects of docking on populations of traditionally docked breeds. The study by Lederer, Bennett and Parkin (2014) looked at the working dog population in Scotland during the 2010/11 shooting season, and separated the dogs by date of birth into two groups: those born before and those born after the Scottish ban on tail docking (including working dogs) that came into effect in April 2007. Among the respondents to the survey, it was found that for working Spaniels, a breed that has traditionally been docked, there had been a drop in the number of dogs born in Scotland from 79.5% (495) before to 51.5% (265) after the introduction of the ban. The drop in the number of Spaniels born in Scotland is assumed to reflect an increase in the number imported from England and other places where docking of working dogs was allowed. However, at the same time, the relative number of working Spaniels in Scotland that were undocked had risen from 8.4% of those born before the ban to 31.7% of those born after the ban.

The Council of Docked Breeds (2010c) posts (unsourced) statistics on Australian litter registrations of various breeds. These show significant drops in litter registration for traditionally docked breeds such as Airedales and Dobermans after a docking ban was implemented. However, these statistics do not include all traditionally docked breeds, nor any undocked breeds. We do not therefore know, for instance, whether litter registration fell for all docked breeds, or whether it rose for some; nor how much year-on-year fluctuation there is in breed registration; nor whether registration of some traditionally undocked breeds also fell.

In Denmark, tail docking of dogs was banned in 1991, except for certain named breeds of hunting dogs. Data provided by Vibeke Knudsen of the Danish Kennel Club, (personal communication) on the number of puppies of four previously docked breeds, registered between1990 and 2013, show that none of the breeds went out of fashion. Of the four breeds – Cocker Spaniel, Boxer, Schnauzer and Doberman Pinscher, the most significantly affected breed – the Cocker Spaniel – has seen a lasting drop in registrations of about 30%. Based on these data at least, there does not seem to be a reason to believe that a ban on tail docking will lead to a disappearance of otherwise popular dog breeds.

However, suppose for the sake of argument, that docking did result in the loss of breeds, or more likely in the decline of numbers of animals of specific breeds. Would this matter? There has certainly been widespread concern about the loss of breeds of domesticated *agricultural* animals. Such 'heritage' breeds may be regarded as valuable genetic pools that can be drawn upon in future to diversify the genetic stock of commercial agricultural breeds, should new breed traits be needed to respond to changing climate or new diseases. They may also have cultural and historical significance (rather like heritage buildings, or familiar landscapes). A similar argument could be made in the case of dogs: genetic material from one breed could be a valuable resource in dog breeding more generally, so preserving it could be important. Equally, people may value the continuing existence of certain breeds, and, for instance, judge a world without Dobermans to be a poorer place. But it is surely reasonable to question how deep the attachment to a breed actually is, if possessing a complete tail is sufficient to render it valueless. Moreover, as these preferred 'looks' are relatively recent, it would actually seem more traditional to value dog breeds with uncropped ears and tails (Bennett & Perini, 2003).

Whatever one thinks of these arguments, the world of dog breeds is never stagnant. As we saw in Chapter 7, breeds such as German Shepherds have changed substantially in appearance over the years; new breed standards can be created to include uncropped ears and tails. Breeds such as Alpine Spaniels and the English White Terrier have become extinct over time, while new breeds, such as the Cesky Terrier, are now recognised. As Herzog (2006) notes, dog breeds undergo extreme 'booms' and 'busts' in popularity, as measured by registrations at the American Kennel Club at least. It is possible that some people will prefer certain breeds when they see them without cropped ears and docked tails. So, while bans on docking and cropping may have effects on specific breeds, these effects are just one factor among many in the changing appearance of existing breeds, the decline of old breeds and the adoption of new breeds.

11.3.7 Professional veterinary ethics

The four surgical procedures considered in this chapter are all carried out by vets (although in some countries, tail docking is also carried out by people with no veterinary training). In countries where such convenience procedures are permissible, it is usually left to the discretion of the individual vet to decide whether or not to perform them, and the matter is divisive within the profession. Banfield, the largest corporate veterinary practice in the United States with more than 800 hospitals and 2000 vets, has banned tail docking, ear cropping and debarking (Weise, 2009).

However, vets may have a number of reasons for carrying out such surgeries. In a letter published in the *Journal of the American Veterinary Medical Association*, one vet makes the point that 'like it or not, ear cropping has a tremendous economic benefit to society, often helping vets pay employees as well as the rent', and maintains that breeders and the breed-related economy also make a profit by selling dogs that are more distinctive (Stone, 2000). Similar financial justification may be offered in the case of declawing: a veterinary practice is, after all, a business (see Chapter 2). If one veterinary practice refuses to carry out the procedure, the client may go to another vet that will – thus depriving the first practice of the business (and perhaps future business from the same client) without there being any gains for the animal. Vets may also take the view that, as Sandøe *et al.* (2008b) comment, they are not hired by animals, but by the people owning the animals. They may consider that it is not their job to take the 'moral high ground' with their clients, and that animals' owners should be free to choose what to do with the animals, as long as it is within the law.

In contrast, other vets strongly adhere to the 'paediatrician' model, considering their primary role to be one of patient advocacy, and promoting the course of action that is best for the patient, irrespective of any other factors (Fettman & Rollin, 2002; see also Chapter 2). On this model, none of these surgeries could be routine, but nonetheless, there may be occasions where vets might determine that procedures such as declawing a cat or devocalising a dog might be best for that particular animal in its specific circumstances.

There is at least one ethical responsibility that it is reasonable to maintain all vets have however: to ensure that owners clearly understand what the procedures involve, and the short- and long-term risks they pose to the animal. Only then can owners give truly informed consent. This is particularly true of declawing, where cat owners may not realise the nature of the surgery involved, especially if told by a vet that it is routine. Jefferson (2011) recommends the avoidance of 'euphemistic' language and asks whether clients would be less likely to request '*declawing*' if they were clearly informed by their cat's 'trusted doctor' that it involved multiple, painful *amputations* of bone, is ethically very controversial, illegal in many countries and several US cities, and may produce permanent negative physical and behavioural effects.

Whatever one thinks of each of the convenience surgeries, ensuring that owners are well informed about the nature and likely effects of the procedures, and the possible alternatives, is of clear ethical significance.

Key Points

- Four convenience surgeries were considered in this chapter: tail docking, ear cropping and debarking of dogs and declawing of cats. These convenience surgeries – with the possible exception of some cases of tail docking – do not have direct medical benefits to the animal.

- All of the procedures cause some pain and discomfort to the animals, limit their ability to engage in natural behaviours to varying degrees, and may have longer-term complications. There are some direct benefits to owners, which could bring indirect benefits to the affected animals, including in a few cases avoiding relinquishment.

- A utilitarian, however, is likely to argue that overall the direct costs to animals of convenience surgeries outweigh the combined direct benefits to owners and indirect benefits to animals, and that this may justify legal bans of such surgeries.

- For ethical approaches on which animals' bodily integrity should be respected or is a right, all of these procedures are highly ethically problematic.

- Banning tail docking and ear cropping may have a negative impact on breed populations, and on some views, this would be ethically problematic. However, so far, there is little evidence either way of the effects of bans on breed populations in countries where such restrictions have been implemented.

- In countries where these procedures are allowed, they are usually performed by vets. Some vets maintain that their primary responsibility is to their business and to human clients, others to their animal patients. In either case, vets should clearly inform clients what these procedures involve, and what alternatives are available.

References

American Kennel Club (2010) *Canine legislation position statement: debarking.* [Online] Available from: http://images.akc.org/pdf/canine_legislation/position_statements /Debarking.pdf [Accessed: 22 July 2014].

American Kennel Club (2012) *Canine legislation position statement: ear cropping, tail docking and dewclaw removal.* [Online] Available from: http://www.akc.org/pdfs /canine_legislation/position_statements/Ear_Cropping_Tail_Docking_and_Dewclaw_ Removal.pdf [Accessed 22 July 2014].

AVMA (n.d.a) *Ear cropping and tail docking of dogs.* American Veterinary Medical Association. [Online] Available from: https://www.avma.org/KB/Policies/Pages/Ear -Cropping-and-Tail-Docking-of-Dogs.aspx [Accessed 22 July 2014].

AVMA (n.d.b) *Declawing of domestic cats.* American Veterinary Medical Association. [Online] Available from: https://www.avma.org/KB/Policies/Pages/Declawing-of -Domestic-Cats.aspx [Accessed: 12th August 2014].

AVMA (2013) *Revised policy on canine devocalization.* American Veterinary Medical Association. [Online] Available from: https://www.avma.org/About/Governance /Documents/2013W_Resolution4_Canine_Devoc.pdf [Accessed 22 July 2014].

Bennett, P.C. & Perini, E. (2003) Tail docking in dogs: a review of the issues. *Australian Veterinary Journal* 81 (4), 208–218.

British Veterinary Association (n.d.). *Tail docking of dogs.* [Online] Available from: http://www.bva.co.uk/atoz/Tail_docking_of_dogs.aspx [Accessed 22 July 2014].

Cameron, N., Lederer, R., Bennett, D. & Parkin, T. (2014) The prevalence of tail injuries in working and non-working breed dogs visiting veterinary practices in Scotland. *Veterinary Record* 174 (18), 450.

Council of Docked Breeds (2010a) *The case for tail docking.* [Online] Available from: http://www.cdb.org/case4dock.htm [Accessed 22 July 2014].

Council of Docked Breeds (2010b) *German docking ban introduced 1st June 1998.* [Online] Available from: http://www.cdb.org/countries/germany.htm [Accessed 22 July 2014].

Council of Docked Breeds (2010c) *Australian litter registration: before and after their tail docking ban.* [Online] Available from: http://www.cdb.org/News/news35.htm [Accessed 22 July 2014].

Diesel, G., Pfeiffer, D., Crispin, S. & Brodbelt, D. (2010) Risk factors for tail injuries in dogs in Great Britain. *Veterinary Record* 166 (26), 812–817.

Dolnick, S. (2010) Heel. Sit. Whisper. Good dog. *The New York Times* 2 February 2010. [Online] Available from: http://www.nytimes.com/2010/02/03/nyregion/03debark. html?pagewanted=all [Accessed 22 July 2014].

Fettman, M.J. & Rollin, B.E. (2002) Modern elements of informed consent for general veterinary practitioners. *Journal of the American Veterinary Medical Association* 221 (10), 1386–1393.

Gross, T.L. & Carr, S.H. (1990) Amputation neuroma of docked tails in dogs. *Veterinary Pathology* 27, 61–62.

Gumbrell, R.C. (1984) Canine ear cropping. *New Zealand Veterinary Journal* 32 (7), 119.

Herzog, H. (2006) Forty two thousand and one Dalmatians: fads, social contagion and dog breed popularity. *Society and Animals* 14 (4), 383–397.

Houlton, J.E.F. (2008) A survey of gundog lameness and injuries in Great Britain in the shooting seasons 2005/2006 and 2006/2007. *Veterinary Comparative Orthopaedics and Traumatology* 21, 231–237.

Jankowski, A.J., Brown, D.C., Duvall, J., Gregor, T.P., Strine, L.E., Ksiazek, L.M. & Ott, A.H. (1998) Comparison of effects of elective tenectomy or onychectomy in cats. *Journal of the American Veterinary Medical Association* 213, 370–373.

Jefferson, E. (2011) *The ethics of convenience.* Humane Society Veterinary Medical Association. [Online] Available from: http://www.hsvma.org/ethics_of_convenience# .UCp8i2BgJi4 [Accessed 22 July 2014].

Justitsministeriet (1991) *Bekendtgørelse om halekupering af visse hunderacer, BEK nr 627 af 29/08/1991.* [Online] Available from: https://www.retsinformation.dk/Forms/R0710. aspx?id=57727 [Accessed 22 July 2014].

Landsberg, G.M. (1991) Feline scratching and destruction and the effects of declawing. *Veterinary Clinics of North America Small Animal Practice* 21, 265–279.

Leaver, S.D.A. & Reimchen, T.E. (2008). Behavioural responses of *Canis familiaris* to different tail lengths of a remotely-controlled life-size dog replica. *Behaviour* 145, 377–390.

Lederer, R., Bennett, D. & Parkin, T. (2014) Survey of tail injuries sustained by working gundogs and terriers in Scotland. *Veterinary Record* 174 (18), 451.

Martinez, S.A., Hauptmann, J. & Walshaw, R. (1993) Comparing two techniques for onychectomy in cats and two adhesives for wound closure. *Veterinary Medicine* 88, 516–525.

Morgan, M. & Houpt, K.A. (1989) Feline behavior problems: the influence of declawing. *Anthrozoos* 3 (1), 50–53.

Neumann, S. (2008) Cosmetic surgery: customer service or professional misconduct. *Canadian Veterinary Journal* 49 (5), 501–504.

Noonan, G.J., Rand, J.S., Blackshaw, J.K. & Priest, J. (1996) Behavioural observations of puppies undergoing tail docking. *Applied Animal Behaviour Science* 49, 335–342.

Patronek, G.J. (2001) Assessment of claims of short- and long-term complications associated with onychectomy in cats. *Journal of the American Veterinary Medical Association* 219 (7), 932–937.

Pickett, L. (2012) *Ask the vet's pets: declawed cats risk chronic pain.* Reading Eagle 5 May 2012. [Online] Available from: http://readingeagle.com/article.aspx?id=388930 [Accessed 22 July 2014].

Pollari, F.L. & Bonnett, B.N. (1996) Evaluation of postoperative complications following elective surgeries of dogs and cats at private practices using computer records. *Canadian Veterinary Journal* 37, 672–678.

Rutgers, B. & Heeger, R. (1999) Inherent worth and respect for animal integrity. In: Dol, M., van Vlissingen, M.F., Kasanmoentalib, S., Visser, T. & Zwart, H. (eds) *Recognising the intrinsic value of animals: beyond animal welfare.* Assen, Van Gorcum & Comp., pp. 41–53.

Sandøe, P., Christiansen, S.B. & Kristensen, A. (2008a) Companion animals. In: Sandøe, P. & Christiansen, S.B., *Ethics of animal use.* Oxford, Blackwell Publishing, pp. 119–136.

Sandøe, P., Christiansen, S.B. & Morgan, C. (2008b) Role of veterinarians and other animal science professionals. In: Sandøe, P. & Christiansen, S.B. *Ethics of animal use.* Oxford, Blackwell Publishing, pp. 49–65.

Stone, R.W. (2000) More on ear cropping and neutering (letter to the editor). *Journal of the American Veterinary Medical Association* 216 (2), 174.

Tobias, K.S. (1994) Feline onychectomy at a teaching institution: a retrospective study of 163 cases. *Veterinary Surgery* 23 (4), 274–280.

Walker, S.M., Tochiki, K.K. & Fitzgerald, M. (2009) Hindpaw incision in early life increases the hyperalgesic response to repeat surgical injury: critical period and dependence on initial afferent activity. *Pain* 147, 99–106.

Weise, E. (2009) *Banfield pet hospitals ban tail docking, ear cropping on dogs. USA Today 12 August 2009.* [Online] Available from: http://www.usatoday.com/news/nation /2009-07-30-dog-tails_N.htm [Accessed 22 July 2014].

Wilkinson, S. & Garrard, E. (1996) Bodily integrity and the sale of human organs. *Journal of Medical Ethics* 22, 334–339.

Treating Sick Animals and End-of-Life Issues

<big>**12**</big>

12.1	Introduction	186
12.2	Treating Sick Animals – Modern Veterinary Medicine	187
12.3	End-of-Life: Palliative Care and Euthanasia	189
12.4	Ethical Issues Relating to Veterinary Treatment	191
	12.4.1 Using animals to help other animals: blood, bone marrow and organ donation	193
	12.4.2 Prolonging the life of sick animals	194
	12.4.3 End-of-life decisions	196

12.1 Introduction

As we saw in Chapters 1 and 3, many people who keep animals as companions consider them to be family members, and often see them as being irreplaceable (Milligan, 2010). Owners of dogs and cats therefore, not only provide for the animals' basic requirements (food, water, shelter), but also take care of their health and comfort. The owner's relationship to a companion animal can become even more complex as the animal ages, or becomes ill; many owners are willing to go to great lengths and spend large sums of money caring for their animal companions, in sickness and in health.

As a result, difficult veterinary consultations may involve counselling owners to stop treatment of terminally ill animals (in contrast to previous decades, where vets more often had to discourage owners from euthanasing healthy companions). This is in part driven by advances in modern veterinary medicine making it possible to prolong the life of chronically ill or old animals, sometimes irrespective of their quality of life, or

Companion Animal Ethics, First Edition. Peter Sandøe, Sandra Corr and Clare Palmer.
© Universities Federation for Animal Welfare 2016.

chances of recovery. The human attachment to a companion animal can be strong and highly emotionally charged, making it very difficult for some owners to be objective when it comes to making decisions about their companion's treatment. Equally, professional, or financial, interests may motivate vets to recommend and undertake advanced investigations, or prolong treatments, even when the prognosis for the animal is poor.

Even with modern treatment advances, however, the average lifespan of companion animals remains much shorter than that of humans, with cats living around 12–16 years, and canine lifespan varying with size (average 8.5 years for a Great Dane, to 14 years for a Yorkshire Terrier). As a result, most people will experience the death of one or more of their companion animals. In some cases, the owner will actually have to take the decision to end the life of their companion animal; a uniquely stressful and at times, ethically challenging decision.

In this chapter, we begin by describing how modern veterinary medicine can extend the quality and quantity of animals' lives, through preventative health measures such as vaccination, access to pain medication and antibiotics, and more advanced treatments such as chemotherapy, blood donation and organ transplantation. We then consider veterinary aspects of palliative care of chronically or terminally ill animals, and euthanasia. Finally, we explore a number of ethical issues that arise as a result of the availability of veterinary treatment, including when the treatment may not be in the best interests of the individual, or other animals, and the option of euthanasia for ill animals.

12.2 Treating Sick Animals – Modern Veterinary Medicine

Advances in veterinary medicine over the last decade enable many animals to be treated that would previously have suffered, died, or been euthanased. Treatment may be preventative (e.g. vaccination), curative, or palliative (relieving the symptoms, but not curing the underlying condition).

Much of general veterinary practice involves providing preventative health care for animals, including regular vaccinations, worming, dietary advice and dental care, as well as treating sick pets. Owners are encouraged to take their pets to the vet for annual vaccination, and a general health check: routine vaccination against common diseases such as canine distemper and parvovirus, and feline leukaemia, has enabled millions of vaccinated animals to live longer and healthier lives. Neutering of young animals that are not going to be bred from is, in some parts of the world, widely promoted as another aspect of responsible pet ownership (see Chapter 10). In addition, many practices provide services aimed at educating clients in responsible pet ownership, by running puppy socialisation classes and training classes (see Chapter 9) and by offering behavioural advice, and other support, such as obesity clinics (see Chapter 8).

When presented with ill animals, modern vets have access to a wide range of drugs to treat chronic diseases such as heart failure, diabetes, osteoarthritis and renal disease, improving the quality and length of life of sick animals by many years. Many drugs that were previously only available for people are now routinely used to treat animals, including powerful painkillers, such as non-steroidal anti-inflammatory drugs and opioids, and antibiotics. Life-saving procedures such as blood transfusions are also now routinely performed in cats and dogs in general practice in the United States, Europe and Australasia. In some places, people typically 'volunteer' their pet as a donor animal, in others, colonies of dogs and cats are kept as donors in University hospitals. Commercial pet blood banks also exist. Donor animals receive regular health checks, and although the procedure is minimally invasive, the donor must be fasted, sedated, have a cannula inserted into the jugular vein in the neck, and be restrained while the blood is collected; this tends to be better tolerated by dogs than cats. In addition, there may be welfare costs involved in housing colonies of donor animals in kennels or catteries.

When cases are complex, or require advanced investigations or treatments, vets, like their medical colleagues, have the option to refer animals to specialists in fields such as orthopaedics, oncology and critical care. Such specialists have undergone several years of postgraduate clinical training in their chosen field. Within specialist practice, veterinary patients may undergo advanced investigations using computed tomography (CT) and magnetic resonance imaging (MRI), previously only available for people. Many previously fatal diseases can also now be routinely treated in companions, for example, using chemotherapy and radiation to manage many types of cancer, based on protocols adapted from human medicine. Where medical treatments fail, advanced surgical treatments such as hip and elbow joint replacements, or heart valve replacements, are available for companions whose owners can afford them, in many specialist veterinary centres throughout the developed world (Figure 12.1(a) and (b)).

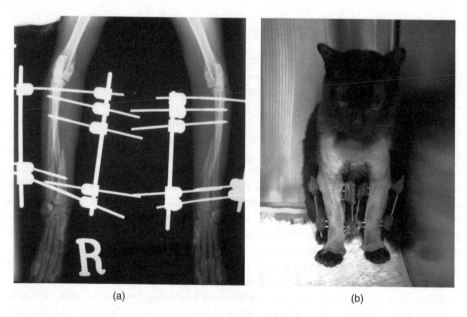

(a)   (b)

Figure 12.1   Advances in veterinary care mean that surgical techniques previously only available for humans are now routinely used in animals. This young Burmese cat suffered severe fractures of both front legs (a), but was comfortable and walking the following day, after having bilateral external skeletal fixators applied (b). (*Images used courtesy of Sandra Corr.*)

In more extreme cases, an animal's life may be saved when it is given an organ from another animal. In renal transplantation, a healthy kidney is surgically removed from a healthy donor animal, and implanted into a recipient animal with renal failure. The donor is often a stray animal from a rehoming shelter, and the usual policy is that the owner of the recipient animal must then adopt and care for the donor for the rest of its life, although this is difficult to enforce.

Renal transplantation is legal in many countries, but the procedure is controversial; it has mainly been performed in the United States, and to some extent in Australia. In the United Kingdom, RCVS (2013) guidance on renal transplantation is at the time of writing suspended, pending review. The first Renal Transplantation Program was started in the University of California (Davis), in 1987, and in 2004, it had the capacity to perform around 24 transplants each year, with success rates of 75–80% in cats and 40% in dogs (although 'success' is not defined; UC Davis, 2004). Studies have reported that up to 29% of cats receiving renal transplants die before discharge, and the remainder have median survival times of 365–613 days (Matthews & Gregory, 1997; Schmiedt *et al.*, 2008). No studies have reported the fate of the donor cats.

12.3 End-of-Life: Palliative Care and Euthanasia

Palliative care is treatment that relieves the symptoms of a disease or condition without curing the underlying cause; examples include giving painkillers to manage cancer pain, or administering nutrition via a feeding tube to an animal that is unable to eat. Palliative care is well established in human medicine, and is a growing field in veterinary medicine, particularly in the United States (where funeral homes and memorial services are also increasingly offered for animals). Palliative care of human patients may enable them to gain a little time, for example, to spend with their children, or to survive for a significant occasion (Löfmark, Nilstun & Ågren Bolmsjö, 2007). In the case of companion animals, it is the owners who often require the extra time to come to terms with losing their pet.

With advances in both human and veterinary medicine, concern is increasingly raised over whether prolongation of life at all costs is in the best interests of the patient. As most countries do not currently permit active euthanasia or assisted suicide of people (the exceptions include the Netherlands and Switzerland), the most difficult decision in human end-of-life care usually involves the point at which transference from curative to palliative care is made (Löfmark, Nilstun & Ågren Bolmsjö, 2007). In veterinary medicine, where euthanasia of incurably ill animals is the norm, the difficult decision often involves deciding *when* to perform the euthanasia.

In its broadest sense, euthanasia is defined as 'the action of inducing a gentle and easy death' (OED, 2014), where death is intended, or at least foreseen. Here we are concerned with active euthanasia (killing) rather than passive euthanasia (letting die when one could keep alive). Normally, active euthanasia refers to killing for the benefit of the one killed, such as would be the case with very ill and dying animals. (There is some controversy about using the term to describe the painless killing of healthy but unwanted animals – see Chapter 13.) The practice of active euthanasia is perhaps the most significant difference between human and veterinary medicine, and the claim is often made, in this context, that animals are in this respect treated better than humans.

In companion animals, euthanasia is most commonly performed by administering an overdose of an anaesthetic drug intravenously into a catheter placed into a vein in the animal's leg, which causes cardiac arrest (usually within 1 minute). Other than the catheter placement, the procedure is painless and appears to cause minimal distress to the animal. Most vets will arrange for cremation of the body, either individually (with many owners requesting return of the ashes), or as a group cremation with other deceased animals, although some owners elect to take the body home for burial (where local laws permit this) (Figure 12.2).

For some people, the decision to euthanase an animal is straightforward, either on financial, convenience, or compassionate grounds. In many cases, however, the owner's

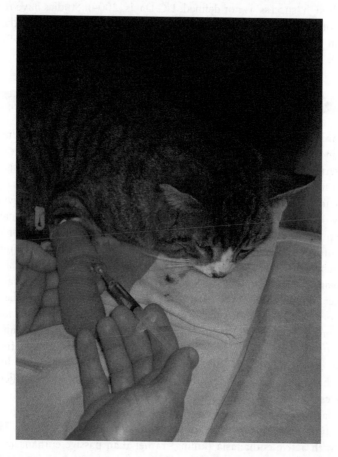

Figure 12.2 Euthanasia of a stray cat with severe head injuries. The cat was initially given first aid; however, the owner could not be found, and due to the severity of the injuries, the cat was euthanased the following day. An injection of Euthatal (Pentobarbital sodium) is being administered via an intravenous catheter into the cephalic vein. (*Image used courtesy of Sandra Corr.*)

attachment to a companion animal means that the decision to undertake euthanasia is often a difficult and protracted one (see Section 12.4.3). In some European countries, for example, Denmark, legislation requires that incurably ill animals should be euthanased if a prolonged life will lead to unnecessary suffering; and it is a legal offence for a vet not to act on such a case (Ministeriet for Fødevarer, 2014: § 20). Different ethical issues are raised by the euthanasia of healthy animals: these are considered in Chapter 13.

12.4 Ethical Issues Relating to Veterinary Treatment

As developments in veterinary medicine keep pace with human medicine, owners and vets have to make increasingly complex decisions about medical treatments. As animals cannot communicate preferences about their own treatment, they must rely on their caregivers – owners and vets – to make decisions, each of whom may have a different agenda (Yeates, 2010). One area of difference is likely to concern whether the interests of the animal, the owner, or even the veterinary surgeon, should take priority, and to what extent. Our inability to decide how, or *if*, a sick animal would want to be treated – or even whether an animal can form a preference – resembles the situation with people who cannot make or express informed decisions, such as the very young, the mentally impaired, or comatose patients. In such cases, the principle of 'best interests' is usually applied, choosing the action that is likely to produce the greatest balance of benefit over harm for the individual, with best interests described as:

> being free of distressing physical symptoms, being free of excessive psycho-
> logical, emotional and existential suffering, to have dignity preserved and
> to live in a state that is generally regarded as not worse than death.
>
> (Berger, 2011)

Perhaps not all of these interests can straightforwardly be attributed to animals, but the underlying principles can inform decision making.

Taking 'best interests' as a goal also implies that the interests of the animal are paramount, and does not necessarily take into account those of the owner or other interested parties. This focus on the animal is adopted by those who favour 'patient advocacy', a view promoting the treatment most likely to provide the greatest benefit with least risk to the animal, irrespective of the owner's wishes and financial constraints.

Other views – perhaps from a more human-centred, contractarian perspective – emphasise the ways animals matter to their owners, rather than being directly concerned about the animals themselves. As many of those who live with animal companions are very attached to them, this more indirect view would still normally result in animals receiving appropriate veterinary treatment. But strong attachment can also have nega-tive consequences for the animal, if an owner keeps a suffering companion animal alive, because euthanasing it would cause her or him (the owner) emotional or psychologi-cal distress. Conversely, from this perspective, it would be acceptable for an owner to euthanase an animal for any reason, no matter how trivial, as the focus is on human desires, not animals' interests.

Vets may, therefore, face significant ethical challenges, as they try to serve the sometimes incompatible interests of both the animals and their owners. Trying to find a
'middle ground' between the best care available and what the owner is willing or able
to spend on treatment can create significant conflict. While some owners choose to spend
little or no money on treating their sick animals, others insist that 'everything must be
done', requesting 'heroic' treatments that may have little chance of success.

So, what motivates owners so differently with regard to the treatment decisions they
make about their companions? Important 'external' influences include the particular
disease and likelihood of recovery, the cost of treatment, and the advice given by the vet.
Internal influences will include the owner's level of attachment to the animal, and their
own particular ethical framework(s). For example, an owner may be more attached to
an animal they have had for a long time, especially if that animal is a link to something
in the past that no longer exists, for example, a deceased partner (Hart, Hart & Mader,
1990). The relation may become more complex when the animal becomes ill, as Sandøe
& Christiansen (2008) discuss: an animal's illness may strengthen the attachment (as the
owner cares for the animal), or weaken it (if the animal can no longer fulfil the role the
owner requires of it). This was explored further in a recent paper by Christiansen *et al.*
(2013), who found that while some owners considered it rewarding to look after their
sick pet, others felt a sense of loss, while others expressed sadness, frustration and guilt.

Veterinary attitudes can be equally diverse. Some vets, in pursuing academic satisfaction or profitable business, may be biased in advising owners to undertake major costly
treatments, which can make owners feel guilty if they do not pursue them, overwhelmed
with choices, or unaware that they can refuse the treatment. Yeates (2010) highlights
this relatively recent change in veterinary-focused motivations towards profit, career
development, 'heroism', public relations and avoiding litigation (e.g. if a client feels
that the vet did not do 'everything possible' to save their animal). In other cases, vets
may be reluctant to stop treatment or recommend euthanasia, because they feel that by
doing so, they are somehow failing the animal and/or the client.

Whatever decision about treatment is made, it is ultimately the client who determines
what happens to their animal, as by law, the animal remains the property of the owner
(see Chapter 16). Only in cases where an animal has a severe injury that cannot be
treated, or a terminal illness, such that to allow it to go on living would cause unnecessary suffering, can the vet in some countries (but not everywhere) disregard the owner's
wishes, and have legal protection. Nonetheless, respect for the autonomy of the client
varies, and Fettman & Rollin (2002: p. 1391) state that:

> the challenge for veterinarians is to provide enough information and
> recommendations to facilitate adequate informed consent from the owner
> without compromising the health of the patient, nor imposing personal
> preferences that may impose acceptance of a level of risk against the client's
> own inclinations.

In the next section, we consider veterinary treatments where the interests of *other*
animals are involved, and then explore in more depth the ethical issues relating to continuing veterinary treatment versus euthanasia.

12.4.1 Using animals to help other animals: blood, bone marrow and organ donation

Using animals to treat other animals, such as through blood transfusions, bone marrow or organ transplants, raises interesting ethical questions about who benefits and who is harmed, and about the impossibility of acquiring consent from the donor (or the recipient).

Take blood donations as an example. From a perspective such as contractarianism, on which human desires are of primary importance, animal-to-animal blood donation would be supported, inasmuch as it would reduce the distress of the owner of a sick companion, and enable the owner of the donor animal to feel that they and their companion had done a good thing. From a broadly utilitarian perspective, blood donations could in theory be justified where the benefits to the recipient animal significantly outweigh the costs to the donor animal (and the human owners). As blood donation, though stressful to some animals in the short term, is unlikely to seriously impair the donor's health, while potentially saving the recipient's life, it looks as though blood donation will in practice frequently be justified on utilitarian grounds. Overall, it is also likely, from this perspective, that the establishment of blood banks can be ethically justified; bone marrow transplants could probably be similarly justified, although, unlike blood donations, these require the donor to undergo a general anaesthetic, minor surgical procedure, and some post-operative discomfort.

Objections to this generally permissive view flow from ethical positions that maintain, for different reasons, that it is 'wrong to take blood from one individual to give to another' (Ashall, 2009); for instance, because animals have rights not to be harmed, or because they cannot give consent. Ashall (2009) proposes that the owners of blood donor animals usually desire to help animals, and may be motivated by anthropomorphism, believing that their animal would like to help others too (this sounds like a kind of *implied* consent). However, there is obviously no reason to attribute this motivation to animals. A better reason might be that, in the case of a blood bank, at least, a donor animal might at some time in the future benefit from being able to use it; if the animal has a chance of a significant benefit later, perhaps the idea of implied consent to the lesser harm now becomes more plausible.

Mullan (2010) considers whether any non-utilitarian ethical arguments used to permit children who are too young to consent, to donate to siblings, could also work for animals. But, as she notes, successfully transferring such arguments to animals is difficult. Animals, for instance, unlike siblings, will not later derive psychological benefits from being donors, nor gain from later association with the recipient sibling (though if the donor animal lives with the recipient animal, it could gain benefits later). The idea that a child has a duty to its family to donate (doubtful even in the human case) also does not easily transfer to animals; this would require extending 'family' to include the whole species, which, Mullan notes, would at least dilute any putative duty. On the other hand, it is also true that animals would not be traumatised later by discovering they had been used as donors, which could happen in the case of a human child.

These worries are more problematic in the case of organ donation, where there are significant adverse effects, and no direct benefits, for the donor animal. In the United

States, the donor is often a stray animal sourced from a shelter. In the United Kingdom, a leading animal charity – the RSPCA – clearly states as policy that it:

> is opposed to the killing or use of live animals for organ donation to other animals … and will not provide animals as donors for such transplant surgery, except for blood transfusion as an emergency procedure.
>
> (RSPCA, 2013)

Organ donation would be permissible from a broadly contractarian perspective, for the same reasons as blood donation. From a utilitarian perspective, organ donation may be permissible in some cases. For instance, if a donor animal is in a shelter and, as a consequence of the donation, is adopted, treated well, and would otherwise remain unadopted, it is likely to benefit over the course of its life (and it would not suffer the psychological difficulties a human in this situation would), while the recipient is likely to benefit from the donation, for a while at least. This seems to maximise benefits (though it might be argued that given the high cost of organ donation, using the money to improve shelter animal welfare instead, for instance, would increase overall benefit even more). A more contextual ethical approach, such as an ethic of care, would also likely accept organ donation in some cases – where the relation between the owner and the recipient animal is retained or strengthened, and a new relation of care and appreciation could be established with the donor animal.

From animal rights and other deontological perspectives, though, companion animal organ donation seems ethically unacceptable. The donor is subject to significant harm without his or her consent, and their bodily integrity is violated. It is very difficult to argue that the recipient animal is 'owed' a transplant, which might defeat these other concerns; while it can be argued that a donor animal has a right not to be harmed, no one argues that animals (or indeed humans!) have a general 'right' to be recipients of complex and expensive transplant surgery.

So, using animals to help other animals will often be acceptable to ethical approaches that consider only the interests of the involved humans, such as contractarianism, or that focus on bringing about best consequences, such as utilitarianism, though utilitarians will take a case-by-case approach. However, some ethical perspectives, such as animal rights views, will raise significant moral concerns about animal-to-animal donation; and these concerns become more intense the greater the risk or harm to the donor animal.

12.4.2 Prolonging the life of sick animals

The benefits of improved health care for companion animals are clear, but the *quality* of an animal's life during and after treatment must be weighed against its increased lifespan. As an example, we can consider the management of dogs and cats with terminal cancer, such as osteosarcoma. Osteosarcoma is the most common bone tumour of dogs and cats. Previously, most animals would have been euthanased at or soon after diagnosis, as without treatment, they would live 2–3 months in severe pain. There are now many different treatment options available for this type of cancer; however, none will cure the animal, and the animal will ultimately be euthanased as a result of unmanageable pain, local recurrence of the tumour, or secondary metastases.

Currently, the most effective and commonly practised treatment in dogs is limb amputation and chemotherapy, which gives a median survival time of around a year, with a quality of life as an amputee that most owners and vets judge to be acceptable; that is, the animal is seen to have a life still worth living, where the dog's good states (such as enjoyment) are not outweighed by its bad states, such as suffering, or frustration. Some owners do not want their animal to undergo such major surgery, however, and request other palliative treatments such as painkillers, or radiotherapy, which may relieve the pain for several weeks or months. From every ethical perspective on which animal suffering matters, the quality of life of the animal during the period of palliation is a crucial issue. If an animal's life seems to be not worth living, then the question of whether it should be euthanased is raised. The difficulty is, of course, in determining when an animal's life becomes no longer worth living; a subject explored in depth by Jessica Pierce in *The Last Walk* (Pierce, 2012).

Further ethical issues are raised when life is prolonged using treatments that might be considered novel or 'heroic', alternatively described as innovative, experimental, unproven, or 'high risk'. Examples include heart valve replacements and renal transplants (discussed previously) both of which are performed in cats and dogs (though rarely). In human medicine, such procedures, now relatively routine, were also once experimental, often resulting in the death of the patient. A significant difference between human and veterinary medicine now is that human medical research and innovation – essential for progress – is closely regulated and audited, and while similar regulation exists in universities and veterinary research institutes in most Western countries, vets in practice can undertake novel treatments with little or no regulation, if they gain owner consent. Agich (2001) points out that any deviation from standard care involves a degree of experimentation, and this requires procedures to be in place to protect the rights and welfare of the subjects. These requirements may not be met in practice, presenting modern vets wishing to be at the cutting edge with ethical challenges – for example, undertaking novel investigations or treatments to advance veterinary knowledge, but at the risk of compromising the welfare of the individual patient.

Another area of ethical concern relates to possible *overtreatment*, as veterinary medicine becomes increasingly specialised and more people have pet insurance. 'Overtreatment' may be defined in a number of different ways, including: a treatment or test that makes no difference to the animal's condition or quality of life, a treatment that results in them being worse off than having no treatment at all or being euthanased, or a treatment that is chosen in favour of a cheaper but equally effective treatment (James Yeates, personal communication). Here, the most relevant notion of 'overtreatment' is the second of these, that is, treatment undertaken against the best interests of the affected animal. Potential overtreatment of this kind may be most frequent in certain specialties, such as geriatric medicine, or critical care/emergency medicine, where the lives of seriously ill animals can be saved, but where they may be left with a life that is not worth living, where the negative experiences of continuing to live outweigh any positive experiences the animals may have.

Ethical concerns about overtreatment in the other senses will depend on the nature and extent of what occurs. Running unnecessary, expensive tests on a blood sample has financial implications for the owner; but while this could negatively impact on the owner's welfare if resources are tight, and would be morally unacceptable for other reasons from almost all ethical perspectives, it would not cause significant pain to the animal, nor impact in other ways on the animal's welfare. In contrast, performing a highly invasive experimental procedure, when there are simpler proven methods of achieving the same result, could have direct, avoidable, adverse consequences for the animal. This kind of overtreatment would be problematic from every ethical perspective we have considered. From a broadly contractarian view, the financial and perhaps emotional cost of such a procedure to the owner would very likely be substantial and therefore count against performing it. For a utilitarian, the risk of unnecessary suffering would be increased, while an animal rights theorist would maintain that the animal's rights not to be seriously harmed could be violated. So, overtreatment may, in some cases, pose a significant ethical problem.

12.4.3 End-of-life decisions

Difficult ethical decisions face both owners and vets when companion animals are in significant pain or distress from incurable injuries and illnesses. Vets may offer palliative care, relieving animals' pain to some degree, but this raises the question for how long palliative care is appropriate, and *whether* and *when* an animal should be actively euthanased (i.e. given drugs that will actively kill it, rather than passively allowing it to die).

We will first consider whether it is ethically acceptable to allow a sick animal to die without intervening. Some owners, when told that their animal has a terminal illness, express a desire for the animal to die 'naturally' at home, with, or without, palliative care. This may be motivated by a moral objection to taking a life, an inability or unwillingness to end *their* companion's life, or for financial reasons, to avoid paying for euthanasia to be performed. From a contractarian perspective, in which only the owners' interests matter, this would be acceptable, irrespective of the reason. However, a study of pet owners found that those who had decided to let their pet die naturally subsequently expressed guilt for allowing what was sometimes a slow and painful death (Quackenbush & Glickman, 1984). From most other ethical perspectives, allowing an animal to die naturally, when it would likely involve suffering, would be ethically unacceptable, and, in some countries, also illegal.

If the idea of allowing the animal to die naturally is rejected, there are two other sorts of ethical concerns to consider: in principle, questions about when (if ever) euthanasia of companion animals is ethically acceptable (or required); and more practical questions, concerning the actual decisions taken by owners and vets about an animal's future.

On a view on which only humans matter ethically, euthanasia of companion animals is only of moral significance inasmuch as it impacts on those humans who care about those animals. From other ethical perspectives, however, animals matter in themselves. But, as we discussed in Chapter 5, this does not necessarily mean that *killing* them is always morally wrong. For a hedonistic utilitarian, for instance, killing an animal is only problematic when it reduces pleasure, or increases pain, in the world. Painlessly killing an animal that has a future containing only unremitting and unending suffering would *reduce* pain in the world, and it is very unlikely that an owner's desire to keep the animal alive could outweigh the animal's suffering. Euthanasia would likely be morally required on this view.

A preference utilitarian, even one who believed dogs and cats to be self-conscious (see Chapter 5) with preferences to go on living, would also think that euthanasia is acceptable in this kind of case. While a dog or a cat could not *express* a preference to die, it does not seem far-fetched to attribute either an unexpressed or a hypothetical preference to die, in circumstances of unremitting and unending suffering.

While, on a rights view, the right to life is usually taken to be an animal's most basic right, where an animal is in severe and incurable pain, we can reasonably assume that – as discussed in Chapter 5 – the animal would waive this right. The animal rights theorist Tom Regan (1984: p. 10), for instance, argues that euthanasia is permissible under certain conditions: the individual must be killed by the least painful means available; the one who kills must believe that the death of the one who is killed is in the interests of the latter, and must be motivated to end the life of the one who is killed out of concern for the latter's interests, good, or welfare.

So, while different ethical interpretations of killing dogs and cats are highly significant in the case of healthy animals that could go on to have good lives, as we will see in Chapter 13, where an animal is undergoing severe pain and distress, with no possibility of relief, virtually every ethical view converges to agree that euthanasia is either acceptable, desirable, or morally required (on many of these views, this is also true of humans in similar states).

However, in practice, decisions about euthanasia can be difficult, and may come in some sense either 'too soon' while an animal has good life left to live with palliative care, or 'too late' when suffering has become intense and quality of life is very poor. This may be due to a lack of knowledge, given the difficulty involved in judging how much an animal is suffering based largely on its behaviour and on medical tests. But other factors may also be significant. Owners may want to euthanase an animal when it could still have good life ahead of it because they cannot afford or do not want to pay for veterinary and palliative care. Other owners may prefer to euthanase an animal sooner rather than later to spare themselves the distress of watching their companion deteriorating, even if the animal's quality of life could be good with palliative care.

On other occasions, owners want to keep animals alive even when palliative care is no longer providing the animal with an adequate quality of life. When the animal is considered a member of the family, making the decision to end its life can be a very distressing, complex and protracted process, often described by owners as the hardest thing they have ever had to do. Because the decision is so difficult and the emotions involved intense, owners may delay euthanasia, then subsequently feel guilty and express regret at having been unable to make the decision sooner (Sandra Corr, personal communication). In a survey, veterinary students reported that one of the most upsetting situations to which they were commonly exposed was witnessing the prolongation of an animal's suffering when an owner was unable to accept that it could not be cured (Herzog *et al.*, 1989). Such scenarios are not uncommon (see Morris (2012) *Blue juice: euthanasia in veterinary medicine*. 'Blue juice' is a colloquial name for the euthanasia drug solution).

Such cases are obviously very difficult for vets, as the patient's interests appear to be in conflict with the client's interests, and the vet is being paid by the client. Vets may take different ethical perspectives, focusing only on the impact on the human client, only on the interests of the companion animal, or attempting to take into account the interests of the owner, the companion animal, other family members, as well as their own interests. Treating severely ill and dying animals often has an emotional cost to the vet as well as the owner, for example, when they are unable to relieve suffering (due to the nature of the illness, or emotional or financial constraints placed on them by the owner), or have to perform euthanasia.

In reality, decisions about *when* to euthanase an animal are influenced by many factors, including: whether the owners were expecting to have to make the decision, their level of denial about the animal's chances of recovery or degree of suffering (both current and future), and the predicted timescales for deterioration; financial factors such as the cost of palliative care; the owners' ability to actually make the decision and the need for other family members to have input into the decision, and other unrelated life events (such as impending family holidays, or current family illness).

Following the loss of a companion animal, most owners suffer similar symptoms of grief to those seen at the loss of a human: anger, guilt, despair, loss of appetite, sleep, longing and withdrawal (Milligan, 2010). As described by Morris (2012), the situation can be made worse by the fact that bereaved pet owners often feel unable to express their grief openly, for fear that other people will not understand, will judge them, or will make comments such as 'it was only a cat/dog – just get another one'. This kind of response, as Sanders (1995) notes, flows from the tension between the ways in which many owners view their animal companions as persons or near-persons, while others see them as non-persons or even as replaceable objects. The complex emotions that many owners feel are highlighted in the following letter, sent to the vet by the owner of a dog euthanased due to serious injuries after being hit by a car (used with permission, and edited):

> On Wednesday I went out for a walk with my two dogs and returned with one. I lost my father too soon in my life and his, and I felt that if I could deal with that pain, you're pretty much armed to take on anything. I was wrong. The range of emotions that I have felt since Wednesday afternoon I am ashamed to admit surpasses any of my life's experiences. The intensity, the shock, the blame, the shame, the grief and the sadness have at times been unbearable.
>
> It was only a dog I have told myself. But she wasn't. She was my naughty little mate, she was the ball of endless energy that I could only dream to be, she was the in house comedian and my own personal trainer and she greeted me every time I came home to an empty house. I suppose I am describing every dog that lives in a loving home but she wasn't every dog, she was our dog. She depended on me and now I realise I depended on her. She left far far too early and she has broken our hearts and we already miss her more than I could ever have imagined.
>
> (S. Starkey, on the loss of his dog, Kiri)

In conclusion, the strong attachment that many people have to their companion animals becomes more complex when the animal becomes ill, or the owner has to make decisions about ending the animal's life. This may be a time when the interests of the owner, the animal and the vet are not fully compatible. Different ethical perspectives will view these possible conflicts of interest differently, but on most ethical views, it is the *quality*, rather than the quantity, of the animal's life that is of the greatest ethical significance.

Key Points

- Most owners of companion animals at some point have to deal with the illness and death of their animal.
- Advances in modern veterinary medicine mean many animals can be saved that would previously have suffered, died or been euthanased.
- The availability of advanced treatments and palliative care raises concerns that animals' lifespan may be extended without due consideration of the *quality* of that additional life.
- The relationship between vet, client and patient is a complex one, and their interests and desires may conflict in terms of the appropriate treatment of sick animals.
- The use of donor animals for blood and organs raises difficult ethical questions about whether benefits to recipient animals can be weighed against the harm to, and lack of consent of, donor animals.
- Unregulated 'novel' treatment, and overtreatment that may not be in the best interests of the animals concerned, are becoming ethical issues.
- Euthanasia of incurably suffering animals raises ethical questions about how death matters ethically for companion animals, and when euthanasia is permissible or desirable.

References

Agich, G.J. (2001) Ethics and innovation in medicine. *Journal of Medical Ethics* 27, 295–296.

Ashall, V. (2009) Everyday ethics: canine blood donor. *In Practice* 31, 527.

Berger, J.T. (2011) Is best interests a relevant decision making standard for enrolling non-capacitated subjects into clinical research? *Journal of Medical Ethics* 37, 45–49.

Christiansen, S.B., Kristensen, A.T., Sandøe, P. & Lassen, J. (2013) Looking after chronically ill dogs: impacts on the caregiver's life. *Anthrozoös* 26 (4), 519–533.

Fettman, M.J. & Rollin, B.E. (2002) Modern elements of informed consent for general veterinary practitioners. *Journal of the American Veterinary Medical Association* 221, 1386–1393.

Hart, L.A., Hart, B.L. & Mader, B. (1990) Humane euthanasia and companion animal death: caring for the animal, the client, and the veterinarian. *Journal of the American Veterinary Medical Association* 197 (10), 1292–1299.

Herzog, H.A., Vore, T.L. & New, J.C. (1989) Conversations with veterinary students: attitudes, ethics, and animals. *Anthrozoös* 2, 181–188.

Löfmark, R., Nilstun, T. & Ågren Bolmsjö, I. (2007) From cure to palliation: concept, decision and acceptance. *Journal of Medical Ethics* 33, 685–688.

Matthews, K.G. & Gregory, C.R. (1997) Renal transplants in cats: 66 cases (1987–1996). *Journal of the American Veterinary Medical Association* 211 (11), 1432–1436.

Milligan, T. (2010) Love for pets. In: Milligan, T. (ed.) *Think now: beyond animal rights: food, pets and ethics*. London, Continuum International Publishing, 106–125.

Ministeriet for Fødevarer, Landbrug og Fiskeri [Ministry of Food, Agriculture and Fisheries of Denmark] (2014). *Bekendtgørelse af dyreværnsloven, LBK nr 473 af 15/05/2014* [Notice on the animal protection law]. [Online] Available from: https://www.retsinformation.dk/Forms/R0710.aspx?id=162911 [Accessed 20 August 2014].

Morris, P. (2012) *Blue juice: euthanasia in veterinary medicine*. Philadelphia, PA, Temple University Press.

Mullan, S. (2010) Comments on the dilemma in the November/December 2009 issue: 'canine blood donor'. *Practice* 32, 39.

OED [Oxford English Dictionary] (2014). [Online] Available from: http://www.oed.com/ [Accessed 20 August 2014].

Pierce, J. (2012) *The last walk: reflections on our pets at the end of their lives*. Chicago, IL & London, UK, The University of Chicago Press.

Quackenbush, J.E. & Glickman, L. (1984) Helping people adjust to the death of a pet. *Health and Social Work* 9, 42–48.

RCVS [Royal College of Veterinary Surgeons] (2013) *Code of professional conduct for veterinary surgeons: renal transplantation (cats)*. [Online] Available from: http://www.rcvs.org.uk/advice-and-guidance/code-of-professional-conduct-for-veterinary-surgeons/supporting-guidance/miscellaneous/ [Accessed 20 August 2014].

Regan, T. (1984) *The case for animal rights*. Berkeley, CA, University of California Press.

RSPCA [Royal Society for the Prevention of Cruelty to Animals] (2013) *RSPCA policies on animal welfare*. [Online] Available from: http://www.rspca.org.uk/ImageLocator/LocateAsset?asset=document&assetId=1232729988566&mode=prd [Accessed 20 August 2014].

Sanders, C.R. (1995) Killing with kindness: veterinary euthanasia and the social construction of personhood. *Sociological Forum* 10 (2), 195–214.

Sandøe, P. & Christiansen, S.B. (2008) *Ethics of animal use*. Oxford, Blackwell Publishing.

Schmiedt, C.W., Holzman, G., Schawarz, T. & McAnulty, J.F. (2008) Survival, complications, and analysis of risk factors after renal transplantation in cats. *Veterinary Surgery* 37, 683–695.

UC Davis Veterinary Medicine [University of California] (2004) *Kidney transplant program helps cats and dogs thrive: veterinarians also investigate techniques to improve long-term survival*. [Online] Available from: http://www.vetmed.ucdavis.edu/whatsnew/article2.cfm?id=1402. [Accessed 20 August 2014]

Yeates, J.W. (2010) When to euthanase. *Veterinary Record* 166, 370–371.

Unwanted and Unowned Companion Animals

13

13.1 Introduction	201
13.2 Why Do Companion Animals Become Unwanted?	202
13.3 Ethical Issues for Owners with Unwanted Companions: Shelters and Abandonment	203
13.4 Euthanasia of Unwanted Healthy Companion Animals	206
13.5 Unowned Animal Populations: Numbers and Relationships	209
13.5.1 Unowned cats: relations to people	210
13.6 Managing Unowned Populations	211
13.6.1 Why manage populations?	211
13.6.2 Ethics of managing unowned cat populations	211

13.1 Introduction

Many dogs and cats live their entire lives under the care and protection of human owners, and most of the ethical questions we have considered so far in this book arise within the context of ongoing companion animal relationships. However, these relationships may fail. Owners' circumstances may change, meaning that they either cannot, or no longer want to, live with their companions. This raises difficult questions about what to do with an unwanted companion; choices include rehoming, abandonment,

Companion Animal Ethics, First Edition. Peter Sandøe, Sandra Corr and Clare Palmer.
© Universities Federation for Animal Welfare 2016.

relinquishment to a shelter, and euthanasia. The decision whether to euthanase a healthy companion raises significant ethical questions for vets and shelter workers, as well as for the owner. We consider ethical questions raised by unwanted companion animals in the first part of this chapter.

Some unwanted companion animals end up homeless, joining existing unowned populations of stray and feral animals. In industrialised Western nations, because of concerns about public health and nuisance, the welfare of the animals themselves, or wildlife protection, these populations are generally managed. But doing so opens up highly controversial ethical issues – for instance, whether to permit or support trap-neuter-return cat colonies. In the second part of this chapter, we consider broader ethical issues raised by managing populations, primarily of unowned cats.

13.2 Why Do Companion Animals Become Unwanted?

Why do owners come to the point of relinquishing, abandoning or euthanasing their healthy companion animals? Studies have mostly been carried out with owners who are in the process of relinquishing animals to shelters for possible adoption or euthanasia. These studies consistently find similar explanations as to why companion animals have become unwanted, though the significance of each reason varies between studies (which may reflect national and cultural differences) and to some degree between dogs and cats. It is worth noting, though, that some researchers, when interviewing people visiting animal shelters to relinquish their animal, found that in the course of in-depth interviews, the initial reason the owner gave for relinquishing their animals changed, or turned out to be only part of the reason for relinquishment (Irvine, 2003). Thus, caution is required when evaluating self-reported reasons for relinquishment.

The main reasons given for relinquishing companion animals at shelters are changes in circumstances (in particular, moving home, new landlords that do not permit animal companions, a new baby, and divorce), 'bad behaviour' (see Chapter 9) and allergies. Other common reasons are that caring for the animal is too time-consuming (especially dogs), that the animal costs too much to maintain, that the owner is having personal problems, or that the owner has too many companion animals already (Scarlett *et al.*, 1999). DiGiacomo, Arluke & Patronek (1998), for instance, found that 27% of animals were relinquished to shelters because of moving home or divorce, that 26.4% of dogs were relinquished for 'bad behaviour', 12% of animals were relinquished because the owners lacked time or money to deal with them, and another 12% because they had 'too many animals'. Economic downturn can contribute to an increase in animal abandonments and relinquishments, especially where owners' properties have been foreclosed (Nowicki, 2011).

New *et al.* (2000) identified certain risk factors for animals being relinquished to shelters: being intact, younger and of a mixed breed; having an owner younger than the age 35, especially a male owner; and not having been owned for very long. Unsurprisingly, one study found that attachment scores (discussed in Chapter 3) were significantly lower for owners relinquishing animals at a shelter in comparison with those bringing animals to a shelter for vaccination (Kwan & Bain, 2013). In the case of dogs, a further risk factor for relinquishment seems to be membership of a breed that is particularly demanding in terms of behaviour or care but that is enjoying temporary fad or status popularity. In the United Kingdom, for instance, acquisitions of wolf-like dogs such as Malamutes, Huskies and Sarloos surged after these dogs' appearance in popular TV shows and films around 2011; but relinquishments soon followed, as these dog breeds can be difficult to live with (Blue Cross, 2012).

13.3 Ethical Issues for Owners with Unwanted Companions: Shelters and Abandonment

The situations described above raise questions as to when it is ethically acceptable to deliberately separate from one's companion, and what options it is acceptable to choose.

In cases where an owner really has no choice but to part with a companion animal – perhaps because a disabling illness renders them unable to take care of the animal – then the separation itself is not an ethical issue. Almost all ethicists accept a principle usually called 'ought implies can' – you can only be required to do something when you are *able* to do it. The situation is less clear-cut when an owner *could* keep an animal, but there are greater (or lesser) pressures to do otherwise, although here, too, much of what is at stake ethically concerns what the options for the companion actually are.

In some cases, it may be possible to find an animal a good home with friends or family, where – although there may initially be distress on both sides – not only will the animal's needs be met, but it will also have good welfare. Some ethicists argue that this kind of arrangement is the *only* ethically acceptable way of parting from an animal companion. So, Burgess-Jackson (1997) argues:

> I have an obligation in such a case to find another home for the animal, and not just someone who will take the dog in. My responsibility is to find someone who will fulfil the dog's primary needs just as I would, if I could.

However, such good homes are often very difficult to find. For many people, the only alternatives may be relinquishing healthy animals to a shelter, abandoning them, or having them euthanased either at the shelter or at a veterinary clinic. So, the first consideration here is whether owners can attempt to overcome the difficulties created by keeping the animal. While financial issues may be tough to resolve, other issues (for instance, behavioural ones – see Chapter 9) may be prevented, or resolved, if help is available – for example, some organisations offer courses for owners and their puppies or young dogs aimed at basic training and socialization. Many veterinary practices (in industrialised Western countries) also offer a variety of services, including holding 'puppy parties' (for early socialisation) and training classes, and arranging consultations for owners with 'problem' pets to receive advice from specialists in animal behaviour. On most ethical views, trying to prevent behavioural problems from occurring, and treating them if they do occur, is the best solution. This prevents predictable suffering or death for the animal, as well as the individual and community costs of abandonment, sheltering, or euthanasing the animal, and it strengthens the attachment of the owner to the animal.

But supposing that the potential problems cannot be overcome, and a good alternative home cannot be identified, what ethical issues are raised by the remaining options: a shelter, abandonment or euthanasia?

The ASPCA (n.d.) estimates that 7.9 million cats and dogs enter shelters each year in the United States, roughly 3.9 million dogs and 3.4 million cats. Of these, according to the ASPCA, about twice as many are picked up and brought to the shelter as are directly owner-relinquished. In the case of dogs, a significant proportion (26%) are returned to their owners (so these are stray, rather than abandoned, dogs) but less than 5% of cats are returned to owners. A study of three animal shelters in Melbourne found that 15.1% of the dogs admitted to the shelter were relinquished by their owners (and 8% of relinquishing owners requested immediate euthanasia for their dog); but all the rest were brought in as strays (Marston, Bennett & Coleman, 2004). These statistics may suggest that more people abandon than relinquish their animals; nonetheless, clearly many people do choose to relinquish to the shelter either for adoption or euthanasia (where this is permitted by the shelter).

When an animal is relinquished to a shelter for adoption, its basic needs in terms of food, hydration and protection are normally met. However, in other respects, it is often difficult for shelters, which are usually constrained in terms of budget, space and staffing, to provide for other aspects of welfare beyond looking after the fulfilment of the animals' physiological needs. Shelter animals are usually confined in small spaces for long periods of time, and may have insufficient social contact of the right kind (with friendly and known humans and members of their own species), or too much social contact of the wrong kind (with unknown humans and hostile animals). A further source of stress is high noise levels within the shelter environment (Coppola, Enns & Grandin, 2006). Research indicates that during their first 3 days in an animal shelter, dogs' cortisol levels (a physiological indicator of stress) 'are almost three times those of normal household dogs' (Coppola, Enns & Grandin, 2010), although these levels diminish over time as the animal becomes, to some degree, acclimatised to the shelter environment. While the impact of the stressors can be reduced by attempts to improve housing, social interaction and environmental stimulation, and reduce noise, for both dogs and cats, a shelter environment is stressful, especially in the first few days (Figure 13.1).

If there is a positive outcome of successful adoption from a shelter, however, this stress appears worthwhile from virtually every perspective: the animal is not killed, it can reasonably be expected to have a good life, and the adopter has a new companion. However, if the animal is not adopted, the future looks less good: the animal may be 'warehoused' (confined for long periods in a small cage), or, if it is in an open access shelter (i.e. a shelter that accepts all animals brought in, rather than accepting only those it can adopt out), the animal may be euthanased. In California, for instance, 81% of cats impounded in open access shelters were ultimately euthanased (Kass, 2005); in 1997, in the United States, it is estimated that 64% of all the animals that entered shelters were euthanased, although some of these may have been sick (AHA, n.d.). These statistics may have changed in the United States recently due to more focus on rehoming shelter animals in so-called no-kill shelters (see more on this below), and they may vary

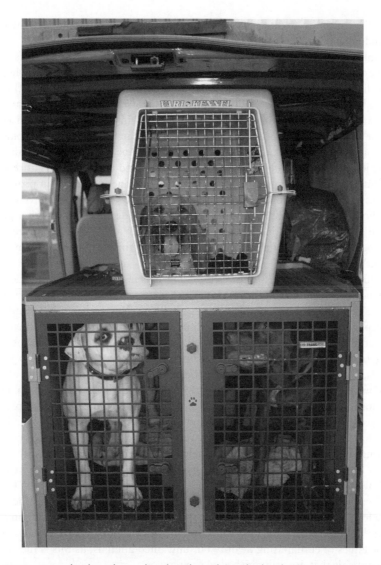

Figure 13.1 Dogs that have been abandoned or relinquished to this Rescue Organisation in the United Kingdom are routinely brought to the local veterinary practice for health checks and neutering, prior to being rehomed. (*Image used courtesy of Sandra Corr.*)

somewhat across nations, but in most countries, more than half of the animals in animal shelters are euthanased. (We will return to the ethical issues raised by euthanasia of healthy but unwanted companion animals shortly.)

Finkler & Terkel (2012) speculate that, in the case of cats at least, knowing about high euthanasia rates in shelters encourages owners to prefer abandonment to shelter relinquishment: 'It is … possible that people also believe it to be more moral to abandon the cat to the street than to relinquish it to a shelter'. Could those who think that abandonment may be better, be right?

It is unlikely that any general conclusion could be drawn here. Which is ethically preferable will depend on whether the animal concerned is a dog or a cat, whether the animal is likely to be 'adoptable', and what kind of history and experience the animal has, as well as broader social and environmental issues (see Chapter 14). It is also worth noting that in many countries, abandonment is illegal. In Western industrialised countries, most abandoned dogs are captured and taken to shelters (although in some North American inner cities and rural areas of southern Europe, especially Italy, abandoned dogs may join feral or semi-feral dog populations). Most dogs have been entirely dependent on human provision and care, and are completely inexperienced in providing for themselves; their welfare following abandonment is likely to be poor. Given this, and the likelihood that they will be captured anyway, relinquishment to a shelter generally looks like a better option than abandonment in terms of dog welfare, even without considering broader social and environmental issues (which are likely to reinforce this judgement).

The situation for cats is less clear. While some cats may have been indoor-only cats, many owned cats have significant outdoor experience, and have hunted and eaten their own prey; they may be more able to support themselves and live independently or semi-independently, and may be able to find a new owner themselves (theoretically, dogs too could find a new owner in this way). Nonetheless, the life of an abandoned cat is a risky one: the animal needs to find sufficient food and shelter, and faces a number of hazards, including contracting diseases, being hit by cars (the major cause of mortality in unowned cats) and being attacked by hostile or predatory animals. In addition, an abandoned cat may be a nuisance or a disease risk to people, as well as preying on wildlife (see the section of this chapter on unowned populations, and Chapter 14). This suggests that in many cases, in terms of the welfare of the cat itself, as well as people and other living things, relinquishment to a shelter is better than abandonment. However, there may be cases where a particular cat is very unlikely to be adopted, plausibly has tolerable welfare if left to support itself, does not pose a significant threat to others, and the only realistic alternative is a period in a shelter followed by euthanasia (the eventual outcome for the majority of cats in shelters). In a case of this kind, abandonment may be preferable. However, what one thinks about this depends on what one concludes about the ethics of euthanasing healthy but unwanted animals, as this is the destiny of so many animals that are relinquished to shelters.

13.4 Euthanasia of Unwanted Healthy Companion Animals

Euthanasia of healthy but unwanted companion animals may be requested by owners at veterinary surgeries or in some cases at shelters; open-access shelters, as we have seen, also euthanase significant numbers of animals that are either thought to be not adoptable, or not adopted after some period of time. This raises ethical issues about when it is permissible to humanely kill a healthy animal, and whether being unwanted and/or unadopted is sufficient reason.

Different ethical perspectives take divergent approaches to humane killing, as was discussed in Chapter 5. A utilitarian with a hedonist approach to welfare, for instance, aims at bringing about best outcomes, measured in terms of maximising pleasures, net of pain. On this view, killing is not *in principle* problematic, but may be ethically questionable when the killing process itself causes pain and distress, and/or when killing would mean more suffering and less pleasure in the world.

It could be argued that, on this view, in many of the cases we consider here killing is permissible. Vets, and many shelters, now kill animals by an intravenous injection that need not cause pain beyond the needle stick involved, though in practice the process may be carried out in ways that do cause some animal distress. Although healthy animals *in principle* could have a good future, this seems doubtful for those that are unlikely to be adopted. Some animals, realistically, face abandonment to a life on the streets with which they cannot cope, or alternatively remaining in a small, noisy cage, with limited exercise and stimulation from interacting with humans, no chance of adoption, and very little positive welfare. Painless death, on a utilitarian view, could be considered a better option than this kind of miserable future life; that is without considering the social and environmental costs to others of abandonment, or the economic costs of keeping an unadopted and miserable animal alive. Of course, for this judgement to be appropriate, it must be a realistic account of the available alternatives; if, for example, someone easily could keep their dog, were the dog only to receive some training to improve its behaviour, euthanasia would *not* be the best outcome among the readily available options.

Research suggests that this broadly utilitarian view, on which euthanasia is the best outcome for an unwanted animal, is commonly taken by those who surrender animals to shelters and those who take unwanted animals to veterinarians for euthanasia. Frommer & Arluke (1999) report that many who surrender animals to animal shelters 'consider euthanization a better solution for their pets than allowing them to live in poor situations … death was preferable to sacrificing the quality of life that the animal deserved and had come to expect'.

Shelter workers may also take a utilitarian approach to cope with being in the 'front line' in terms of euthanasing healthy animals. Studies repeatedly show that shelter workers and companion animal vets face an unusual kind of 'moral stress' (Rollin, 2006). The decision to work with animals usually emerges from a strong sense of caring for animals' welfare. Being required, then, to euthanase healthy animals because no one wants the animal as a companion runs against the grain; they took the job to care, and they ended up killing; what Arluke & Sanders (1996) call the 'caring-killing paradox'.

Vets have the option to refuse to euthanase healthy animals brought to them for this purpose, although in most cases, they will comply with the owner's wishes (usually because they are concerned about what will happen to the animal if they do not – see Morris (2012)). Refusal is more difficult or impossible for shelter workers, faced with a relentless incoming flow of animals with nowhere else to go, and a constant shortage of space. In these circumstances, research suggests, those who work in shelters adopt a form of utilitarian ethical reasoning: that rather than being 'warehoused' the animals are better off humanely killed; and that, as individuals, shelter workers can at least ensure that the animals' death involves as little pain and distress as possible. Shelter workers can, after all, reasonably maintain that the animals' deaths are not their personal moral responsibility; they are merely the instruments for carrying out a policy that is accepted by the 'general public' which is, ultimately, responsible (Arluke, 2003).

A second ethical approach here, also considered in Chapter 5, maintains that on account of their sentience and cognitive capacities, animals such as cats and dogs have *rights*. The most basic and important right any being can have is the right not to be killed. And even if we can suppose – as we discussed in Chapter 12 – that an animal in severe and incurable pain might waive its right to life, we cannot suppose this to be true of healthy but unwanted animals. On this view, killing healthy animals violates their rights, and is therefore wrong: owners should not ask for it, and shelter workers and vets should not carry it out.

Regan (1983) maintains that killing healthy animals is not euthanasia at all, as the term 'euthanasia' should only be used when killing is in the interests of the one killed: it is not in the interests of healthy animals to die. If their options for continued life are so miserable that their life is not worth living, then that is because people have made it so. We would not be impressed with the argument that it would be better to euthanase a human being, because otherwise we will lock them away in miserable conditions for the rest of their lives, making their lives not worth living.

The principle that healthy animals have a right not to be killed underpins the growth in the 'no-kill' shelter movement (usually defined as shelters where 90% or more of admitted animals are not euthanased). The first sentence of the Resolution in the *Declaration of the No Kill Movement*, for instance, is that the 'right to live is every animal's most basic and fundamental right' (No Kill Advocacy, n.d.). While not always phrased in terms of animals' rights, the idea that healthy but unwanted or unowned dogs and cats should not be killed is becoming increasingly widespread. In Italy, unowned dogs and cats may not legally be euthanased unless they are 'severely ill or incurable'. Some municipalities in the United States, for instance, San Francisco, have also declared themselves 'no-kill'. In these legal contexts, *all* animal shelters must be 'no-kill'; in Italy, shelters receive subsidies to pay for the basic upkeep of animals that cannot be killed. Although it is difficult to provide firm evidence here, no-kill shelters may have served to raise awareness about responsible dog/cat ownership, and to publicise the view that potential dog or cat owners should adopt unowned animals from shelters.

However, ethical questions can also be raised about no-kill shelters. As healthy animals are not euthanased, there is often limited room for new animals, so these animals are turned away. No-kill shelters are sometimes called 'closed access', because they do not take in every animal that is brought to them. In addition, although shelters vary, and can be well or poorly resourced, animals may be kept in small spaces, where diseases can spread quickly, for indefinite periods of time. A utilitarian would argue both that a warehoused animal with little chance of adoption would at some point be better off dead, and that there could be a much better use of resources for animal welfare than the long-term confinement of unadopted animals. It is also (controversially) argued that no-kill shelters 'cherry-pick' the most adoptable animals, leaving the unadoptable animals to be euthanased in the open-access shelters (reported by Arluke, 2003). If this analysis were correct, no-kill shelters would function as a substitute source of adopted animals, without raising the total numbers of animals adopted. However, research carried out by

Frank & Frank (2007) suggests that no-kill shelter adoption programmes *do* work to increase overall numbers of adoptions, rather than just being a substitute source of animals for adoption (this is the only empirical study so far explicitly to examine this issue).

Compromise between a broadly utilitarian and a broadly rights-based view about killing unwanted companion animals seems unlikely. However, there are goals that both views could agree on: trying to reduce the numbers of healthy animals being relinquished to shelters for adoption, brought to vets or shelters for euthanasia, or straying from their homes. Policies that might help to achieve this could focus on helping people to access neutering services, so that they do not find themselves with unwanted litters (many animal welfare organisations have been pursuing this strategy); better tracking of animals that stray, for example, through compulsory microchip schemes; reducing the number of human–animal relationships that fail by making educational resources more widely available, along with access to animal behaviourists and psychologists; and trap-neuter-return for feral and unadoptable cat colonies (though this too raises controversial ethical issues; we return to this subsequently).

In fact, the number of animals euthanased in shelters does seem to be falling in a number of countries, including the United Kingdom and United States. Statistics indicate that the number of dogs and cats euthanased each year in the US shelters, for example, has decreased, from 12–20 million to an estimated 3–4 million (HSUS, 2014). Nonetheless, millions of unwanted companion animals are still euthanased every year across the industrialised Western nations.

So far in this chapter, we have focused on companion animals that have become unwanted, and decisions about what to do with such animals. One of the possibilities was abandonment. Abandonment and straying have, however, led to significant populations of unowned animals – primarily cats – living within human communities in industrialised nations. We have not focused on these animals in this book, because our primary concern is with animals that actually are human companions; unowned animals are not normally anyone's companions. However, as the unowned animal population has derived from the owned companion animal population, and unowned cats in particular generate a number of ethical problems, we conclude the chapter with a discussion of unowned animals. This takes us beyond ethical decisions made by individual animal owners or shelter workers to broader ethical questions raised by the management of whole populations of unowned animals.

13.5 Unowned Animal Populations: Numbers and Relationships

There are no reliable statistics on unowned cat and dog populations. Such statistics as there are largely depend on proxy measures, such as the numbers of animals that enter shelters each year (though of course, many unowned animals never enter shelters, and many animals that enter shelters are not unowned). What statistics there are have little historical depth, as animal shelters only recently began systematically collecting data about the animals that enter and whether they are reclaimed, adopted or euthanased (and some shelters still do not do this).

Jessup (2004), in an often cited figure, estimates that there are 60–100 million unowned cats in the United States, but does not support this with evidence. The ASPCA (n.d.) says there are no reliable estimates of the numbers of unowned dogs in the United States; most stray or abandoned dogs are removed to shelters. In the United Kingdom, the Dogs Trust collects records on dogs handled by local authorities every year, either picked up by a dog warden or a member of the public, or relinquished by an owner. Between 31 March 2013 and 1 April 2014, 110,675 dogs were handled by local authorities who answered the survey (GfK NOP Social Research, 2014). A separate study identified 150,000 cats entering the UK animal shelters in 2010 (Stavisky *et al.*, 2012). The main focus of the rest of this chapter is on cats, which almost everywhere in the industrialised Western nations maintain fairly substantial unowned populations; there are far fewer unowned dogs.

13.5.1 Unowned cats: relations to people

Domestic cats can occupy very different relations of closeness to, and dependence on, human beings, compared to dogs. The International Society for Feline Medicine (ISFM) divides domestic cats into four groups: (a) household cats, living with and cared for by humans, typically spending some or all of their time in a human home, who may be kept as single or multiple cats; (b) stray or abandoned cats that have been previously cared for by a human (typically in a home) but are now free-living, have some direct human contact and tolerance and are fed and provided for to some extent; (c) street and community cats that are free-living either as single or as colony cat(s), usually have some direct human contact and tolerance, and are fed and provided for to some extent; and (d) feral cats that are free-living as single or colony cat(s), have generally little or no direct human interaction or dependency and often avoid direct human contact (Sparkes *et al.*, 2013). Feral cats, in particular, are extremely difficult to socialise to human contact after they are around 8 weeks old. This is significant for their management, because they cannot be adopted as companion cats.

Unowned cats are often deliberately supported by human beings. In the United States, a review of studies on feeding unowned cats found it to be a widespread activity crossing socioeconomic strata; between 8% and 12% of people in each study fed unowned cats (Levy & Crawford, 2004). A study in Tel Aviv found that 25% of cat owners also fed unowned cats (Finkler & Terkel, 2012). These high numbers suggest a significant human population that is concerned for the welfare of unowned cats, and has high tolerance for their existence. But attitudes to unowned cats vary significantly, both between individuals and across cultures. In some countries, such as Italy, unowned cats are accepted and legally protected; Rome has around 300,000 unowned cats, with some cat colonies legally designated part of the city's 'bioheritage' (though this policy is controversial, as disputes over the famous Torre Argentina cat shelter in Rome indicate). In most countries, however, unowned cats are legally pests, and can be caught and euthanased, or killed by other means, though even in these countries they also have defenders.

13.6 Managing Unowned Populations

13.6.1 Why manage populations?

Although many countries to a greater or lesser extent tolerate unowned cat populations, most countries and cities nonetheless try to manage these populations. There are a number of reasons for this, which we will note briefly here (many of these are discussed in more detail in Chapter 14).

First, unowned cats pose public health concerns, including rabies, toxoplasmosis (in faeces), fleas, hookworms, roundworms, ringworm and tapeworms. They are also vectors for leptospirosis and cryptosporidiosis and serve as a reservoir for Bartonella infections (implicated in cat scratch disease). Unowned cats may also transmit diseases to companion cats with homes. Second, the predatory behaviour of unowned cats, in particular, may have a substantial impact on wildlife. (These issues are discussed in Chapter 14.) Third, it is often argued that the welfare of unowned cats is very poor: 75% of feral kittens die before they are 6 months old (Stoskopf & Nutter, 2004). Jessup (2004) cites an American Veterinary Medical Association figure of a 2-year average lifespan for unowned cats in comparison for 10 years for owned cats. It is argued that unowned cats face constant hazards from disease, traffic, attacks and accidents. Finally, unowned cat populations can multiply extremely fast. Cats can get pregnant before they are 6 months old, and have up to three litters a year of between two and six kittens, though one or two litters is more common. Despite the low survival rate of feral kittens, these reproductive rates lead to very rapid population growth. The more unowned cats there are, the more the public health, environmental and welfare concerns multiply.

From many ethical perspectives, enhanced risks of human disease, loss of wildlife and poor cat welfare pose challenges, most obviously that they are all likely to increase suffering and reduce pleasure in the world, though they may also threaten other values. These concerns underpin the management of unowned cat populations.

13.6.2 Ethics of managing unowned cat populations

There are two obvious strategies for managing unowned cat populations: reducing the risks posed by the populations, and reducing or eliminating the populations themselves. The first strategy – reducing the risks posed by the population – mostly comprises vaccination programmes. These do not completely eliminate the disease risks from unowned cats, and as many of these diseases are also carried by wildlife such as rats, foxes and coyotes, public health risks would remain unless all wildlife were also vaccinated. However, while vaccination may improve both human and cat welfare by preventing some suffering from diseases, it reduces rather than eliminates welfare concerns, and does not address environmental issues at all.

The second strategy – managing the populations themselves – could involve (a) programmes to routinely neuter members of existing unowned populations (which has some risk-reducing as well as population-reducing effects) and (b) programmes to remove these populations, with the aim of rehoming or placing the cats in a sanctuary if possible, otherwise euthanasing them. Both these policies, for different reasons, are controversial. We will consider neutering first.

Neutering unowned cats does lower risks to public and animal health. It reduces mating fights and roaming, both of which are activities that spread disease and increase the risk of injury; and since in the case of cats, giving birth is a key transmission route for feline immunodeficiency virus (FIV) and feline leukaemia virus (FELV), it removes the risk of passing these diseases on to offspring. However, the main effect of neutering in this context is to reduce population growth (Figure 13.2).

In Chapter 10, we outlined ethical worries about routine neutering of cats and dogs kept confined as companions: the biggest ethical concern was with the health effects of neutering male dogs. The situation is rather different in the context of the routine neutering of unowned cats, however, where the potential health problems from neutering, such as obesity, are less significant because the cats are free-roaming, and the opportunity for reproduction is (almost) unlimited. So, even if one accepts the ethical concerns about neutering we outlined in Chapter 10, they seem less salient here; and on many ethical views, the overall population welfare and other gains made by neutering unowned companions outweigh any concerns that neutering may generate. However, it is worth noting that this does not hold for *all* ethical positions. If neutering is understood to violate an animal's rights, the fact that *other* animals might benefit from the animal being neutered (or that animals who would live short, miserable lives will not come into existence) does not obviously provide an ethical justification for neutering, though as we saw in Chapter 10, some rights theorists can adapt their theory to allow for it.

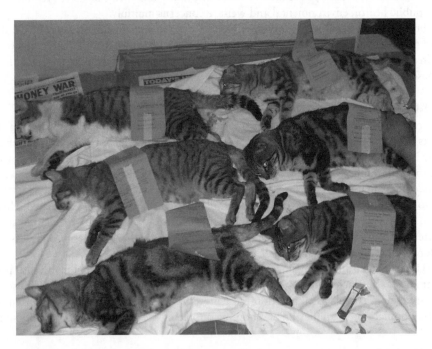

Figure 13.2 Trap-neuter-release program in Portugal. The cats are being monitored during recovery following castration. (*Image used courtesy of Jenny Stavisky.*)

In order to reduce unowned animal populations, some cities and districts (such as Dallas, in the United States) have introduced ordinances requiring almost all animals to be neutered, and offering low-cost spay and neuter programmes to those who cannot otherwise afford it. More commonly, public bodies and many non-profit organisations support trap-neuter-return (sometimes also called trap-neuter-release) (TNR) programmes, which trap, neuter (and usually vaccinate, at least against rabies) unowned populations of cats, and then return them to their original location, removing the tip of their ear to show they have been neutered, and trying to rehome kittens and adoptable strays. Such TNR policies have both very strong support, and significant opposition.

Supporters maintain that TNR is both practically feasible and ethically desirable. It reduces public and animal health risk, and, when combined with vaccination, improves individual animal welfare. Many TNR programmes also require local individuals or communities to commit to feeding the neutered cats and checking on colonies, which again is likely to improve the animals' welfare. It is also argued that there are population-level benefits, as TNR creates colonies with stable or declining populations of familiar animals that (unlike just removing colonies) deters new cats from moving in. Perhaps most importantly, TNR avoids euthanasing feral and otherwise unadoptable cats, whose lives are regarded, on this view, as being valuable. TNR is sometimes combined with no-kill policies. In Italian law, while 'Feral cats have the right to live free; they are protected and cannot be moved from their colony' (Natoli *et al.*, 2006), they may nonetheless be neutered and returned to the colony.

However, there are very strong objections to this view (as discussed in Palmer, 2014). Those who oppose TNR argue that it fails to achieve the goals of population management. First, opponents argue, it does not really reduce populations; at best it stabilises them, and they often increase as people dump new, unwanted, and often unneutered cats into them, thinking that the cat will be cared for as part of the colony. Even if vaccinated for rabies and other cat diseases, cats can still pass diseases such as toxoplasmosis to humans, they still have worms and fleas, and they can still be a nuisance. Unowned cats may still have poor welfare, lack access to vets, and face multiple threats from traffic and predators. Often the key argument in this debate, cats in TNR colonies still prey on wildlife, causing suffering and distress to individual wild animals (see Chapter 14) and possibly threatening species. These factors have persuaded the animal rights organisation, PETA, surprisingly, to reject TNR of unowned cats in favour of euthanasia:

> Homeless cats do not die of old age. Highly contagious diseases are common, as are infected puncture wounds, broken bones, urinary tract infections, brain damage, internal injuries, attacks by other animals or cruel humans, automobile accidents, and terrible living conditions like freezing or stifling temperatures, scrounging for food, and being considered a "nuisance", through no fault of their own. Moreover, free-roaming cats also terrorize and kill countless birds and other wildlife who are not equipped to deal with such predators. Having witnessed firsthand the gruesome things that can happen to feral cats and to the animals they prey on, PETA cannot in good conscience oppose euthanasia as a humane alternative to dealing with cat overpopulation
>
> (PETA, n.d.).

PETA seems to take the view that unowned cats – including those in TNR colonies – have lives not worth living; their experiences are on balance so negative that they would be better off dead. However, the evidence to support this is mixed. Some TNR colonies seem to maintain cats in reasonable health – for instance, a study of TNR colonies on a Florida university campus found that at the end of 7 years, 83% of cats had been there for more than 6 years and were in 'adequate physical condition' (Levy, Gale & Gale, 2003), though this may not be a very typical TNR population. At least in some cases, though, what is being recommended here is the euthanasia of unowned but reasonably healthy cats – and this raises many of the same issues we discussed earlier in the chapter about the euthanasia of healthy, but unwanted, animals.

To conclude: animals may be abandoned, relinquished to shelters, or euthanased for a variety of reasons, some of which are beyond the owner's direct control (such as illness or loss of income), while in other cases, alternative solutions could have been found (e.g. in the case of behavioural issues that could have been addressed by training). Both the issues of abandonment, and the subsequent management of the different populations of unwanted animals, generate some of the most difficult problems in companion animal ethics, from almost every ethical approach.

Key Points

- Healthy companion animals can become unwanted for housing, family, financial or behavioural reasons; owners must then decide what to do with their animals.
- While the best options are finding ways to continue living with the animal, or rehoming it in a caring home, in many cases, the only choices are to relinquish healthy animals to a shelter, abandon them, or euthanase them. All of these present ethical challenges.
- Although successful adoption in a new home is a good outcome, shelter housing is normally stressful, and there is a high likelihood of euthanasia, except in no-kill shelters.
- Euthanasing healthy companion animals raises ethical problems from most ethical perspectives, in particular views on which animals have rights, which have influenced the development of no-kill shelters. Utilitarians, however, permit euthanasia of healthy animals where the realistic alternative is a miserable ongoing life.
- Abandoned animals normally suffer significant welfare loss, and join populations of stray and feral animals, especially cats. These unowned cats pose public health risks, may have poor welfare, and prey on wildlife; for these reasons, their populations are usually managed.
- Management tools for unowned cats, including trap-neuter-return and euthanasia, also raise significant ethical problems, and generate major empirical and ethical disagreements.

References

AHA [American Humane Association] (n.d.) *Animal shelter euthanasia.* [Online] Available from: http://www.americanhumane.org/animals/stop-animal-abuse/fact-sheets/animal -shelter-euthanasia.html [Accessed 21 August 2014].

Arluke, A., & Sanders, C. (1996) *Regarding animals*. Philadelphia, PA, Temple University Press.

Arluke, A. (2003) The no-kill controversy: manifest and latent sources of tension. In: Salem, D.J. & Rowan, A.N. (eds) *The state of the animals II: 2003*. Washington, DC, Humane Society Press, pp. 67–83.

ASPCA [American Society for the Prevention of Cruelty to Animals] (n.d.) *Pet statistics*. [Online] Available from: http://www.aspca.org/about-us/faq/pet-statistics [Accessed 21 August 2014].

Blue Cross (2012) *Worrying surge in abandoned wolf-like breeds*. [Online] Available from: http://www.bluecross.org.uk/2000-105347/worrying-surge-in-abandoned-wolf-like -breeds.html [Accessed 21 August 2014].

Burgess-Jackson, K. (1997) Doing right by our animal companions. *The Journal of Ethics* 2, 159–185.

Coppola, C., Enns, M. & Grandin, T. (2006) Human interaction and cortisol: can human contact reduce stress for shelter dogs? *Physiology of Behaviour* 87 (3) 537–541.

Coppola, C., Enns, M. & Grandin, T. (2010) Noise in the animal shelter environment: building design and the effects of daily noise exposure. *Journal of Applied Animal Welfare Science* 9 (1), 1–7.

DiGiacomo, N., Arluke, A. & Patronek, G. (1998) Surrendering pets to shelters: the relinquisher's perspective. *Anthrozoos* 11 (1), 41–51.

Finkler, H. & Terkel, J. (2012) The contribution of cat owners' attitudes and behaviours to the free-roaming cat overpopulation in Tel Aviv, Israel. *Preventive Veterinary Medicine* 104, 125–135.

Frank, J. & Frank, P. (2007) Analysis of programs to reduce overpopulation of companion animals: do adoption and low cost spay/neuter programs merely cause substitution of sources? *Ecological Economics* 62 (3–4), 740–746.

Frommer, S. & Arluke, A. (1999) Loving them to death: blame-displacing strategies of animal shelter workers and surrenderers. *Society and Animals* 7 (1), 1–16.

GfK NOP Social Research (2014) Stray dogs survey 2014: Summary Report. A report prepared for Dogs Trust. [Online] Available from: https://www.dogstrust.org.uk/whats -happening/news/stray%20dogs%202014%20report.pdf [Accessed 11 December 2014]

HSUS [Humane Society of the United States] (2014) *Pets by the numbers*. [Online] Available from: http://www.humanesociety.org/issues/pet_overpopulation/facts/pet_ownership_ statistics.html [Accessed 21 August 2014].

Irvine, L. (2003) A problem of unwanted pets: a case study in how institutions "think" about clients' needs. *Social Problems* 50 (4), 550–566.

Jessup, D.A. (2004) The welfare of feral cats and wildlife. *Journal of the American Veterinary Medical Association* 225, 1377–1383.

Kass, P. (2005) Cat overpopulation in the United States. *Animal Welfare* 3, 119–139.

Kwan, J. & Bain, M. (2013) Owner attachment and problem behaviors related to relinquishment and training techniques of dogs. *Journal of Applied Animal Welfare Science* 16 (2), 168–183.

Levy, J.K. & Crawford, P.C. (2004) Humane strategies for controlling feral cat populations. *Journal of the American Veterinary Medical Association* 225, 1354–1360.

Levy, J.K., Gale, D.W. & Gale, L.A. (2003) Evaluation of a long-term trap neuter return and adoption program on a free-roaming cat population. *Journal of the American Veterinary Medical Association* 222, 42–46.

Morris, P. (2012) *Blue juice: euthanasia in veterinary medicine*. Philadelphia, PA, Temple University Press.

Natoli, E., Maragliano, L., Cariola, G., Faini, A., Bonanni, R., Cafazzo, S. & Fantini, C. (2006) Management of feral domestic cats in the urban environment of Rome (Italy). *Preventative Veterinary Medicine* 77 (3–4), 180–185.

Marston, L. Bennett, P. & Coleman, G. (2004) What happens to shelter dogs? An analysis of data for 1 year from three Australian shelters. *Journal of Applied Animal Welfare Science* 7 (1), 27–47.

New, J.C., Salman, M.D., King, M., Scarlett, J.M., Kass, P.H. & Hutchison, J.M. (2000) Characteristics of shelter-relinquished animals and their owners compared with animals and their owners in U.S. pet-owning households. *Journal of Applied Animal Welfare Science* 3 (3), 179–201.

No Kill Advocacy Center (n.d.) *Declaration of the no kill movement in the United States.* [Online] Available from: http://www.nokilldeclaration.org/ [Accessed 21 August 2014].

Nowicki, S.A. (2011) Give me shelter: the foreclosure crisis and its effect on America's animals. *The Stanford Journal of Animal Law and Policy* 4, 99–121.

Palmer, C. (2014) Value conflicts in feral cat management: trap-neuter return or trap-euthanize? In: Appleby, M.C., Weary, D.M. & Sandøe, P. (eds) *Dilemmas in animal welfare.* Wallingford, CABI, pp. 148–168.

PETA [People for the Ethical Treatment of Animals] (n.d.) *Trap, neuter, return and monitor programs for feral cats: doing it right.* [Online] Available from: http://www.peta.org /issues/companion-animal-issues/companion-animals-factsheets/trap-neuter-return -monitor-programs-feral-cats-right/ [Accessed 21 August 2014].

Regan, T. (1983) *The case for animal rights.* Berkeley, CA, University of California Press.

Rollin, B. (2006) *An introduction to veterinary medical ethics.* Oxford, Blackwell.

Scarlett, J.M., Salman, M., New, J. & Kass, P. (1999) Reasons for relinquishment of pets in U.S. shelters: lifestyle issues and allergies. *Journal of Applied Animal Welfare Science* 2, 41–57.

Sparkes, A.H., Bessant, C., Cope, K., Ellis, S.L.H., Finka, L., Halls, V., Hiestand, K., Horsford, K., Laurence, C., MacFarlaine, I., Neville, P.F., Stavisky, J. & Yeates, J. (2013) ISFM guidelines on population management and welfare of unowned domestic cats (*Felis catus*). *Journal of Feline Medicine and Surgery* 15 (9), 811–817.

Stavisky, J., Brennan, M., Downes, M. & Dean, R. (2012) Demographics and economic burden of un-owned cats and dogs in the UK: results of a 2010 census. *BMC Veterinary Research* 8, 163.

Stoskopf, M.K. & Nutter, F.B. (2004) Analyzing approaches to feral cat management: one size does not fit all. *Journal of the American Veterinary Medical Association* 221, 1361–1364.

Ethics and Broader Impacts of Companion Animals

14

14.1 Introduction   217
14.2 Public Health and Zoonoses   218
14.3 Companion Animals and Use of Resources   221
    14.3.1 Animal food and human food   221
    14.3.2 The opportunity cost of companion animals 223
14.4 Companion Animals, Sustainability, and the Environment   225
    14.4.1 Resource use and waste   225
    14.4.2 Wildlife competition and predation   228

14.1 Introduction

It is often claimed that companion animals are reservoirs of disease, that they use resources that could otherwise help people or maintain other animals, or that they are environmentally unsustainable. For instance, in *The Guardian* newspaper in 2014, under the heading 'Are pets bad for the environment?', Erik Assadourian of the World-watch Institute disapprovingly noted that 'Two German Shepherds use more resources just for their annual food needs than the average Bangladeshi uses each year in total' and argued that the earth cannot sustain growing populations of companion animals.

In this chapter, we consider claims about such broader impacts of companion animals, and largely focus on the potential *negative* impact that companion animals have

Companion Animal Ethics, First Edition. Peter Sandøe, Sandra Corr and Clare Palmer.
© Universities Federation for Animal Welfare 2016.

on human well-being, other animals, and the environment. We will not consider the broader *positive* impacts of companion animals' relationship with their owners, since these were discussed in Chapter 3; nor will we consider dangerous dogs (see Chapter 9). However, since debates on the topic generally extend to include stray and feral cats and dogs, we will include these animals here (in addition to what has already been said in Chapter 13). Where we discuss companion animals in the context of wildlife (in Section 14.4.2), we will briefly discuss birds kept as companions, since some bird species raise distinctive issues here.

We will begin by considering ethical issues raised by zoonoses (infectious diseases that can be transmitted between non-human animals and humans), and then we will explore a variety of ethical worries about companion animals, resource use, sustainability and the environment. The concern here is not that the companion relationship in itself is ethically questionable (a view we considered in Chapter 5), but rather that problems arise because of the human and/or environmental impacts of companion animals. This does not necessarily mean, though, that we will only take a consequentialist perspective. It is theoretically possible that some impacts are never acceptable, for instance, because they infringe on others' rights.

14.2 Public Health and Zoonoses

It is estimated that 75% of newly reported human infections emerge from a (non-human) animal reservoir (Taylor, Latham & Woolhouse, 2001). Zoonotic diseases carried by companion animals may cause minor ailments such as skin irritation (mange, ringworm) or gastrointestinal upsets (campylobacter or cryptosporidia). However, they can also be fatal; rabies is the best-known example. In some cases, infections can be mild or asymptomatic in normally healthy adults but can have serious consequences in children and the immune-compromised – for example, toxoplasma, a protozoa found in infected cat faeces, can infect the human foetus, causing brain damage or blindness. Some zoonoses are transmitted by direct contact through bites and scratches (e.g. rabies, cat scratch fever (*Bartonella henselae*)), while others are transmitted indirectly via contaminated soil or water (e.g. roundworm in dog faeces). Zoonotic diseases shared with birds, such as psittacosis, may be transmitted through airborne means. Cats and dogs also transmit diseases between themselves; in particular, unowned and feral cats may have higher levels of FIV (the feline version of HIV) than owned cats (Muirden, 2002), and can transmit both FIV and FeLV (feline leukaemia) to owned cats allowed outdoors (Figure 14.1).

Outdoor and feral cats can also transmit disease to wildlife. In California, for instance, high numbers of sea otters are infected with *Toxoplasma gondii*, shed only in the faeces of cats (Dabritz *et al.*, 2006). However, it is worth noting that cats and dogs can be vulnerable to cross-species transmission too. Humans can, for example, infect companion animals with methicillin-resistant *Staphylococcus aureus* (MRSA) and influenza A (H1N1) pdm09 virus (Day *et al.*, 2012).

Acquiring a zoonotic disease from a companion animal normally has a negative impact on human welfare (however welfare is understood); in some cases, the disease

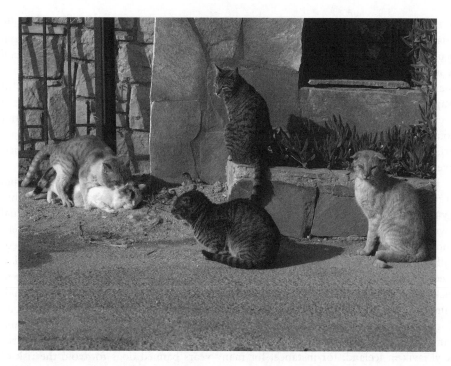

Figure 14.1 Feral cat colony. Many of the cats are in reasonable body condition, although obviously scarred from fighting. (*t-lorien/iStock.*)

can be very severe, or even fatal. And of course, many of these diseases (not least rabies) are also very bad for animal welfare. But is this of *ethical* concern?

One way in which a zoonotic disease may be of ethical concern is when people choose to acquire companion animals that may put themselves, or other people, at risk of disease. This may mean that owners have moral responsibilities to protect others from the possible disease impacts of their dog or cat. A second way in which a zoonotic disease may be of ethical concern is that it normally causes suffering. Utilitarians who aim to minimise suffering should, therefore, try to tackle these diseases, and to reduce their incidence. This raises questions about what strategies should be adopted to achieve this reduction, and by whom – the national government, local communities, individual companion animal owners, or all of these groups? Internationally, strategies have ranged from preventative action, including vaccinations, surveillance, careful husbandry to reduce exposure, and bans on keeping animal companions in urban areas, to wide-ranging animal culls.

Culling is generally the most ethically challenging policy, especially where it involves not only feral animals, but also the animals with whom people actually live. In the industrialised West, few formal culls of companion animals or unowned dogs or cats have been carried out for zoonotic reasons; most severe zoonotic diseases have been controlled by surveillance, vaccination and medication. From some ethical perspectives, such as that of an animal rights theorist, killing – especially of a dog or cat that does not actually have a disease – in order to protect humans or other animals is morally unacceptable (just as culling people in similar cases would be unacceptable). From a utilitarian perspective, however, if there were no plausible alternative, and a cull would likely bring about best overall consequences, it could be ethically justified. In the case of rabies in particular, though, it is sometimes argued that programmes of trapping, neutering, vaccination and release of feral dogs are actually more effective in preventing the spread of disease than outright culls, and so would bring about better consequences (Molento, 2014). Certainly, countries where unowned dogs and cats are primarily controlled by shooting or poisoning *in situ* do not report a reduction in their overall populations (WSPA/RSPCA, 2007).

Ethical concerns about reducing human and nonhuman pain and suffering underpin arguments that individual owners, communities, and governments have a responsibility to prevent the spread of zoonotic diseases from companion animals. For individual owners, this primarily means ensuring that the animal receives relevant vaccinations, and safely disposing of an animal's faeces. However, the safe disposal of faeces is practically problematic in the case of cats (see Section 14.4.1). In the case of dogs, disposal of faeces is easier in principle, but in practice, many people fail to do so safely. Failure to pick up after dogs can spread worm-based disease, as well as create a community nuisance; this has led most public authorities to regulate in this area. Many locations ban dogs (for instance, from beaches) and others have dog fouling bylaws carrying significant financial penalties. Some cities take concerns about zoonoses especially seriously. Reykjavik in Iceland, for instance, for many years banned dogs to avoid the risk of zoonotic disease and dog aggression; while it is now possible to gain a legal exemption (at a price), dogs are still banned from most public places. However, given how much dog ownership matters to many people (see Chapter 3) and the possibility of regulation for various protective measures (such as vaccination and cleaning up dog faeces), from a utilitarian perspective, at least, the costs of such a ban may well outweigh the benefits it provides.

One further concern about the linked nature of human and animal disease is the use of antibiotics in companion animal medicine, where there are worries that 'veterinary use of antimicrobials is contributing to the emergence of resistant bacterial strains in humans' (Bonner, 2014). While the primary concerns here are about the prophylactic (preventative) use of antibiotics in agricultural animal production, veterinary use of antimicrobials in companion animals has recently come under scrutiny, especially in Europe. Since increasingly resistant bacterial strains are likely to increase suffering in people and in animals, different ethical perspectives will largely converge in agreeing that actions that make bacterial resistance more likely should be restricted, both as an ethical practice by individual vets, and, where necessary, by regulation.

The linked nature of many human and animal diseases need not always be regarded negatively. The development of ideas about 'One Health' – defined by the American Veterinary Medical Association as 'the collaborative effort of multiple disciplines – working locally, nationally, and globally – to attain optimal health for people, animals and the environment' (One Health, 2008: p. 13) has emphasised more positive impacts of the closeness between humans and animals. Rabinowitz *et al.* (2008), for example, drawing on the idea of One Health, argue that rather than seeing animals as posing a risk of disease ('Us vs Them'), we should think in terms of *shared* risk, in particular with respect to the effects of environmental hazards. Animals could be regarded as 'sentinels' of disease risks to humans, and as companion animals live so closely with humans, they may be particularly useful for this. For instance, it has been suggested that cancer in dogs linked to lawn chemicals or indoor air pollution 'could be a model for diseases in children sharing the same households' (Rabinowitz, Odophin & Dein, 2008: p. 226). While this approach may appear human-centred (valuing animal diseases as a way of better understanding threats to human public health from disease), it could nonetheless contribute both to human and to companion animal welfare.

14.3 Companion Animals and Use of Resources

Two ethical concerns are popularly expressed about companion animals in the context of human resource use. One is that companion animals are competing for the human food supply. The second is that given global hunger and poverty, spending significant amounts of household resources on animal companions cannot be ethically justified.

14.3.1 Animal food and human food

Concern that companion animals are eating food that humans would otherwise eat has a long history – as we saw in Chapter 1, people reflected on this even in the sixteenth century. The worry may rest on some combination of two different beliefs: firstly, that humans could, and otherwise would, eat what companion animals are consuming, and secondly, that there is an overall shortage of food, so that if companion animals are being fed more, what is available for humans is decreasing, or not increasing as fast as it otherwise would.

We will consider these ideas in turn. Most cats and dogs eat commercially produced food, usually a combination of animal products, water, some kind of grains and starches, binders and thickeners, preservatives, and various supplementary nutrients required for health. The ethical concern here is (usually) that the meat or fish protein (rather than the grains and other products) in cat and dog food otherwise could, and perhaps would, be used to feed people. In order to assess this concern, we need to know what meat and fish actually are in pet food.

Animal products in commercial pet food are usually composed from different sources. The food may contain meat left over from production processes, including what is removed from mechanical deboning, and other meat not usually marketed for human consumption (Nestle & Nesheim, 2010). Most commercial dog and cat food also contains meat by-products, including heads, feet, beaks, viscera, lungs, blood, brains, bones: parts not usually eaten in the industrialised West, but sometimes eaten in other areas of the world. Commercial foods also frequently contain animal meals from rendered ingredients with a variety of sources including '4D' meat (classified as being from animals that were dead, dying, diseased or disabled at the time they were inspected), used cooking oil from restaurants, and expired meat from retail sources, as well as unwanted parts of slaughtered animals. These materials are 'rendered' – ground up, heated, sterilised and dehydrated in a process designed to kill viruses and bacteria, and to prevent disease transmission. The process separates out fat and dried protein solids, both of which are then used in companion animal food. Rendered protein meal provides 5–40% of the protein and fats in most commercial cat and dog foods (Aldrich, 2013); about 25% of rendered material in the United States is used for pet food (the rest is used in non-food products such as soap). Cat and dog food also contains fats, including tallow and lard/white grease, which could be eaten by humans, so 'pet food companies may partially compete in the human edible market for this ingredient' (Aldrich, 2006); however, these fats are in plentiful general supply.

Much commercial cat and dog food, then, contains mostly by-products of slaughtered animals that humans do not usually (but could) eat, and rendered products that are not intended for human consumption. So, the production of this kind of companion animal food does not appear to compete directly with the human food supply, given current tastes about which parts of animals are normally eaten.

However, the situation is different with fish protein. Fish-based cat food is often not only made from fish by-products but also from small pelagic forage fish, such as anchovies, mackerel, herring and sardines. Fishmeal also mostly comes from fish primarily caught to make the meal, rather than from by-products (Nestle & Nesheim, 2010). Although not a significant part of the diet in the industrialised West, these fish are an important protein source in many developing countries, especially in sub-Saharan Africa. Small pelagic fish also constitute about 12–13% of the diet of marine animals and seabirds (Kaschner et al., 2006); so plausibly, an increase in companion animal consumption of small pelagic fish may impact on wild animal welfare. In addition, these small pelagic fish and fish by-products are increasingly used in aquaculture in the form of fishmeal and fish oil (to feed farmed salmon, in particular). Demand for small pelagic fish both from aquaculture and from pet food has led to increased competition for the resource, as industrial fishing companies take substantial catches, reducing their availability to local people who rely on small pelagic fish, and plausibly shifting the allocation of the resource from people (and wild animals) to cats (Tacon & Metian, 2009). At present, although aquaculture is a far bigger consumer of small pelagic fish than the cat food industry, the cat food industry's consumption of fish is growing (though accurate statistics are hard to come by), and so cat food production may also constrain the growth of the human farmed fish supply. In 2002, according to De Silva & Turchini (2008), the cat food industry used 2,478,520 tonnes of raw forage fish – this much fish made into fishmeal, they claim, could have supported a doubling in global farmed salmon production. And an increase in global farmed salmon means more food for people. So, indirectly, wild pelagic fish now fed to cats could feed people, via farmed salmon (although, obviously, expansion of fish farming depends on much more just than availability of fishmeal).

A second issue here is particularly interesting. Some dog and cat owners do not want to feed their animals rendered meals, meat by-products, binders and preservatives: food that they would not eat themselves. Their concern is that the low-grade meat by-product and rendered meat meal in commercial pet foods threaten their companions' health: if pets are family members, it might be argued, they should be fed like the rest of the family. As an alternative to standard commercial foods, then, these owners buy ultra-premium pet foods, or make pet food at home from meat and fish of a quality they are willing to eat themselves. This practice does take food from the human food supply, with the goal of improving companion animal welfare. Of course, it is very unlikely that any particular food item fed to an animal companion would otherwise have been redirected to a human being in need. But direct diversion of food from human beings to companion animals may not be all that is at stake; it is possible, for instance, that an increase in demand for human food for companion animals could lead to an increase in food prices, making food less accessible to those living in poverty.

Thinking about food prices indicates just how complex this issue is (too complex to be considered in any detail here). Underpinning worries about diverting food from the human food supply to companion animals is the concern that there is, or will soon be, an overall shortage of food in the world (if there were no concern about food supply, presumably the diversion issue would not matter). In absolute terms, though, it can be claimed that there is 'enough food in the world today for everyone to have the nourishment necessary for a healthy and productive life' (WFP, 2014). However, this obviously does not mean that no problems exist: some people cannot access sufficient food, others can access it, but cannot afford to buy it; a substantial proportion of it is wasted in production, transportation (or lack of transportation) and in the home, and there are significant concerns about future availability of food with growing human populations. So, even if there is no *absolute* shortage of food, some individuals and communities, now and in the future, will not have enough of it.

Given the complexity of all these factors, though, it is very difficult to say what effect current demand for cat and dog food has on global food markets, nor what effect it might have in the future, not least because what the future holds for global food markets is itself very unclear. As suggested, direct competition between human food and companion animal food is not all that is at stake, as demand for companion animal food could impact the human food market in different ways. Nonetheless, at present, there is no substantial evidence that cat and dog food is in any major way competing with, or having serious impacts on, the human food supply.

14.3.2 The opportunity cost of companion animals

The second concern here is much more general: that, given that so many people are impoverished, the amount that is spent on companion animals by their owners cannot be justified. In support of this claim, the huge cumulative sums spent to support companion animals are often cited, for example, the $53 billion Americans spent on their pets in 2012 (APPA, n.d.). If this money were instead spent on assisting those in poverty, it is argued, *human* welfare could be substantially improved. So, companion animals have, in this sense, a high opportunity cost, in that the money spent on them could instead be spent on making life better for people.

Hadley and O'Sullivan (2009) develop a more systematic version of this argument. Their starting premise is: 'there's an emerging philosophical consensus that people in affluent nations are obliged to help distant strangers in dire need'. Drawing on pioneering work by the philosopher Singer (1972), they argue that just as someone who sees a child drowning in a nearby pond should rescue it, so a reasonably affluent person should rescue a child starving in a distant country, as neither method of death (drowning rather than starving), nor physical distance, is relevant to our moral obligations. We should give, Hadley and O'Sullivan argue, at least a 'reasonable amount' to those in need – which means diverting money from alternative spending on luxuries. Here, Hadley and O'Sullivan do not argue that companion animals should not be kept at all, but rather that our spending on them should be confined to meeting their basic needs. First, they argue, animals cannot appreciate luxury goods, so spending on these goods cannot be justified. And secondly, they maintain (adopting a view we discussed in Chapter 5) that while dogs and cats are conscious and can feel pain, they are not *self*-conscious, so death (as the end of self) does not matter to them. Given this, expensive veterinary care to keep companion animals alive cannot be ethically justified, as the animals themselves do not have an interest in it; if they are in incurable pain, they should be euthanased.

> When considerations of animal cognition are taken into account, veterinary expenditure which extends an animal's life, at considerable cost, can be cast as just another example of luxury expenditure designed to satisfy the preferences of the purchaser.
>
> (Hadley & O'Sullivan, 2009: p. 369)

As this quotation suggests, the goal here is not to pick out spending on companion animals as different and less justified than other kinds of luxury spending, nor is this an argument against keeping companion animals at all (though it is easy to see how this could be a logical extension of their view). Hadley and O'Sullivan work from a basically utilitarian premise that much more benefit overall could be gained by helping to relieve distant human suffering, than in preserving the life of an animal that has no sense of its own self anyway.

Obviously this argument, and others like it (with respect to spending on food, drugs, etc. for companion animals), is controversial in a number of ways. As was noted in Chapter 5, on some views, death does matter to cats and dogs; but while affirming this would undermine Hadley and O'Sullivan's argument against expensive life-preserving veterinary care, it would not counter their objection to general 'unnecessary spending' on animal companions. Some ethicists deny that we have duties to help those who are in dire need, unless we are in some way responsible for that neediness; or that even if we have such duties, giving aid is not the best way of performing them. So, they would reject the basic ethical premise, even if they accepted the empirical one. Yet others will argue that there are plenty of other areas on which people could target spending reductions (such as on car ownership or alcohol consumption) rather than on life-saving medical interventions for companion animals. From a utilitarian perspective, cutting down spending on companion animals is unlikely to be the most efficient way to generate more utility, given that many other objects of expenditure are less likely to generate positive utility – and may even generate negative utility. Most pragmatically, it might be argued that as it is unlikely that most affluent people would otherwise give this money to assist the distant poor (and might spend it on other consumer goods!), they may as well spend it on veterinary care for their companion animals.

Inasmuch as arguments like Hadley and O'Sullivan's encourage affluent individuals to consider their spending priorities, they are important. However, in targeting companion animals, these arguments seem problematic, in particular as they do not fully take on board the significance of human attachment to companion animals (see Chapters 3 and 12). That many owners seriously consider expensive life-saving surgery for their companions flows from the intensity of their attachment to them. A world in which owners would cheaply euthanase their sick or injured companion animals would be a world in which the attachment humans typically feel towards their companion animals was considerably weaker. Such weaker attachment would likely have other implications for companion animal welfare that Hadley and O'Sullivan would themselves find problematic.

14.4 Companion Animals, Sustainability, and the Environment

A further set of ethical worries concerns the *environmental* impacts of companion animals. There are different kinds of concerns here, and the concerns vary with respect to cats and dogs, and companion birds (see Section 14.4.2). We divide these concerns into two groups: one relating to resource use and waste, and the other to predation on wildlife. A significant feature of these environmental concerns is that attempting to resolve some of them either exacerbates other concerns, or creates potential risks for human or companion animal welfare.

14.4.1 Resource use and waste

Worries that the pet food industry competes with, or negatively impacts, the human food supply, as we have seen, are only partially justified, as much of the animal-based content in popular commercial pet food brands is not normally consumed by people. However, other concerns around pet food focus on its *environmental* sustainability. Does the production of pet food, for instance, have a high carbon footprint or draw on particular non-food resources that are scarce and non-renewable? Concern about these questions has been most strongly voiced in Robert and Brenda Vale's book *Time to eat the dog? The real guide to sustainable living* (Vale & Vale, 2009). Here the authors attempted to calculate the environmental cost of feeding pets of different sizes in terms of their 'eco footprints' – the amount of land that would be needed to support them. The *New Scientist* summarised this:

> The Vales analysed the ingredients of common brands of pet food. They calculated, for example, that a medium-sized dog would consume 90 grams of meat and 156 grams of cereals daily in its recommended 300-gram portion of dried dog food. At its pre-dried weight, that equates to 450 grams of fresh meat and 260 grams of cereal. That means that over the course of a year, Fido wolfs down about 164 kilograms of meat and 95 kilograms of cereals. It takes 43.3 square metres of land to generate 1 kilogram of chicken per year –far more for beef and lamb – and 13.4 square metres to generate a kilogram of cereals. So that gives him a footprint of 0.84 hectares. For a big dog such as a German shepherd, the figure is 1.1 hectares.
>
> (Ravilious, 2009: p. 46)

A cat, they calculated, has a lower (but still fairly substantial) eco-footprint of 0.15 hectares.

These figures, though, are somewhat misleading (as the Vales note in passing) as they imply that the animal products in commercial cat and dog food are, as it were, animal products specially produced for cats and dogs. But the rendered meat products and meat by-products fall into a different category. The National Renderers Association in the United States claims that rendering in fact converts inedible animal by-products and other materials into 11 billion pounds of reclaimed animal fat annually, and comments:

> The use of rendered fat is a concentrated source of energy for animal and poultry feeds as well as a high quality feedstock for biodiesel. Undoubtedly, the rendering process provides the most logical and environmentally acceptable approach for recycling animals and inedible material into usable commodities.
>
> (National Renderers Association, n.d.)

On this basis, the eco-footprint for animals eating these kinds of commercial foods is significantly lower than the Vales' calculations suggest, as using rendered animal products, and meat by-products in pet food, does not create new demand. But (as with competition with the human food supply) this is not true of animals eating ultra-premium foods or home-made diets; even regular commercial foods have some meat, fish and other ingredients such as cereals that do put pressure on the environment. There is also the energy cost of manufacturing, packaging and transporting pet food to consider. These are not the only environmental costs of looking after pets on a day-to-day basis – waste is another concern.

While keeping cats indoors may, as we suggest subsequently, protect significant environmental values, and reduce the transmission of disease, indoor cats must use cat litter, and the production of most litters has negative environmental impacts. Traditionally, and still most popularly, cat litter is made from bentonite clay or fuller's earth that is strip-mined, and then processed at high temperatures. But reclamation and re-vegetation of these strip-mined sites have been very difficult to achieve (Schuman, 1999). The silica for silica gel cat litter, a common alternative cat litter, is also mined in damaging ways. More recent 'green' litters are made from organic substances such as reclaimed sawdust, corn, wheat and recycled paper. These are in origin less environmentally problematic, but still need processing and transportation.

In addition to production, disposal of both litter and faeces of indoor and outdoor cats is problematic. As discussed previously, cat faeces is a potential source of infectious organisms and zoonotic diseases, such as *Toxoplasma gondii* – so, flushing and composting of cat faeces are environmentally problematic. The alternative is to seal cat faeces and contaminated litter in a plastic bag, put in the trash and send it to landfill. Once encased in plastic, though, even organic cat litter that is in principle biodegradable does not degrade; given the millions of cats in Europe and North America, this creates a significant waste burden. So, different environmental concerns – zoonotic disease versus the burden of waste – point towards different actions. In the United States at least, the welfare risk from disease is usually argued to outweigh the waste burden of putting feline waste in the landfill. Dog faeces, which does not carry *Toxoplasma gondii,* can normally be flushed or digested in a small dog waste disposal system.

Cats and dogs, then, clearly use resources that add to global environmental problems such as habitat destruction and climate change. They also create waste that is environmentally damaging. This is without considering the environmental impacts of the rest of the pet market: collars, leads, baskets, balls, cages, toys, treats, dog apparel, fences, pharmaceuticals, food supplements, shampoos, brushes, scratch posts, burial caskets. It is this combination of food, waste production, and consumer goods that Erik Assadourian has in mind when commenting:

> With a human population of 7.2 billion and a dog and cat population now in the hundreds of millions (it's estimated at 179m in the US alone), the Earth cannot sustain these populations – especially as a growing percentage of pets live their lives as ravenous consumers.

> (Assadourian, 2014)

This claim, though, seems extreme. Certainly, companion animals have environmental impacts (though the environmental impacts of an additional cat or dog pale into insignificance in comparison with the environmental impacts of adding an additional human being, in the industrialised Western nations, at least). While cats and dogs obviously need to eat and defecate, if owners choose, the environmental impacts of both these activities can be reduced, especially in the case of dogs. Much of the commercial market in pet merchandise is not necessary, and could be reduced or eliminated – there is no reason why animal companions should be 'ravenous consumers'; though if cats are kept indoors (see the following subsection), the provision of toys and scratching posts does become more important for welfare. However, it is also worth pointing out that if people reduce or stop spending on companion animals, they would presumably spend their freed-up resources on something else; there is no obvious reason to think that the alternatives would be more 'environmentally friendly'.

In summary, then, ethical arguments that we should not keep companion animals at all, because the practice is unsustainable and the environmental costs too high, seem somewhat overblown, especially given the environmental impacts of other common practices such as driving cars or going on vacations overseas. That is not to say there would not be environmental benefits from, for instance, more companion animal sharing schemes, choosing smaller, less resource-intensive dogs, considering the environmental impacts of purchasing and waste disposal decisions, and cutting back consumer spending on animal companions. All of these could mitigate the environmental impacts of animal companions, though they would only bring overall environmental benefits if the money saved was not spent on alternative consumer goods instead.

However, there is one further, important area of environmental concern to consider here: negative impacts of animal companions on wildlife, other than contributing to the spread of disease. We consider two aspects of this concern here: more briefly, the impact of former animal companions that compete with native wildlife for resources and, more extensively, companion animal wildlife predation, in particular by outdoor cats.

14.4.2 Wildlife competition and predation

One key concern in current wildlife conservation is human-introduced animals that compete with, or prey on, native wildlife. Cats, and to a much lesser extent dogs, are of key concern here, but we will first say something about other companion animals.

Some of the most problematic animals in terms of competition with, and predation on, native wildlife have been snakes, fish, and turtles, acquired as juveniles and then abandoned in the wild as adults, when their substantial size and care requirements become apparent. As these animals are rarely kept as companions in the sense discussed in this book, we will not focus on them here. However, one group of companion animals that can be problematic in this respect is companion birds. As we will discuss in Chapter 15, a wide variety of birds, especially parrots, macaws and parakeets are often kept as companions. But some companion birds, when released or escaping into environments in which they are not native, establish populations that impact on native wildlife. In London, UK for instance, rose-ringed and monk parakeets, from escaped or released companion populations, have established significant feral colonies. Researchers from Imperial College, London, found that the presence of rose-ringed parakeets had negative impacts on native bird populations, noting that 'Parakeet presence significantly reduced feeding rates and increased vigilance among native birds compared with our control treatments' (Peck *et al.*, 2014). This is not only problematic for the native birds; the presence of rose-ringed parakeets in London discourages popular native birds from feeding at bird tables, which is disliked by many people accustomed to feeding them.

Given these negative impacts, from most ethical perspectives, it would be preferable if rose-ringed parakeets and other non-native birds had not become established in these new habitats. On the other hand, eliminating them, once established, is both practically, and ethically, difficult. They are usually most effectively removed by being killed, but it is hard to simultaneously avoid killing non-target species. In addition, a high proportion of the population must be killed to resolve the problem (and this will not work if more animals are released by owners). Killing, or wounding but failing to kill, individual sentient birds also raises significant ethical questions; from an animal rights perspective, doing so would be impermissible, and from a utilitarian view, there would have to be benefits to other humans and animals that really would outweigh the costs of culling in terms of suffering of the birds themselves. From some contextual approaches to ethics, it might be argued that as humans deliberately imported these birds into an alien environment, and in many cases deliberately released them there, there is a special responsibility to care for them, rather than to kill them. What is more, many people have become attached to these non-native bird species and like to see them in their parks and gardens, so proposing to cull them provokes both distress and public protest, making pursuing these policies practically very difficult.

While former companions such as parakeets raise problems of competition with wildlife, the effects of dogs, and especially cats, on wildlife are much more dramatic. Dogs harass and hunt rabbits, squirrels, deer, kit foxes, and wild turkeys in the United

States (Young *et al.*, 2011) and beach-nesting birds and koalas in Australia (Lunney *et al.*, 2007; Williams *et al.*, 2009). However, there are far fewer free-roaming owned or feral dogs than cats in Western industrialised societies, and cats are a much bigger predation concern. So, we focus here on outdoor cats and wildlife.

All cats perform chasing, pouncing and hunting behaviours. In principle, any cat with unsupervised outdoor access may spend time actually hunting, although not all cats do. Unowned and feral cats hunt, even when they are part of a human-supported colony. A study using 'kitty cams' (cameras worn around cats' necks) found that 44% of owned cats with outdoor access actively engaged in hunting (Loyd *et al.*, 2013). Research shows that cats will hunt even when they are well fed; experimental evidence indicates that they prioritise hunting over eating even preferred foods (Adamec, 1976). Cats' main prey is small mammals, in particular mice and rabbits; however, they also catch birds, reptiles, and invertebrates. In Australia and New Zealand, cats also prey on small marsupials.

Why is cat predation on wildlife thought to be so important? Two kinds of values seem to be at stake. The first is a concern about the suffering and death of individual wild animals. There is no doubt that cats kill large numbers of small mammals, birds and lizards wherever they roam (see, for instance, Woods, McDonald & Harris, 2003). Loyd & colleagues (2013) found that of the 44% of cats that hunted in Athens, Georgia, the average success rate was two items a week, mostly lizards. David Jessup claims (though without providing substantiating evidence) that overall in North America:

> Free-roaming and feral cats yearly kill hundreds of millions, perhaps as many as a billion, native North American birds, mammals, reptiles, amphibians and fish … they are maimed, mauled, dismembered, ripped apart, and gutted while they are still alive, and even if they survive the encounter they often die of sepsis because of the virulent nature of the oral fauna of cats.
>
> (Jessup, 2004: pp. 1377–1378)

Cats may also cause disturbance, alarm and fear to wildlife, even when they fail successfully to catch their prey. As we noted in Chapter 5, those who value subjective animal welfare are likely to find the negative experiences of fear, pain and suffering that cats' predation generates ethically troubling (though it is also likely that many of these animals would anyway die unpleasant deaths, for instance, in cold winters). Those who value the lives of conscious beings may also be concerned about cats' *killing* of animals, independently of any suffering caused. As the focus of these concerns is individual wild animal welfare and individual lives, the concerns apply wherever cats are hunting; the suffering and death of a common backyard mockingbird would matter just as much from this perspective as that of an endangered sandpiper.

The second value – or cluster of values – concerns not so much the individual wild animal, as the loss of environmental values that cat predation may cause. Two values in particular are usually emphasised here – the value of species, and the value of healthy, functioning ecosystems. On this view, when cats prey on members of threatened species, or their predation impacts on ecosystems, there is a significant loss of environmental value. So, while a cat hunting a common backyard mockingbird does not threaten any significant loss of ecological or species value, a cat hunting an endangered sandpiper in a small colony that has an important function in the ecosystem would be highly problematic. Research clearly shows that in some locations – such as where cats have been introduced to oceanic islands with endemic and vulnerable populations – their predation can have major effects (Nogales *et al.*, 2004). This is also true where cats are located close to endangered species of ground-nesting birds or rodents. However, cats' effects on wildlife in other locations, such as urban and suburban areas, are more difficult to assess. Some conservationists argue that gardens and parks in urban and suburban areas can be key stopping places for migratory bird populations, so cat predation there will be in some cases highly problematic (Jessup, 2004; Lepczyk *et al.*, 2010; Longcore *et al.*, 2009). Others conclude that 'the direct effect of cats on native fauna will be secondary to the more dramatic effects of loss of native vegetation by the suburbs themselves' (Dickman, 2009: p. 45).

Cat predation, then, looks troubling from a number of different value perspectives. But these concerns are complex. For instance, someone who values subjective animal welfare is likely to be concerned about cat welfare as well as wild animal welfare. It is very plausible that being able to roam and hunt is good for cat welfare (see Chapter 4). So, how should these competing welfare concerns be weighed? A hedonistic utilitarian would argue for something like maximising pleasure, net of pain. As one hunting cat causes intense suffering to many animals, that seems like an argument to stop cats from hunting. But this view has other potentially unwanted implications. If one is concerned about wild animal suffering, then perhaps all predation is problematic – after all, domestic cats are not the only animals that cause suffering and death to their prey. (McMahan, 2010 defends the view that it would be better if we could reduce wild predation.) But most people do not want to be committed to the view that we should eliminate predators, or even that there is something wrong with predation. It is also possible that stopping cat predation would not much reduce wild suffering and death anyway. Some argue that cats prey on wildlife that would not otherwise have lived a good life –the 'doomed surplus' (Smith, 2009); if this is the case, the animals caught by cats would likely die in some other way soon anyway.

From ethical positions other than utilitarianism, as we saw in Chapter 5, being concerned about the welfare of all animals does not necessarily mean that we have the same obligations to all animals. On ethical views that emphasise context and relationship, we could, as individuals or communities, have special obligations for the welfare of our own animal companions, or members of companion animal species, because of our special relationships or history with them, without these obligations extending to wildlife. On a rights view, while it may be argued that a companion cat has a basic right not to be confined by people, birds and mice do not have any rights against cats, as cats are not moral agents, the kinds of being we can hold morally responsible for anything, including rights protection. So, while cats may have a right to liberty of movement, on a rights view, there is no reason why we should protect wild animals from them. These possible positions show how a diversity of different ethical conclusions is possible here, even among those who take welfare to be valuable.

However, even if a wildlife welfare argument against predation is difficult to maintain, there clearly are cases where cats can contribute to threatening species or diminishing ecosystem functioning – though this does not seem true of all actively hunting cats everywhere. What are the ethical options where this is the case? Where cats are homed, it is possible to restrict roaming and make hunting more difficult, for instance, by putting a bell on the cat, confining the cat to certain safe outdoor spaces, supervising all outdoor access, or by keeping cats permanently indoors. Supervising and belling are not very effective (as anyone who has tried to supervise a cat who wants to hunt outdoors knows)! As we saw in Chapter 4, keeping cats indoors is very divisive, with ongoing disagreement over whether it is, or is not, better for cats' welfare, while confined outdoor spaces raise practical, aesthetic and economic difficulties for many households. Where cats are stray or feral, the options are more limited. Relocation to a less-sensitive environment is possible, but practically difficult; trap-neuter-return policies may stabilise colony size, but are slow to affect numbers of animals being preyed upon; rehoming is possible but only for cats that are or can be socialised; and there are, anyway, currently insufficient homes. The only remaining practical alternative is to euthanase the cats. As discussed in Chapter 13, euthanasia of healthy animals raises significant ethical challenges, and when adopted as policy often causes a substantial public outcry.

The impact of cat predation on wildlife, especially by cats without homes and where threatened or endangered species are involved, is a highly contested ethical issue. (See Palmer, 2014; Palmer & Sandøe, 2014 for further discussion.) It brings together – and into conflict – ethical concerns about animal welfare, the value of animal lives and the environment, in a context where some people, at least, have very deeply held attachments and commitments; in situations of this kind, no easy or universal resolution is possible.

Key Points

- Companion animals may infect humans with zoonotic diseases; these can be very serious or even fatal, though this outcome is rare in industrialised Western nations.
- The diseases can be controlled in animals in various ways including vaccination, medication, surveillance and culls; but culls are controversial, both in terms of effectiveness and ethical acceptability. An alternative way of thinking about these issues is one of 'shared risk'.
- It is sometimes claimed that pet food competes with the human food supply. However, the animal products found in most commercial pet food would not be consumed by people. But the inclusion of pelagic fish in cat food, and the move to ultra-gourmet pet food, may have an impact on human food supply and possibly wild animal welfare.
- It is also sometimes claimed that the amount spent on companion animals, including for expensive veterinary care, cannot be justified given global human poverty, but this argument is problematic in a number of ways.

- Companion animals do use resources and create waste, but there are ways in which the impact of this can be mitigated; the environmental impacts do not seem sufficient to support arguments that living with companion animals cannot be justified for environmental reasons.
- Companion animals can compete with and prey on native wildlife. This may occur when feral populations of former companions (e.g. parakeets and feral cats) become established, or where owned animals have outdoor access.
- Cat predation impacts on animal welfare and can have significant environmental impacts. This is a very difficult and complicated ethical problem, especially as significantly reducing predation from unowned cats would require euthanasing them.

References

Adamec, R.E. (1976) The interaction of hunger and preying in the domestic cat (*Felis catus*): an adaptive hierarchy. *Behavioral Biology* 18, 263–272.

Aldrich, G. (2006) Rendered products in pet food. In: Meeker, D.L. (ed.) *Essential rendering: all about the animal by-products industry*. Arlington, VA, Kirby Lithographic Company, pp. 159–177. [Online] Available from: http://www.nationalrenderers.org/nutrition/pet-food/ [Accessed 22 August 2014].

Aldrich, G. (2013) *Rendered ingredients in pet food*. Presentation. [Online] Available from: https://d10k7k7mywg42z.cloudfront.net/assets/511a48238ad7ca3a92000ce9/Greg_Aldrich___Rendered_Ingredients_in_Pet_Foods.pdf [Accessed 22 August 2014].

APPA [American Pet foods and Products Association] (n.d.) *Pet industry market size & ownership statistics*. [Online] Available from: http://www.americanpetproducts.org/press_industrytrends.asp [Accessed 22 August 2014].

Assadourian, Erik. (2014) Are pets bad for the environment? *The Guardian* 1 May [Online] Available from: http://www.theguardian.com/sustainable-business/reduce-pets-sustainable-future-cats-dogs [Accessed 22 August 2014].

Bonner, J. (2014) *Dispensing microbial drugs*. [Online] Available from: http://www.bsava.com/Portals/4/knowledgevault/resources/files/Dispensing_antimicrobial_drugs.pdf [Accessed 22 August 2014].

Dabritz, H., Atwill, E., Gardner, I., Miller, M. & Conrad, P. (2006) Outdoor fecal deposition by free-roaming cats and attitudes of cat owners and non-owners toward stray pets, wildlife and water pollution. *Journal of the American Veterinary Association* 229 (1), 74–81.

Day, M.J., Breitschwerdt, E., Cleaveland, S., Karkare, U., Khanna, C., Kirpensteijn, J., Kuiken, T., Lappin, M.R., McQuiston, J., Mumford, E., Myers, T., Palatnik-de-Sousa, C.B., Rubin, C., Takashima, G. & Thiermann, A. (2012) Surveillance of zoonotic infectious disease transmitted by small companion animals. *Emerging Infectious Diseases* 18 (12). DOI: 10.3201/eid1812.120664

De Silva, S.S. & Turchini, G.M. (2008) Towards understanding the impacts of the pet food industry on world fish and seafood supplies. *Journal of Agricultural and Environmental Ethics* 21, 459–467.

Dickman, C.R. (2009) Housecats as predators in the Australian environment: impacts and management. *Human-Wildlife Conflicts* 3 (1), 41–48.

Hadley, J. & O'Sullivan, S. (2009) World poverty, animal minds and the ethics of veterinary expenditure. *Environmental Values* 18, 361–378.

Jessup, D.A. (2004) The welfare of feral cats and wildlife. *Journal of the American Veterinary Medical Association* 225, 1377–1383.

Kaschner, K., Karpouzi, V., Watson, R., Pauly, D. 2006. Forage fish consumption by marine mammals and seabirds. In: Alder, J., Pauly, D. (eds) *On the multiple uses of forage fish: from ecosystems to markets*. Fisheries Centre Research Reports 14 (3). Fisheries Centre, University of British Columbia.

Lepczyk, C., Dauphine, D., Bird, D., Conant, S., Cooper, R., Duffy, D., Hatley, P., Marra, P., Stone, E. & Temple, S. (2010) What conservation biologists can do to counter trap-neuter-return: response to Longcore et al. *Conservation Biology* 24 (2), 627–629.

Longcore, T., Rich, C. & Sullivan, L.M. (2009) Critical assessment of claims regarding management of feral cats by trap-neuter-return. *Conservation Biology* 23 (4), 887–894.

Loyd, K.A.T., Hernandez, S.M., Carroll, J.P., Abernathy, K.J. & Marshall, G.J. (2013) Quantifying free-roaming domestic cat predation using animal-borne video cameras. *Biological Conservation* 160, 183–189.

Lunney, D., Gresser, S., O'Neill, L.E., Matthews, A. & Rhodes, J. (2007) The impact of fire and dogs on koalas at Port Stephens, New South Wales, using population viability analysis. *Pacific Conservation Biology* 13 (3), 189–201.

McMahan, J. (2010) The meat-eaters. *New York Times* 19 September. [Online] Available from: http://opinionator.blogs.nytimes.com/2010/09/19/the-meat-eaters/ [Accessed 22 August 2014].

Molento, C.F.M. (2014) Public health and animal welfare. In: Appleby, M.C., Weary, D.M. & Sandøe, P. (eds) *Dilemmas in animal welfare*. Wallingford, CABI, pp. 102–123.

Muirden, A. (2002) Prevalence of feline leukaemia virus and antibodies to feline immunodeficiency virus and feline coronavirus in stray cats sent to an RSPCA hospital. *Veterinary Record* 150 (20), 621–625.

National Renderers Association (n.d.) *The environmental impact*. [Online] Available from: http://www.nationalrenderers.org/environmental/ [Accessed 22 August 2014].

Nestle, M. & Nesheim, M. (2010). *Feed your pet right*. New York, Free Press.

Nogales, M., Martin, A., Tershy, B.R., Donlan, C.J., Veitch, R., Puerta, N., Wood, B. & Alonso, J. (2004) A review of feral cat eradication on islands. *Conservation Biology* 18, 310–319.

One Health Initiative Task Force (2008) *One health: a new professional imperative*. American Veterinary Medical Association. [Online] Available from: https://www.avma.org/KB/Resources/Reports/Documents/onehealth_final.pdf [Accessed 22 August 2014].

Palmer, C. (2014) Moral conflict in feral cat management: trap-neuter-return or trap-euthanize? In: Appleby, M.C., Weary, D.M. & Sandøe, P. (eds) *Dilemmas in animal welfare*. Wallingford, CABI, pp. 148–168.

Palmer, C. & Sandøe, P. (2014) Captive cats: should cats be routinely confined indoors for their own good? In: Gruen, L. (ed.) *Ethics of captivity*. Oxford, Oxford University Press, pp. 135–155.

Peck, H.L., Pringle, H.E., Marshall, H.H., Owens, I.P.F. & Lord, A.M. (2014) Experimental evidence of impacts of an invasive parakeet on foraging behavior of native birds. *Behavioral Ecology*. 25(3) 582–590.

Rabinowitz, P.M., Odophin, L. & Dein, F.J. (2008) From "us vs. them" to "shared risk": can animals help link environmental factors to human health? *Ecohealth* 5, 224–229.

Ravilious, K. (2009) How green is your pet? *New Scientist* 24 (October), 46–47.

Schuman, G.E. (1999) Reclamation of abandoned bentonite mined lands. In: Wong, H. (ed.) *Remediation and management of degraded lands.* Boca Raton, FL, CRC Press, pp. 77–88.

Singer, P. (1972) Famine, affluence and morality. *Philosophy and Public Affairs* 1 (3), 229–243.

Smith, R. (2009) *Cats: warm furry friends or natural born killers?* Expert comment. University of Huddersfield. [Online] Available from: http://www.hud.ac.uk/sas /comment/display/?articleid=rhs090909 [Accessed 22 August 2014].

Tacon, A.G. & Metian, M. (2009) Fishing for feed or fishing for food: increasing global competition for small pelagic forage fish. *Ambio* 38 (6), 294–302.

Taylor, L.H., Latham, S.M. & Woolhouse, M.E. (2001) Risk factors for disease emergence. *Philosophical Transactions of the Royal Society B: Biological Science* 356, 983–989.

Vale, R. & Vale, B. (2009) *Time to eat the dog? The real guide to sustainable living.* London. Thames & Hudson.

Williams, K., Weston, M., Henry, S. & McGuire, G. (2009) Birds and beaches, dogs and leashes: dog owners' sense of obligation to leash dogs in Victoria Australia. *Human Dimensions of Wildlife* 14, 89–101.

Woods, M., McDonald, R.A. & Harris, S. (2003) Predation of wildlife by domestic cats *Felix catus* in Great Britain. *Mammal Review* 33 (2), 174–188.

WFP [World Food Programme] (2014) *Hunger: frequently asked questions (FAQs).* [Online] Available from: http://www.wfp.org/hunger/faqs [Accessed 22 August 2014].

WSPA/RSPCA (2007) Stray Animal Control Practices: Europe. [Online] Available from: http: //www.fao.org/fileadmin/user_upload/animalwelfare/WSPA_RSPCA%20International% 20stray%20control%20practices%20in%20Europe%202006_2007.pdf [Accessed 23 August 2014].

Young, J.K., Olson, K.A., Reading, R.P., Amgalanbaatar, S. & Berger, J. (2011) Is wildlife going to the dogs? Impacts of feral and free-roaming dogs on wildlife populations. *Bioscience* 61 (2), 125–132.

Other Companions

15

15.1 Introduction   235
15.2 The Welfare of Other Companions   236
    15.2.1 Small rodents (mice, gerbils, rats, guinea pigs, hamsters)   237
    15.2.2 Rabbits   238
    15.2.3 Birds   239
15.3 Wild-Caught Birds and the Pet Trade   241
15.4 Ethical Approaches to Other Companions   242
15.5 Should Ownership of Some Species Be Restricted, or Completely
    Prohibited?   246

15.1 Introduction

This book has focused on dogs and cats, as our typical animal companions: three-quarters of those households that choose to live with animals, choose dogs and/or cats. Other animals are, of course, kept in the home or garden, but not usually as companions. Aquarium fish are, for example, commonly kept for their aesthetic appeal or their psychologically relaxing effects, rather than for companionship. However, other animals that we have not so far considered can be kept as companions, though less often than cats and dogs – in particular rabbits, birds and small rodents (e.g. hamsters, rats and guinea pigs).

Defining a companion species is not straightforward, though, as different people will keep the same species for different reasons. For example, macaws could be kept either for companionship, or purely for their aesthetic appeal, while some people might turn to their tarantula or goldfish for mutual play or comfort. And keeping any animal in a

Companion Animal Ethics, First Edition. Peter Sandøe, Sandra Corr and Clare Palmer.
© Universities Federation for Animal Welfare 2016.

household may raise ethical issues, not just those kept as companions. However, here we will maintain this book's focus on companionship, and consider the central ethical issues raised by what we call the 'other companions', with a focus on small mammals, rabbits and birds.

These 'other companions' may be acquired for various reasons, for instance, if people are not allowed to keep dogs or cats in rental properties, or are not physically able to care for them, owing to illnesses, disabilities or allergies. But there are also positive motivations for acquiring other companions: some people may always have lived with animals of a particular kind, and be loyal to the species (Serpell, 1981). They may just enjoy, or find otherwise rewarding, interacting with animals of that kind. In addition, many of the animals in this category may be acquired for children, perhaps with the goal of teaching responsibility and care, or because the child asked for a pet (Fifield & Forsyth, 1999).

In this chapter, we first consider welfare challenges posed by these other companions, some of which are not raised, or not raised to the same degree, by keeping dogs and cats. We then also consider one broader concern – the companion bird trade – that not only raises major welfare issues for birds, but also has broader social and environmental impacts. We then move on to consider different ethical approaches to these welfare issues and to the wild bird trade. In the final section of the chapter, we reflect on whether ownership of some kinds of companion animals is normally unethical, and should be restricted or prohibited altogether.

15.2 The Welfare of Other Companions

One starting point for thinking about the welfare of other companions is to return to the Five Freedoms we have discussed before (Chapter 4): the freedom from hunger and thirst; the freedom from discomfort (including the provision of an appropriate environment); the freedom from pain, injury and disease; the freedom to express normal behaviour (including sufficient space and appropriate social interaction); and the freedom from fear and distress. However, as we also discussed in Chapter 4, these freedoms, while important, are all rather negative, focusing on freedom from what is bad, such as suffering and restrictions on normal behaviour. In addition, we should also think about *positive* welfare, where companions have good lives, with opportunities to flourish, and to carry out enjoyable, engaging and challenging activities.

Many of the welfare issues we have discussed in the case of cats and dogs may also affect other companions – for instance, they may become obese due to inappropriate diet and lack of exercise. However, other companions are often kept in ways that also generate some distinct welfare problems. For example, most other companions live in cages, and do not generally have freedom to move about the house. They may be allowed to run or fly indoors or outdoors on occasions, but most of the time they are closely confined, which (as we will discuss below) raises questions about their ability to perform key normal behaviours. Relatedly, partly on account of being confined (and in some cases, also nocturnal), other companions run the risk of being neglected and forgotten by their owners. While, as Sainthouse (2011) notes, cats and dogs can and do loudly pester their owners if they are hungry and thirsty, small mammals, rabbits and birds normally lack this ability. More generally, especially where other companions are small, and do not interact much with their owners, any health problems they have may be less noticeable than in the case of cats and dogs.

Another common factor shared by at least some of the other companions (mainly the small mammals and rabbits) is that, as noted in the Introduction, they are often recommended and acquired for children as 'starter pets' because they are supposed to be easy to care for (the ASPCA (n.d.), for instance, recommends guinea pigs as an excellent 'starter pet' for older children). As we will note next, however, it is not that easy to care for these animals well; the difficulties of doing so are exacerbated if, in order to teach children responsibility, the animals are left largely or solely to children's care, which rarely happens with cats and dogs.

Finally, a major issue shared by most of the other companions concerns social contact with conspecifics. Cats and dogs are usually socially integrated into their human households, and have significant interactions with their owners. Cats may do well, or better, as solitary felines within a household; while dogs normally benefit from contact with other dogs, they are typically taken out for walks and play in dog parks where these conspecific socialising opportunities exist. However, many of the other companions, including some of the large birds, are frequently kept alone, even though they are often highly social. As we will discuss, even though they may have some contact with their owners, being kept alone means that they lack any opportunity to express important social behaviours with conspecifics.

Many different species of animals may be kept as companions, and we are unable to discuss them all here; for instance, we will not be discussing chinchillas, ferrets, and semi-wild/wild companions (such as wolf-dogs, monkeys, and exotic or tamed wild mammals), as the numbers of these animals kept as companions are comparatively small. We will focus here on the most common of the other below: small rodents, rabbits and birds.

15.2.1 Small rodents (mice, gerbils, rats, guinea pigs, hamsters)

Small rodents – sometimes called 'pocket pets' – have particular needs that, if not met, may lead to welfare problems; we will focus on three here: environment, social contact and veterinary care.

All these small rodents are normally kept indoors in cages (though guinea pigs are sometimes kept outside in hutches). However, caged environments that promote good welfare are difficult to establish and to maintain. Cages are often too small, even when their occupants, such as golden hamsters, are themselves small. Studies indicate, for instance, that the smaller the cage in which a hamster is housed, the more stereotypic behaviour such as wire-gnawing it performs (Fischer *et al.*, 2007). As well as being large enough for their occupants to exercise, cages also need to be kept clean, as the animals urinate and defecate throughout; failure to clean cages can lead to disease. Yet, while it is important to keep cages clean, given the opportunity, small mammals such as gerbils create intricate tunnels that they continually modify; rats and mice can become stressed as a result of having scent marks and olfactory clues constantly removed (Sayers & Smith, 2010); Syrian hamsters prefer 14 days old to new bedding (Veillette & Reebs, 2010). So, while cage cleanliness is important, small rodents also seem to prefer familiarity, and materials they can manipulate in their environment; both appear to be important to welfare. Environmental enrichment, through adding toys, hides, food treats, and bedding materials to the cages, encourages the animals to forage and exercise (but may also compromise cleanliness).

Another element of the ability to perform 'normal behaviour' involves achieving an appropriate amount of social contact with conspecifics. Rats, mice, gerbils and guinea pigs, for instance, are very social: guinea pigs form lasting bonds with conspecifics, and keeping them alone is widely thought to cause significant welfare problems (Hillyer, Quesenberry & Donnelly, 1997). In fact, in recognition of the welfare importance of conspecific companionship, in 2008, Switzerland implemented a law requiring that social species, including guinea pigs, should have regular interaction with a member of the same species (Swissinfo.ch, 2008). But this need for social contact with conspecifics is not universal among small rodents. Syrian hamsters are solitary; being housed with or even near to another hamster is stressful, while male mice are territorial and fight if caged together. Thus, where suitable social housing requirements are not met, welfare is likely to be compromised.

Finally, although these species are fairly common companions, research suggests they are not often taken to vets (Keown, Farnworth & Adams, 2011), and, therefore, vets are likely to be less familiar with their health issues than they are in the case of cats and dogs. Keown, Farnworth & Adams (2011) surveyed vets in New Zealand on their familiarity with treatments for, and their willingness to treat, guinea pigs and rabbits. They concluded that in New Zealand at least, 'there is a relative paucity of information regarding pain recognition, and anaesthetic and analgesic protocols for rodents and lagomorphs [here, rabbits] outside laboratories' (Keown, Farnworth & Adams, 2011: p. 305). This may mean that these animals are not receiving adequate relief from pain, especially post-operatively.

15.2.2 Rabbits

Rabbits are, in some countries, the third most popular companion animals after cats and dogs; there are estimated to be 3.2 million companion rabbits in the United States (AVMA, 2012), and around 1.7 million companion rabbits in the United Kingdom (PDSA, 2013). We will consider a couple of the most significant issues affecting rabbit welfare here.

The first is diet. Wild rabbits' main diet is grass, which is important for nutrition and digestion; and because rabbits' teeth grow continuously, high-fibre diets (grass and hay) are necessary to grind the teeth down. While most domestic rabbits are usually given access to some hay or grass, they are often also fed commercial mix foods that are selectively eaten. Selective feeding commonly leaves rabbits with too little calcium in their diet, contributing to dental disease. In a study of 102 fairly young pet rabbits, Mullan & Main (2006) found that 29.4% had dental disease, some in an advanced state. Rabbit mix foods may also be high in protein, fat and carbohydrate, which can cause obesity, digestive problems and diarrhoea.

These problems are compounded because owners often do not understand key issues about rabbit health – in the Mullan & Main (2006) study, most owners were unaware that their rabbits had dental disease – and infrequently took them to see a vet. According to a survey of UK pet owners, only 56% of rabbit owners are registered with a vet, and while 64% check their rabbit's teeth at least monthly, 12% of owners never check their rabbits for maggots – leaving 200,000 rabbits at risk of 'fly-strike' (where maggots eat the rabbit's flesh, causing severe suffering, and, in some cases, death) (PDSA, 2013).

The second issue is environment – both social and physical – as, although companion rabbits have been domesticated, research suggests that domestication has not significantly changed their behavioural repertoire (Edgar & Mullan, 2011). In the wild, rabbits live in burrow systems with many other rabbits, and even when on the surface, they tend to remain within 10 metres of another individual 40–50% of the time (Cowan, 1987). However, many rabbits kept in the home are kept in solitude. A study in the Netherlands found that 48% of households kept solitary rabbits (Schepers, Koene & Beerda, 2009); while studies in the United Kingdom found 56% (Mullan & Main, 2006) and 65% (PDSA, 2013) of rabbits were kept alone. Schepers, Koene & Beerda (2009) concluded that this solitary housing could be a contributing factor in the short lifespan of the rabbits studied (4.2 years on average, rather than a potential 13 years). It is sometimes mistakenly thought that housing a rabbit with a guinea pig meets both animals' needs for social contact; but only conspecifics make suitable companions (PDSA, 2013).

Access to sufficient space is also a concern. Wild rabbits have a home range of 7000–20,000 m^2. Mullan & Main (2006) found that in the United Kingdom, 84% of rabbits were kept in hutches smaller than those recommended by animal welfare groups (which were themselves far smaller than the usual range of a wild rabbit); just over 20% were kept in cages smaller than those recommended even for laboratory rabbits. A more recent study in the United Kingdom found that only 40% of rabbits had access to a run, only 23% dug in the garden on a daily basis, and 18% had no access to exercise on a daily basis (PDSA, 2013).

As with the other small mammals, rabbits are often thought of as an easy companion for children to keep; however, they are especially vulnerable to a variety of welfare problems if their housing and husbandry are suboptimal. In an article in the UK newspaper *The Observer* entitled 'Pet rabbits are cruelly neglected and mistreated in Britain', RSPCA inspector Tony Woodley is quoted as saying:

> If you ask any RSPCA officer which animal they feel most sorry for, it's usually the poor, forgotten rabbit sitting in a tiny hutch without the proper food, or any food at all, and some dirty water. It might once have been loved for a brief time by some child, but it has quickly been forgotten and it's a very sad sight that I have seen countless times.

(McVeigh, 2011)

15.2.3 Birds

The category of 'birds' is rather broad one. Many different species of birds are kept in households, from relatively small budgerigars to large birds such as macaws, though the majority of companion birds are in the *Psittaciforme* (parrot) order. While budgerigars live on average 8–10 years, some of the larger parrots may live for 50–80 years, making these animal companions the most long-lived of all those we are considering in this book: they can frequently outlive their human owner.

As we noted in Chapter 1, the popularity of birds kept as companions has decreased as the popularity of cats and dogs has risen; but many millions of birds are still kept as companions in households worldwide. According to the AVMA (2012), there are 8.3 million birds kept as companions in the United States; the European Pet Food Industry Federation estimates that more than 42 million caged birds are kept in the European Union (FEDIAF, 2011).

Most of the birds kept as companions are not regarded as domesticated; some are still acquired directly from the wild (see Section 15.3), and others are only one or two generations from wild birds (especially parrots, given their longevity – see Meehan & Mench, 2006). Engebretson (2006: p. 263) notes that 'many of the bird species that are bred and traded as companion animals remain physically indistinguishable from their wild counterparts'. Given the difference between the lives of wild birds and caged companion birds, we might expect significant welfare issues to arise from keeping them in the home; we can only consider these briefly here (see Meehan & Mench, 2006 for further details on parrot welfare, in particular). Key areas of welfare concern, as with other companion animals we have considered here, are diet and disease, lack of social interaction with conspecifics, and being kept in environments that are too small and barren to allow them to perform normal behaviours.

First, with respect to diet and disease: captive birds, like rabbits, are selective eaters. Many of them are fed seed diets in the home; but these diets are high in fat and lack nutrients. According to Harrison (1998), around 90% of all clinical conditions seen by avian practitioners are caused by malnutrition. So, while birds may be provided with diets that would be at least minimally adequate if not selectively eaten, in practice, the birds may not get the nutrition they need; this makes them vulnerable to various diseases, including fungal infections (Engebretson, 2006). Although birds may have a number of health problems, research suggests that birds kept as companions are rarely offered veterinary care – strikingly less so than dogs, and, to a significantly lesser degree, than cats. In the United States, in 2006, 82.7% of owned dogs and 63.7% of owned cats had been taken to the vet at least once, but only 13.9% of bird-owning households used the services of a vet (Shepherd, 2008).

Companion birds also often lack sufficient space to perform normal behaviours, including flying, even though some nations and US states legislate a minimum cage size. The US state of Colorado, for instance, regulates cage size for birds:

> The cage must be large enough to provide full body extension without contact with the confines. The cage must be wide enough in at least one direction to accommodate completely stretched wings.
>
> (Born Free USA, n.d.)

The UK Wildlife and Countryside Act (1981) likewise requires cages to be of a suitable size to allow birds to extend their wings in every direction. Even so, this does not give birds sufficient room to fly, or to perform other normal behaviours. Engebretson (2006: p. 265) reports that in the case of parrots, post-mortems often reveal stress-related lesions, which, it is postulated, are because of 'physical and behavioural restrictions imposed by standard captive environments'. Birds that are unable to perform normal behaviours because of confinement may also perform stereotypic behaviours, or develop habits such as feather-picking (Hawkins, 2009, Meehan & Mench, 2006).

Many bird species kept as companions are social, and evidence suggests that time spent with conspecifics is important to their welfare. However, even here, social inter-action may work differently between species; while new budgerigars can be fairly easily integrated with existing budgerigars as budgerigar flocks are not strongly hierarchical, other parrots require much slower introductions to new conspecifics (Hawkins, 2009). For some members of the parrot species, being housed alone is thought to be particularly stressful. African Gray parrots, for instance, live in flocks of from 20–30 to several thousand birds in the wild; keeping them singly 'inevitably leads to psychological problems of fear and aggression' (Girling, 2009: p. 128).

Before moving on to look at some ethical responses to these welfare concerns, we will consider one more issue that is important for bird welfare, but that also has other impacts: wild-caught birds and the pet trade.

15.3 Wild-Caught Birds and the Pet Trade

Some birds kept as companions are captured from the wild. The international trade in wildlife – for purposes such as food, traditional medicine, entertainment or pets – is huge. Precise figures specifically relating to the pet trade are difficult to obtain, because captive-bred and wild-caught animals are often not separately identified, or are wrongly identified, and a significant proportion of the market is illegal under CITES (the Convention on International Trade in Endangered Species) and so is not formally reported at all. Much of the wild-caught pet trade concerns animals beyond the scope of this book, including primates, reptiles, snakes and fish. However, the trade in wild-caught birds destined to become companion animals is relevant here.

Originally, all companion birds were wild caught. However, many species (such as budgerigars) are now largely or wholly captive bred, and some captive breeding takes place in all companion bird species. But certain breeds of parrots and macaws are still, to some degree, illegally captured from the wild, and illegally traded, and become available on the companion bird market (although it is, for instance, illegal to import wild-caught parrots into the United States for the pet trade).

The capture, transportation and export of wild-caught birds have very negative welfare implications. Capture is stressful (for instance, birds are often caught in nets or glue traps) and may cause death through trauma or exhaustion, or diseases such as capture myopathy, a degeneration of skeletal muscle (Engebretson, 2006). Surviving birds are then usually transported in overcrowded conditions, often receiving insufficient food and water, and diseases spread quickly. Mortality rates among wild-captured birds are very high. For instance, recent research estimates the mortality rate of wild-captured grey parrots in Congo to be 45–65% from capture to market in Kinshasa (Hart, 2013).

However, this trade benefits some humans' welfare; for example, the economic benefits to often impoverished communities from collecting and selling wild birds can be significant. A study in the Peruvian Amazon of the illegal harvest of parrot nestlings found that doing so 'represented an important source of income for local families during the flood season, when fish and agricultural products are more scarce' (González, 2003). Yet these benefits may be short lived: González (2003) goes on to suggest that the parrots are being driven to extinction because too many are collected, and the collection methods frequently destroy nesting trees. If the parrots disappear, then so will the benefits: not only will people not be able to collect nestlings, but future costs could be substantial, if for instance, an ecotourism industry based on bird watching might otherwise have been established.

This raises other factors that, while not directly of welfare concern, might be relevant to thinking ethically about the capture of wild birds as companions: the effects on wild animal populations, species and ecological systems, rather than on *individual* wild animal welfare. Removing birds can significantly deplete wild populations, reduce genetic diversity, and potentially threaten whole species (although it can be difficult to distinguish the effects of the pet trade from other more general threats, e.g. from habitat destruction). The ways in which members of the target species are captured may also damage ecosystems and cause the deaths of members of other, non-target, species. This is particularly a concern with respect to Amazon bird species, where the problem can self-reinforce:

> individuals who greatly value rarity will often increase the economic incentives to capture increasingly rare species, thus creating a positive feedback loop with uncommon species being more valuable and therefore more sought-after.
>
> (Fernandes-Ferreira *et al.*, 2012: p. 231)

One way of avoiding the problems of the wild bird trade is to buy only captive-bred birds. But while this may be easy enough when acquiring budgerigars or canaries, it is much more difficult to be sure of the provenance of birds such as Amazon parrots and macaws. Wild-caught birds may be sold more cheaply, or they may be labelled as captive-bred and laundered through breeding farms (Schuppli, Fraser & Bacon, 2014); so a purchaser may not be sure of exactly what he or she is acquiring. For this reason, Engebretson (2006: p. 273), among others, argues that as long as people are permitted to keep parrots as companions, the smuggling of parrots for the pet trade is likely to continue.

The wild capture of birds that ultimately (even if illegally, or purchased in ignorance) end up as companions, raises a wider set of value issues alongside both human and animal welfare. These issues need to be considered in taking a broader ethical view of keeping other companions, as we suggest in the following section.

15.4 Ethical Approaches to Other Companions

Keeping animals other than cats and dogs as companions raises a wide range of welfare problems, primarily for the animals, but in some cases, also for people; and where birds are wild caught, environmental impacts may also be significant. What should we think about this in ethical terms?

We begin with human-centred ethical approaches such as contractarianism (see Chapter 5) where human interests and concerns are of primary importance and animal welfare and the environment matter only in as much as they matter to people. Even from these approaches, the issues raised here are of ethical significance. An unsuitable companion animal (such as a nocturnal hamster for a child, that bites when woken in the day) or a companion animal that is listless, performs stereotypical behaviours, or is fearful or aggressive because its welfare is poor, can cause its owners' distress, and is likely to reduce their enjoyment in having an animal companion. An owner may be upset when, because he or she does not know what a companion needs to flourish, significant welfare problems or premature death occur. On most human-centred ethical views, it would be better if these outcomes were avoided by improved welfare for the animal.

It is worth noting, though, that in some cases animals may suffer welfare problems without them having noticeable behavioural effects in the early stages – as with dental disease in rabbits, or some forms of malnutrition in birds. Here, as the welfare issues do not impact on human relationships to the animals, they do not matter ethically from a human-centred perspective. In other cases, improving an animal's welfare sufficiently to avoid problems for the animal may entail sacrifice by an owner – for instance, of house-hold space – that the owner does not want to make. From a human-centred perspective, if the owner values household space more than their companion's welfare, then there is no ethical responsibility to give the space up.

The market in wild-caught birds is also of ethical concern from a human-centred perspective. While people who engage in the trade benefit from it, as noted earlier, these benefits are unlikely to be sustainable; while much of what owners enjoy about keep-ing birds as companions could be equally well produced by captive-bred birds, which also carry less risk of disease transmission to people. So, the human gains from the trade, in the long term, are small, if they exist at all. Meanwhile, many people value bird species, ecosystems, and the biodiversity they partly comprise, because they are extremely useful in providing long-term services to people (for instance, they may con-tribute to new drugs, they help to purify freshwater and so on) and/or because they subjectively value their existence (what economists sometimes call 'existence value') and deplore their loss. From this human perspective, the wild-caught bird trade is ethically unacceptable. Human-centred ethical views of this kind underpin international laws banning the capture of many species of wild birds, and national laws forbidding the importation of wild-caught birds for the companion animal market.

Other ethical approaches take animal welfare directly into account. A utilitarian might begin by asking whether, in any particular case, better welfare overall could be achieved by changing the way an animal companion is cared for – for instance, by giving animals more space, a better diet, environmental enrichment, or a companion. These changes may cause less suffering and enrich animals' lives, and may also improve the owner's enjoyment in the companion, especially if the change comes at minimal cost to the owner, such as switching from all seed to pelleted food for parrots. However, other changes – such as sacrificing household space for the companion – may come at a greater cost to the owner. Utilitarianism, unlike human-centred approaches, then must weigh the owner's feelings of inconvenience, negative aesthetic experience and so on, against the benefits to the animals' welfare. In most cases, although changes in space or companionship may be a nuisance for an owner, they make major differences to the welfare of an animal, and so the benefits to the animal will usually outweigh the costs to the owner.

One difficulty with the weighing process from the perspective of a utilitarian is that, (as we noted in Chapter 4), in practice, it is hard to work out what 'good welfare' actually is, even when there is agreement on how to define and measure welfare. This is because different aspects of welfare can be in conflict (as in the case of letting a cat outdoors). For example, keeping a cage very clean may reduce an animal's risk of disease, and so make suffering less likely, something a utilitarian cares about. But it may also create a barren environment for an animal, lacking sufficient interest and enrichment, leaving the animal bored and frustrated – and a utilitarian cares about these negative experiences too. So, a utilitarian not only has to weigh human interests in relation to animal interests, but also to make a judgement about what would actually be best overall for the animal or animals concerned.

A utilitarian approach would also be concerned about the wild bird trade, in as much as it impacts on human and animal welfare. Suffering inflicted on the traded birds and other animals would be of high significance, as would the overall benefits to humans (those engaged in the trade) and the costs to humans (where welfare is impacted by the loss of the services ecosystems provide, or people are distressed by the suffering of birds or the loss of species and systems). It is worth noting that from a utilitarian perspective, the loss of species (for instance) only matters inasmuch as it impacts on human or animal welfare; it is not ethically important in itself. Given the high level of bird suffering the wild companion bird trade produces (likely to be much more than birds would experience in the wild; certainly mortality rates are higher), and other negative outcomes, from a utilitarian perspective, the trade is almost certainly unethical (though there is certainly room for debate about the best practical and policy responses to the trade).

Contextual approaches to ethics, such as an ethics of care, are concerned with questions about what is owed to a companion animal, given the animal's relationship to the owner, and how to make the relationship between the animal and owner more fulfilling and mutually engaging. Most contextual approaches to ethics will maintain that once an animal is in the home, it has been made dependent on the owner, and as the owner has placed it in this situation of dependence, there is a moral responsibility to care for the animal and to ensure that its needs are met.

For contextual views on which the flourishing of relationship matters, given that poor welfare can lead to fear, aggression and stereotypic behaviours that inhibit flourishing, the animal will need to have good welfare (although this may not be true of welfare compromises that do not have behavioural manifestations). One particularly interesting issue here concerns bird rearing and companionship. It has traditionally been argued that both hand-rearing companion birds (which means early maternal separation, and in parrots, a higher risk of disease (Romagnano, 2003)) and keeping social birds singly, encourage birds to bond with their human owner. If this were correct, there might be a conflict between the ethical goal of developing a strong bond between the owner and the bird, and a goal of good, species-specific welfare. However, recent research suggests that, in the case of parrots at least, parent-rearing, with some human handling, creates birds just as tame as does hand-rearing (Aengus & Millam, 1999); while housing in same-sex pairs improves, rather than undermines, bird–owner relationships (Meehan, Garner & Mench, 2003).

Finally, we will consider a rights view. First, it is clear that an animal rights view would unequivocally condemn the trade in wild birds, as it infringes on every right a bird might be thought to have, and no benefits to humans could be thought to outweigh such rights infringements. Assuming that a rights view claims, most basically, that animals have negative rights such as a right not to be seriously harmed, and not to be imprisoned, concerns about keeping other companion animals also exist. Keeping rabbits in small hutches and birds in small cages are likely to be seen here as rights infringements, and significant adjustments called for in order to provide companion animals with basic liberties. As an example of a view like this, we could consider the House Rabbit Society (HRS), an organisation committed to protect the rights of companion rabbits and, more generally to ensure that they have good lives.

The HRS rests on a clearly outlined ethical position, on which all domestic rabbits are valuable as individuals; they 'should be afforded at least the same individual rights, level of care, and opportunity for longevity as commonly afforded to dogs and cats who live as human companions'. As domestic rabbits have been produced by humans and are dependent on them, it is a 'human responsibility that these animals be cared for in a manner appropriate to their needs' (HRS, 2013). Interestingly, this view combines a rights perspective with a contextual ethic of special responsibility for animals produced and owned by humans. Among the ethical responsibilities that the organisation defends are neutering rabbits (though there is recognition within the HRS that neutering is an ethically serious decision), ensuring that they receive veterinary treatment, keeping them in groups of two or more, and providing spaces and opportunities for their mental and physical stimulation. This last responsibility may require significant adaptation of human homes for rabbits, either creating very large and complex interior cage structures, or allowing rabbits freedom to roam within some, or all, of the home.

Julie Smith, founder of a chapter of the HRS in Wisconsin, proposes what she calls a 'performance ethics' of living with rabbits in the home, where to the greatest extent possible with continued human occupation, 'physical and mental space' is made available for 'animal agency' (Smith, 2003). For Smith, this meant significant changes to her physical domestic environment:

> Rabbit-proofing meant that most of the furniture was made of metal, electrical cords were fastened behind furniture or covered in hard plastic or metal tubing, and protective wood strips were tacked on to wood baseboards and wood trim around closets and windows. In addition, linoleum replaced carpet – or the carpet was abandoned to shredding – and fencing enclosed bookcases. So-called "litterbox training" primarily meant capitalizing on the rabbit habit of urinating consistently in one or two places. We simply put litterboxes where the rabbits decided to eliminate.
>
> (Smith, 2003)

This description of making a home suitable for the free movement of rabbits is just one example of how difficult it can be to live with many other species in the ways we usually live with cats and dogs. In addition, in the case of rabbits, as with cats, there are also questions about the freedom to have outdoor access.

From all of these ethical perspectives, then, even human-centred, contractarian ones, it is normally better if the animals we keep as companions are cared for in ways that protect and promote, rather than undermine, their welfare. For some of the animal species discussed earlier, good welfare is possible, but the owner may have to be more accommodating to the animals' needs than is often recognised. However, achieving good welfare, in the case of some species, just may not be possible in an average home. This raises the question whether some species should not normally be kept as companion animals at all, or whether ownership of some species should be restricted (through a ban or by requiring a licence).

15.5 Should Ownership of Some Species Be Restricted, or Completely Prohibited?

We have seen so far in this chapter that keeping companion animals other than cats and dogs can raise significant welfare and conservation concerns. Previously in the book, we also considered other issues, such as the spread of zoonoses and companion animal invasiveness (Chapter 14), and aggression, particularly in dogs (Chapter 9), which can also be problematic in the case of other companions. If an animal combined enough of these characteristics (being aggressive, being a member of a threatened species, wild caught, a carrier of zoonotic disease, potentially invasive, and very difficult to keep in a state of good welfare) or manifested even one of the characteristics in a sufficiently extreme way, we might think that keeping it as a companion is unethical, and should not be legally permitted. For example, domestic ownership of some big cat and primate species is not permitted in some countries.

Schuppli & Fraser (2000), and Schuppli et al. (2014), have developed a useful framework for assessing the ethical suitability of different species as companion animals. They suggest a series of questions that should be asked about each species, concerning knowledge about a species' welfare and the difficulty (or otherwise) of achieving good welfare in the home, the impacts on the welfare of others (human and non-human) from attack and disease, and the environmental risks posed both by procuring and releasing the animal. They then propose a rough categorisation of pets and animal companions into (see Box 15.1) the following groups, reflecting the required level of owner commitment and expertise.

Schuppli & Fraser (2000) place golden hamsters and mice into Category A (though as we have seen, even these animals can pose welfare challenges, and, according to Schuppli & Fraser (2000), require enriched cages and regular handling). Most cat and dog breeds are placed into Category B: cats and dogs are fairly demanding in terms of welfare, can create problems of noise, disease, and injury, but they can be procured from responsible

---

Box 15.1 Categories of animal species classified according to their degree of suitability as companion animals.

Category A: Species whose use for companionship is generally positive for the animal and the owner, whose needs are easily met, whose procurement and transportation raise no appreciable problems, and whose use involves no apparent risks to the community or the environment.

Category B: Species that require significant commitment of time and/or resources in order that their use be positive for the animal and the owner, but where ownership is unproblematic with regard to procurement, transportation and effects on the community and the environment. Substantial owner education may be needed for such species.

Category C: Species that have complex or demanding requirements needing skilful and knowledgeable owners who are prepared to commit significant time and/or resources to animal ownership, but where ownership is unproblematic with regard to procurement, transportation and effects on the community and the environment. Control of ownership (e.g. ownership only by qualified persons) may be appropriate for such species.

Category D: Species where there is insufficient knowledge (e.g. regarding procurement, transportation, environmental impact or the animal's needs) to allow a confident assessment of its suitability as a companion animal. Use of these species might be acceptable in the future if knowledge becomes adequate and any necessary safeguards are in place.

Category E: Species that are unsuitable as companion animals because of undue harm or risk of harm to one or more of: the animal, the owner, the community, or the environment.

Reproduced from Schuppli & Fraser (2000: p. 366) with permission from the authors and from Universities Federation for Animal Welfare (UFAW), United Kingdom. Copyright UFAW 2013

---

sources, are reasonably well understood, many people have expertise in caring for them, and they thrive as companions. Rabbits and guinea pigs probably fall into Category B too, as they do not pose environmental hazards nor strong zoonotic threats, their procurement is not a problem, and they can have good welfare as companions, though this does require 'substantial' owner education.

In contrast, significant ethical problems are raised by keeping animals in Categories D and E; as such, private ownership of species falling into these categories should be restricted or prevented. From what we have discussed earlier, it is likely that many parrot species should fall into at least Category D. We saw in Chapter 14 that some parrot species are invasive; we have seen in this chapter that their procurement may pose environmental threats; they may carry zoonotic diseases; achieving good welfare, especially for larger birds, is extremely difficult; and their longevity means that they may well out-live their human owner. In fact, these features, together with being flock animals, cause Engebretson (2006) to place parrots into Category E. This is a particularly striking eth-ical conclusion, because, as noted earlier, there are more than 42 million caged birds in the European Union alone, many of whom are parrots; this suggests that some serious ethical rethinking may be required about keeping parrots as companions (Figure 15.1).

A more recent paper by Warwick *et al.* (2014) focuses on a narrower problem: how to assess animals' suitability as pets or companions based on ease or difficulty of keeping them in the home (so, leaving aside broader ethical questions about procurement and invasiveness, and focusing wholly on human and animal welfare). The authors call this the EMODE (Easy, Moderate, Difficult, Extreme) system; it is a system intended to be accessible for a layperson thinking of acquiring a pet, and for legislators who lack specialised knowledge of animal welfare. 'Easiness' in terms of animal welfare, they suggest, is directly related to how straightforward it is to satisfy the 'five freedoms' (discussed earlier); easiness in terms of human welfare concerns risk of zoonotic disease transmission or physical attack, how easily any risk is managed, and whether there is good professional knowledge and advice available. On this basis, some companion animals, including some dogs and cats score as Easy, and some as Moderate, Difficult or Extreme (though no dogs and cats are Extreme). However, no birds are Easy; not many are Moderate; most are classed as Difficult or Extreme, along with unusual mammals and primates.

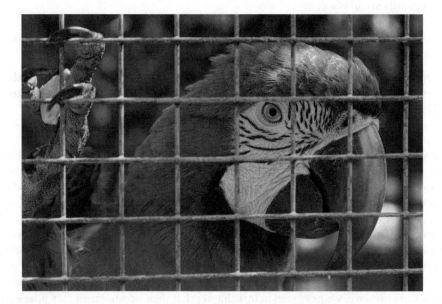

Figure 15.1 Large parrot (Macaw) in a cage. Parrots are gregarious birds, living in the wild in large flocks. They are very popular pets, but are rarely kept in suitable environments. (*Micha Klootwijk/Shutterstock.com.*)

Both Schuppli & Fraser (2000) and Warwick *et al.* (2014) make very clear the significant ethical challenges posed by keeping companion animals other than cats and dogs. Some species pose health risks to their owners or others, and their capture, escape or release can damage ecosystems that humans need. This is problematic even from human-centred ethical perspectives that focus wholly on the value of human welfare and human lives. Some animals, including such commonly kept birds as parrots, cannot easily, or cannot at all, achieve good welfare in human homes; keeping them is problematic, in different ways, from all the ethical approaches we have considered.

Key Points

- Rabbits, small rodents and birds, especially parrots, are also kept as companions, although their numbers are lower than cats and dogs.
- These animals are usually kept confined in cages or hutches, in a house or garden, and are less able to express their needs to their owners than cats and dogs.
- Welfare problems can arise when these other companions have insufficient space to perform normal behaviours, have nutritionally inadequate diets, lack contact with conspecifics (where this is important), live in barren environments, or receive little appropriate veterinary care.
- The wild bird trade causes additional welfare issues for some bird species, and has significant environmental impacts.
- These welfare issues, and the wild bird trade, are undesirable from almost every ethical perspective considered, as they have negative impacts on humans, animals and the environment.
- Some species of animal may present such significant welfare challenges in the home, or contribute to other problems to such a degree, that they would be better not kept as companions at all.

References

Aengus, W.L. & Millam, J.R. (1999) Taming parent-reared orange-winged Amazon parrots by neonatal handling. *Zoo Biology* 18, 177–187.

ASPCA [American Society for Prevention of Cruelty to Animals] (n.d.) *Small pet care*. [Online] Available from: http://www.aspca.org/pet-care/small-pet-care [Accessed 22 August 2014].

AVMA [American Veterinary Medical Association] (2012) *U.S. pet ownership statistics*. [Online] Available from: https://www.avma.org/KB/Resources/Statistics/Pages/Market-research-statistics-US-pet-ownership.aspx [Accessed 22 August 2014].

Born Free USA (n.d.) *Current law and suggested approaches to improving captive bird welfare: Colorado*. [Online] Available from: http://www.bornfreeusa.org/b4a2_birdwelfare.php [Accessed 25 August 2014].

Cowan, D.P. (1987) Group living in the European rabbit (*Oryctolagus cuniculus*): mutual benefit or resource localization? *Journal of Animal Ecology* 56 (3), 779–795.

Edgar, J.L. & Mullan, S.M. (2011) Knowledge and attitudes of 52 UK pet rabbit owners at the point of sale. *Veterinary Record* 168, 353.

Engebretson, M. (2006) The welfare and suitability of parrots as companion animals: a review. *Animal Welfare* 15, 263–276.

FEDIAF [European Pet Food Industry Federation] (2011) *Facts and figures 2010*. Brussels, FEDIAF.

Fernandes-Ferreira, H., Veiga Mendonça, S., Albano, C., Silva Ferreira, F. & Nóbrega Alves, R.R. (2012) Hunting, use and conservation of birds in North East Brazil. *Biodiversity and Conservation* 21, 221–244.

Fifield, S.J. & Forsyth, D.K. (1999) A pet for the children: factors related to family pet ownership. *Anthrozoos: A Multidisciplinary Journal of The Interactions of People & Animals* 12, 24–32.

Fischer, K., Gebhardt-Henrich, S.G. & Steiger, A. (2007) Behaviour of golden hamsters (*Mesocricetus auratus*) kept in four different cage sizes. *Animal Welfare* 16, 85–93.

Girling, S. (2009) The welfare of captive birds in the future. In: Duncan, I.J.H. & Hawkins, P. (eds) *The welfare of domestic fowl and other captive birds*. Dordrecht, Springer, pp.115-136.

González, J.A. (2003). Harvesting, local trade, and the conservation of parrots in the Northeastern Peruvian Amazon. *Biological Conservation* 114, 437–446.

Harrison, G.J. (1998) Twenty years of progress in pet bird nutrition. *Journal of the American Veterinary Medical Association* 212 (8), 1226–1230.

Hart, T. (2013) *Watching Congo's grey parrots perish*. [Online] Available from: http://www.bonoboincongo.com/2013/09/26/watching-congos-grey-parrots-perish/ [Accessed 26 August 2014].

Hawkins, P. (2009) The welfare implications of housing captive wild and domesticated birds. In: Duncan, I.J.H. & Hawkins, P. (eds) *The welfare of domestic fowl and other captive birds*. Dordrecht, Springer, pp. 53–102.

Hillyer, E., Quesenberry, K. & Donnelly, T. (1997) Biology, husbandry, and clinical techniques of guinea pigs and chinchillas. In: Hillyer, E. & Quesenberry, K. (eds) *Ferrets, rabbits, and rodents: clinical medicine and surgery*. 2nd edition, St. Louis, MO, Saunders, pp. 232–244.

HRS [House Rabbit Society] (2013) *HRS philosophy*. [Online] Available from: http://rabbit.org/house-rabbit-society-philosophy-2/ [Accessed 26 August 2014].

Keown, A.J., Farnworth, M.J. & Adams, N.J. (2011) Attitudes towards perception and management of pain in rabbits and guinea pigs by a sample of veterinarians in New Zealand. *New Zealand Veterinary Journal* 59 (6), 305–310.

McVeigh, T. (2011) *Pet rabbits are cruelly neglected and mistreated in Britain, survey finds. The Observer* 21 May. [Online] Available from: http://www.theguardian.com/world/2011/may/21/pet-rabbits-cruelly-neglected-mistreated [Accessed 25 August 2014].

Meehan, C.L., Garner, J.P. & Mench, J.A. (2003) Isosexual pair housing improves the welfare of young Amazon parrots. *Applied Animal Behaviour Science* 81 (1), 73–88.

Meehan, C. & Mench, J. (2006) Captive parrot welfare. In: Luescher, A.U. (ed.) *Manual of parrot welfare*. Ames, IA, Blackwell, pp. 301–318.

Mullan, S.M. & Main, D.C.J. (2006) Survey of the husbandry, health and welfare of 102 pet rabbits. *Veterinary Record* 159, 103–109.

PDSA [The People's Dispensary for Sick Animals] (2013) *The state of our pet nation 2013: PDSA animal wellbeing report.* [Online] Available from: https://www.pdsa.org.uk/pet-health-advice/pdsa-animal-wellbeing-report [Accessed 22 August 2014].

Romagnano, A. (2003) Problems associated with improper hand feeding. *Hartz. Exotic Health Newsletter* 2, 3.

Sainthouse, P. (2011) *Small pet welfare issues.* [Online] Available from: https://suite.io/paula-sainthouse/4w962dx [Accessed 22 August 2014].

Sayers, I. & Smith, S. (2010) Mice, rats, hamsters and gerbils. In: Meridith, A. & Johnson-Delaney, C. (eds) *BSAVA manual of exotic pets: a foundation manual.* Gloucester, British Small Animal Veterinary Association, pp. 1–27.

Schepers, F., Koene, P. & Beerda, B. (2009) Welfare assessment in pet rabbits. *Animal Welfare* 18, 477–485.

Schuppli, C.A. & Fraser, D. (2000) A framework for assessing the suitability of different species as companion animals. *Animal Welfare* 9 (4), 359–372.

Schuppli, C.A., Fraser, D. & Bacon, H.J. (2014) Welfare of non-traditional pets. *Review of Science and Technology* 33 (1), 221–231.

Shepherd, A.J. (2008) Results of the 2007 AVMA survey on pet owning households regarding use of veterinary services and expenditures. *Journal of the American Veterinary Medical Association* 233 (5), 727–728.

Serpell, J. (1981) Childhood pets and their influence on adults' attitudes. *Psychological Reports* 49 (2), 651–654.

Smith, J.A. (2003) Beyond dominance and affection: living with rabbits in post-humanist households. *Society and Animals* 11 (2), 181–197.

Swissinfo.ch. (2008) *Life looks up for Swiss animals* [Online] Available from: http://www.swissinfo.ch/eng/life-looks-up-for-swiss-animals/6608378 [Accessed 11 December 2014].

UK Wildlife and Countryside Act (1981) *Chapter 69* [Online] Available from: http://www.legislation.gov.uk/ukpga/1981/69 [Accessed 26 August 2014].

Veillette, M. & Reebs, G. (2010) Preference of Syrian hamsters to nest in old versus new bedding. *Applied Animal Behaviour Science* 125 (3), 189–194.

Warwick, C., Steedman, C., Jessop, M., Toland, E. & Lindley, S. (2014) Assigning degrees of ease or difficulty for pet animal maintenance: the EMODE system concept. *Journal of Agricultural and Environmental Ethics* 27, 87–101.

Companion Animals and the Future

16.1 Introduction   252
16.2 Changing Ethical and Political Frameworks   253
16.3 Changing Legal and Public Policy Frameworks   255
    16.3.1 The legal status of companion animals   256
    16.3.2 Potential specific laws and policies   257
16.4 Changing Markets and Pressures on the
Veterinary Profession   261
16.5 In Conclusion: What Might an Ethical Future Life with
Companion Animals Look Like?   265

16.1 Introduction

The companion animal sector has changed dramatically since World War II, as discussed in Chapters 1 and 2. The total number of cats and dogs kept as companions in North America, Europe and Australasia has grown dramatically, a growth that, more recently, has extended to some Asian countries, including South Korea (Podberscek, 2009) and China, where about 10% of urban households are estimated to have dogs (Heady, Na & Zheng, 2008). This growth in the number of animal companions may have been caused by a change in attitudes towards dogs and cats over time, where they became increasingly seen as companions and family members rather than, for instance, primarily as guards or mousers.

The ways in which people care for and manage companion animals have also changed substantially since the 1940s; for instance, commercial food is used almost universally

Companion Animal Ethics, First Edition. Peter Sandøe, Sandra Corr and Clare Palmer.
© Universities Federation for Animal Welfare 2016.

in the wealthier parts of the world; in many countries, neutering is routine, as are vaccination and regular veterinary care; and dog training is common, as is the indoor confinement of cats. These changes have, in some respects, led to better welfare for cats and dogs, although some of these changes, as well as highly selective breeding in dogs, may also increase risks of certain diseases, and of obesity (see Chapters 7 and 8).

Beyond these changes in the demand for companion animals and the ways they live with their owners, other concerns and interests are currently impacting, or are likely to impact, the lives of companion animals, and the people who keep them. Besides growing concerns about animal welfare and respect for animals (Chapters 1, 4 and 5), these include concerns about zoonotic diseases, sustainability and environmental protection (Chapter 14), 'dangerous dogs' (Chapter 9) and the expansion of the market for companion animal-oriented goods and services.

These changing interests, concerns, attitudes and practices pull the companion animal sector in different – and sometimes opposing – directions. In particular, they stimulate initiatives at all levels, from the local to the global, to develop new ethical, legal and policy proposals with respect to companion animals. In this concluding chapter, we explore some ideas about the possible future for companion animals, and their role and place in modern human life, focusing on ethical, legal and policy proposals that we think will be of significance, and considering these in the context of the markets related to companion animals.

We will begin by looking at several recent approaches in ethical and political theory that we think will be developed in the future, and then consider some important legal and policy initiatives that may lead to future changes in the governance of companion animals. In the light of these proposals, we will discuss some plausible changes in the markets related to companion animals, and finally outline some thoughts on what a future ethical life with companion animals might look like. Inevitably, much of this chapter will be somewhat speculative, although we will draw on the most state-of-the-art, up-to-date research from previous chapters to inform our thinking about these future possibilities.

16.2 Changing Ethical and Political Frameworks

As we saw in earlier chapters, there are currently very diverse views about the ethics of keeping animals as companions, the role of animal companions in human societies, and how we should live with them. There seems little likelihood of a general convergence between these views, but we do think that political and ethical theorists will in future work these positions out more carefully, and explore their practical implications.

One view that seems likely to persist, and to be developed, is the view that keeping companion animals is unethical *in principle*. In Chapter 5, we briefly outlined the animal rights philosopher Gary Francione's (2012) argument that the existence of companion animals is *intrinsically* ethically problematic, because it involves creating animals that are fundamentally dependent on people. The worry here is not about animal welfare – how life feels to the companion animals, the frustration or satisfaction of animals' desires, nor whether they can perform natural behaviours. It is about creating beings to be dependent by nature, and applies 'however well we treat our nonhuman companions' (Francione & Garner, 2010: p. 79). On this view, we should not create beings that cannot survive, or at least cannot flourish, without constant human support; either because dependence means vulnerability to exploitation, or more basically based on the belief that being autonomous and self-supporting, as wild animals are here thought to be, is in principle the only morally acceptable state. While many new ethical and political frameworks for thinking about animals reject this view, we do expect that in-principle objections like this one to keeping companion animals (and perhaps domesticated animals more generally) will play a significant role in future ethical discussions.

Alongside *in principle* objections, there has also been a growth of *in practice* objections to keeping so many cats and dogs in industrialised Western nations, on the grounds of sustainability and environmental impact (see Chapter 14). We expect these more practical ethical arguments to become increasingly widely expressed, as the human population grows, and concerns about carbon emissions, loss of biodiversity, the reliability of global food supply (and so on) intensify. It is possible that these kinds of objections to keeping companion animals may become part of the resurgence of a more human-centred, contractarian ethics, in which human interests in acquiring resources are seen as having much higher priority than the provision of resources for companion animals.

While these two views are very different – one based on the view that breeding and keeping animals as companions is in some way demeaning to the animals, the other on the view that keeping companion animals is essentially frivolous – together they could constitute a future ethical backlash against the growth in numbers of, and expenditure on, companion animals.

In contrast, other very different proposals maintain that the high significance of companion animals in society should be publicly recognised, and that they should be much more systematically integrated into our social, political and even architectural decision making. One reason for proposing this is essentially human-centred, based on the view that, as companion animals are so ubiquitous, and they matter so much to so many people, we should formally, rather than just implicitly, recognise their importance. But most of those developing such proposals also take the interests of companion animals themselves very seriously, and argue that these interests should be better represented in political debate. The focus here, as Kimberly K. Smith makes clear in her book *Governing Animals* (2012: p.xiii), is not so much 'the moral duty we have as private individuals' towards animals, but rather 'whether and how the state … can defend animal welfare' and what we should take to be our political responsibilities as citizens towards animals, including companion animals.

Sue Donaldson and Will Kymlicka have made an important contribution to this discussion in their book *Zoopolis* (2012). They propose that we should integrate companion animals into the political frameworks we use for human citizenship, arguing that, as companion animals, and domesticated animals more generally, are sentient (and therefore in their view, of ethical importance), have been brought into our society, and do not have other possible forms of existence, we should include them in our social and political arrangements 'on fair terms' (Donaldson & Kymlicka, 2012: p. 101). Citizenship, they argue, is the appropriate social and political framework for companion animals: they should be granted residency as citizens, and they should be given certain rights as citizens, including appropriate mobility rights and a presumption against confinement (p. 132); certain kinds of protections (e.g. from fires and floods); and provision of some basic health care (p. 142). Interestingly, Donaldson & Kymlicka (2012: p. 83) explicitly reject the worry about creating animals to be dependent. After all, humans are 'highly dependent and vulnerable beings' too; some people with disabilities are highly dependent on others all of the time. But this does not mean, they argue, that people dependent in these ways cannot be citizens; rather they need assistance in being able to communicate their interests and preferences so that these can be fully taken account of in policymaking. Animals, too, they maintain, should be granted such assistance.

One of the difficulties a citizenship model presents, as Donaldson and Kymlicka accept, is that assigning citizenship freedoms and entitlements to companion animals may be in tension with certain interpretations of what is in their own welfare, and with the welfare of other humans and non-humans. We have seen examples of this kind of tension throughout this book. For instance, arguing that a cat should have liberty rights to roam may impact negatively on the cat's own welfare (in terms of exposure to disease or traffic accidents, for instance), as well as on the welfare of small wild mammals, birds and reptiles on which a roaming cat might prey. As we have seen, assigning companion animals reproductive rights may be in tension with the welfare of the puppies and kittens produced by unneutered dogs and cats, and with the welfare of the owners of these unneutered animals. Even without accepting the details of Donaldson and Kymlicka's argument, how tensions like these may best be addressed, both ethically and in policy terms, will surely be one of the key problems for the future.

While Donaldson and Kymlicka's arguments rest on a theoretical view about companion animal citizenship that is itself unlikely to be widely accepted any time soon, many of the more practical issues they raise, such as the responsibility to rescue companion animals in the context of disasters such as storms, floods and fires, are likely to be an important element of future companion animal policy, as we suggest in the next section.

16.3 Changing Legal and Public Policy Frameworks

Related to debates about the appropriate ethical and political frameworks for thinking about companion animals are ongoing discussions about the development of companion animal law and policy, found in most industrialised Western nations (and elsewhere). These include very broad debates about the proper legal status of companion animals, and much more specific discussions about concerns such as compensation to owners for the loss of companions, the treatment of stray and unowned animals, allowing cats outside, rescue of companion animals in disasters, dangerous dogs, dog waste, leash laws and pet trusts. It is worth noting that many of these specific legal and policy concerns are about protecting humans, usually from the impacts of their own, or others', companion animals, rather than about protecting animals for their own sake.

16.3.1 The legal status of companion animals

In many countries, such as the United States, companion animals are legal property. Technically, this means that owners can 'buy or sell them, bequeath them in … wills, give them away, or choose to "destroy" them' (Hankin, 2007: p. 321), although most states and nations have some anti-cruelty and animal welfare statutes that mean owners have an obligation to look after the basic needs of the animals in their care. Some countries, particularly in Europe, exert greater legal control than the US over what owners may do to their companion animals, for example, through banning declawing and other forms of 'convenience surgery' (see Chapter 11). So, even if companion animals are property, there may still be significant legal requirements concerning how their owners may treat them.

Property status for companion animals has been widely challenged, for two reasons. One reason concerns what, it is argued, is owed directly to the animals themselves: as companion animals are independent beings with their own interests, they are not appropriately thought of as 'just property'. This position has already been endorsed in some countries; for instance, the Norwegian Animal Welfare Act (2010) states: 'Animals have an intrinsic value which is irrespective of the usable value they may have for man'; in 2014, France recognised companion animals as no longer just 'moveable goods' but 'living beings capable of feelings' (Bacchi, 2014); and the European Union as of 2009 recognised animals as '*sentient beings*' (EU, 2007).

The second reason for the challenge is that where animals are legally mere property, arguing that their owners are owed substantial damages when a companion is harmed or killed is legally very difficult or impossible. In the United States, this issue came to a head during a pet food recall in 2007, when owners sought damages from pet food companies after thousands of animals died from eating contaminated food. As the animals were classified as being property, the owners were only entitled to claim 'reasonable economic damages'. More generally, when a companion is harmed or killed, an owner who files a lawsuit for damages is only entitled to claim 'fair market value' for the animal, which may of course be very little, especially if the animal is of a mixed breed. As long as animals are mere property, no straightforward legal entitlement to damages for emotional harm or loss of companionship exists (although in a very few cases, such awards have nonetheless been made (see Roukas, 2007)). However, if companion animals' legal status changes, making them something other than mere property, more substantial claims for damages become possible.

One of several systematic proposals to change companion animals' legal status in those countries where they remain mere property has been developed by Favre (2010), who suggests that companion animals be placed in a new category of what he calls 'living property'. In one sense here, the animals are still property: they can be kept, owned and used. However, the idea of 'living property' recognises that companion animals also have their own interests, and should, therefore, be assigned some legal rights – for instance, to sufficient space, not to be harmed, and to be cared for, as animal welfare legislation in some countries already requires. Favre suggests that the owners of animal companions should have similar legal responsibilities to meet their animals' basic needs as parents do to their own children. This means that 'the rights of owners will have to be limited to some degree to accommodate some of the interests that their property asserts against them'; that those who do not own companion animals will still have some duties towards other people's animal companions; and that companion animals will have some rights themselves (Favre, 2010: p. 1053). As Smith (2012: p. 85) notes, in making this proposal, Favre takes advantage of a distinction between what is known as legal title and equitable title. If a person has legal title, he or she has control of the property; but someone who has equitable title should benefit from it. Thus, the holder of legal title (here, the human owner) has a legal duty to take the interests of the holder of equitable title (the owned animal companion) into account.

In countries where companion animals are now solely legal property, a future legal status change to something like 'living property' seems plausible. As we have seen, there is already precedent for this in many European countries, and it would reflect the widespread shift in attitudes towards viewing companion animals as family members. However, such a change is likely to be opposed. Some groups will argue against it on the basis that this would be the first step on a slippery slope to extend similar protections to other animals, including agricultural and laboratory animals, who have similar levels of sentience and who are similarly dependent on human provision. Others, including some vets and pet food manufacturers, may be worried about the potential cost to them of a legal status change, for instance, in terms of how much they might be sued. Yet others would oppose such a change on the grounds that it does not go far enough – that companion animals should not be regarded as property, living or otherwise, but rather as independent legal persons, rather like human beings (NHRP, n.d.). However, the latter proposal seems far less likely to gain legal acceptance than the more restricted idea of them becoming some form of legal living property.

16.3.2 Potential specific laws and policies

A huge array of laws and policies pertaining to companion animals are currently under discussion, or have been implemented in some places and are likely to be implemented elsewhere. Some of these directly protect or promote the welfare of the animals themselves, some aim to benefit or protect their owners, and some aim at both; others aim to protect other people, other animals, or the environment from the impacts of companion animals. We will just consider a few of these here.

One group of initiatives aims at better representing the interests of companion animals in political processes, policymaking, and a variety of legal contexts. (This is something that philosophers such as Donaldson and Kymlicka, with their idea of companion animal citizenship, would welcome.) This can take several forms. For example, in terms of political representation, the Netherlands currently has a political party, the Party for the Animals, that aims to represent animals' interests in elected bodies, including the national parliament; the party claims that its 'highest goal is animal welfare and the respectful treatment of animals' (Party for the Animals, 2014). In policymaking terms, in California, some neighbourhood councils have appointed Directors of Animal Welfare to represent animals' interests in the construction of local policies (Smith, 2012). In a legal context, the canton of Zurich in Switzerland appointed a lawyer to the position of animal advocate, to represent the interests of animals in particular cases (though in 2010, the Swiss voted not to extend this form of animal representation more widely across the nation). While representing animals in all these ways is both conceptually and practically complicated (see Smith, 2012), increased representation seems to be a plausible part of the future of the companion animal sector. Discussion of representation and other issues relevant to companion animal law can be found in a multiplicity of journals, including in the United Kingdom, *The Journal of Animal Welfare Law* published by the Association of Lawyers for Animal Welfare, and in the United States, a number of journals including the *Journal of Animal Law* and the *Stanford Journal of Animal Law and Policy*.

There is also currently a proliferation of local, city and state and national government codes of practice and policies about companion animals kept within their jurisdiction. For example, the state of Victoria in Australia has a 'Code of Practice for the Private Keeping of Cats' that aims to provide 'minimum standards of accommodation, management and care' of cats (some of which reflect legal requirements) as well as outlining what constitutes 'best practice', for example, that cats should wear quick-release collars. Some countries or cities have more stringent and enforceable policies. For example, a number of European states have laws requiring dogs to be kept on leash or otherwise under the strict control of the owner in urban areas (see e.g. Ministeriet for Fødevarer, 2013). The city of Winnipeg in Canada passed a complex series of bylaws in 2013, including requiring the sterilisation of all dogs and cats over 6 months old unless they have an exemption license, and that both dogs and cats when outside and off the owner's property must be kept on a leash not more than 20 feet long, and 6 feet on a street (City of Winnipeg, 2013). It seems likely that more cities and countries will adopt such codes of practice and bylaws (Figure 16.1).

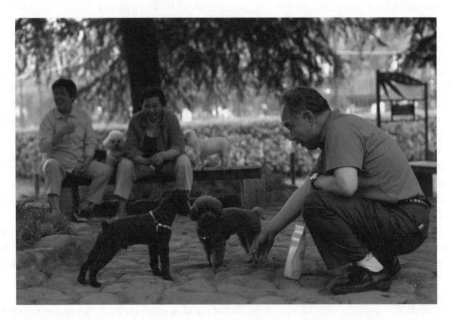

Figure 16.1 A man playing with dogs at a park in Shanghai, China. In an effort to control the soaring pet population and control rabies, the city is slashing its steep fees for dog registration and setting a limit of one dog per family. (*AP, reproduced with permission from Polfoto.*)

Other likely changes aim to benefit both animals and their owners, and may have wider economic benefits. For instance, some cities, states and countries are making micro-chipping of cats and dogs compulsory: by making it easier to reunite lost companions with owners, this aims to protect both parties; and by reducing the number of animals in shelters, should also produce economic benefits. In some countries, including the United States, there is now provision for owners to establish Pet Trusts, 'a legally sanctioned arrangement that provides for the care and maintenance of one or more pets in the event of their owner's disability or death' (Bressant-Kibwe, n.d.). These trusts are increasingly popular, and may benefit both the companion animal by legally protecting its ongoing care, and the owner by providing peace of mind that their animal will be provided for after they die.

The rescue of companion animals before, during, and after major disasters is another area of recent legislative concern. In the United States, prior to Hurricane Katrina, there were no laws requiring animals to be evacuated, rescued or sheltered in an emergency (Hodges, 2011). However, many people either refused to be evacuated without their companions, endangering their own lives; or re-entered danger areas subsequently to rescue them (even so, it is estimated that 250,000 companion animals may have died in Katrina; Figure 16.2). This led to the passing of the Federal Pets Evacuation and Transportation Act of 2006 requiring US states' emergency plans to take account of pets; by 2011, 30 US states had done so. This legislative change is particularly interesting, because its clear goal is to protect human welfare in disasters; but as people endanger their own welfare to remain with their companions, the law must extend to take companion animals into account too. For philosophers like Donaldson & Kymlicka, this might be seen as the right law for the wrong reason; companion animals should be assisted because they are non-human citizens, not because human citizens will endanger themselves otherwise.

One further area in which laws have already changed in some countries (such as France) concerns the custody of companion animals when co-owners divorce. As companion animals become increasingly regarded as family members, even where they are still technically property, some courts decide the custody of animal companions similarly to that of children, rather than as the division of property. In the United States, for instance, in some cases: 'Courts have considered the best interest of the pets in determining who gets custody of them. They have also awarded shared custody, visitation, and alimony payments to the owners' (McLain, 2009). This, of course, leads to highly complex outcomes. It is very likely that in the future, in many countries, formal processes will be created to deal with the custody of animal companions in divorce cases, directly taking into account the animals' own interests.

Finally, other key areas of law and policy likely to be created or extended in many countries concern protection *from* animal companions, for people, other animals and the environment. For example, laws against the so-called dangerous dog breeds may be extended or introduced where they do not currently exist. Relatedly, some cities and states are considering introducing mandatory third-party insurance for those owning large dogs, in order to provide a fund for compensation if the dog attacks a third party. (If enforced, this might have an impact on large dog ownership.) These changes do not

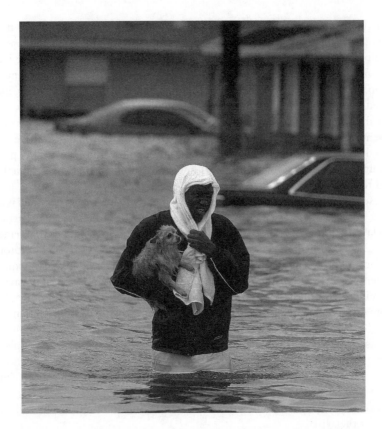

Figure 16.2 Hurricane Katrina hit the Gulf Coast on 29 August 2005, killing an estimated 250,000 animals, and causing $108 billion worth of damages. Many pet owners refused to leave without their pets: this owner risked his own safety to rescue his dog. (*AP, reproduced with permission from Polfoto.*)

directly benefit animals' welfare, but third-party insurance could benefit owners (as well as, obviously, costing the owners) and certainly is likely to benefit other people.

Laws and policies about environmental protection have so far focused on pollution from faeces (about which many cities have bylaws) and predation (mainly by cats). Bylaws that require cats to be confined in order to protect wildlife, either at night, or all the time, will probably be very widely adopted in the future, especially in places with threatened indigenous wildlife. The State of Victoria's code includes as 'best practice' that cats should be kept indoors at night and preferably all the time; cat curfew and cat confinement bylaws are under discussion in municipalities across Australia and New Zealand. Interestingly, where such bylaws are being discussed, they are often presented as win–win: good for wildlife, and good for cats' welfare. However, as we saw in Chapters 4 and 5, the latter conclusion, at least, may be challenged.

16.4 Changing Markets and Pressures on the Veterinary Profession

Whether companion animals are property, or some form of living property, or 'family members', they can still be bought and sold. Alongside the market for companion animals themselves, there is also a growing market for the products and services that surround them – most notably the pet food industry, but also the industries producing accessories and toys, the veterinary and other companion animal professions, and companion animal pharmaceutical products. This market is likely to continue to expand, as animals are increasingly being kept as companions globally, including in Russia, Mexico, the Philippines, China, and Brazil, where the average combined increase for all these countries in dog and cat ownership between 2002 and 2012 was estimated to be 34% (USDA, 2013).

This growth in demand raises questions about supply: how will companion animals be sourced in the future? From commercial breeding establishments, shelters, or small 'responsible breeders'? How will they be fed?

As we saw in Chapter 6, there has recently been an expansion of welfare regulations applying to commercial breeding establishments in Europe and the United States and some restrictions on selling puppies and kittens in pet shops. It is likely that this trend will continue, although such regulations may result in only marginal welfare gains. Beyond the industrialised West, companion animals are commonly acquired from unregulated commercial breeding establishments, where animals may have significant welfare and disease problems. On a global scale, it is likely that commercial breeding establishments will increase rather than decline, given the rising demand for companion dogs and cats.

In the United States, Europe and Australasia, a significant number of animals are now adopted from shelters (according to the HSUS (2014); in the United States, in 2012, this was 20% of owned dogs and 26% of owned cats). It is possible that more animals will be acquired from shelters in future, as adoption is perceived as an ethical thing to do. The HSUS (2014), for instance, currently promotes shelter adoptions with the slogan 'Adopt, don't shop', claiming that 'If you adopt, you'll save a life'. However, as the number of animals coming into shelters, in some places at least, is dropping (see Chapter 13), it could take longer to acquire a companion from a shelter, especially if the prospective owner has particular requirements (for a puppy or kitten, or for an animal of a particular breed). It may also become necessary to move animals between shelters to meet differing demand levels, for example, from areas with high numbers of unowned animals to areas where long winters mean short breeding seasons and fewer kittens and puppies. An alternative to an increase in shelter adoption (or perhaps a parallel process) is growth in the market for healthy animals derived from 'responsible breeders' for whom breeding is not primarily a commercial enterprise, as discussed in Chapter 6.

In countries in Asia and South America, in particular, where the demand for companion animals is increasing rapidly, there is room for significant expansion in adoption from animal shelters. Most of these countries have huge populations of unowned cats and dogs, and where shelters exist, they are full. Little formal research on the current situation for shelter adoption exists, but informal evidence suggests that adoption rates are low on account of negative perceptions of shelters. So, for instance, the animal welfare society Together for Animals in China (2014) claims that:

> The low adoption rate is largely due to the low public opinion of shelter animals. The common misunderstanding of shelter animals is that they are cheap, dirty and damaged. The current underdeveloped state of animal shelters in China has further reinforced such opinion.

If this is right, some attitudinal shifts may be needed (as happened in Europe and the United States) if shelter adoptions are to increase in future.

The markets surrounding companion animals have massively grown in the last couple of decades: in the United States, $17 billion was spent on pets in 1994, in comparison to an estimated $58.51 billion in 2013, with consistent year-on-year growth (APPA, 2014). The estimated breakdown of these 2013 sums are: $22.62 billion on food; $13.72 billion on supplies and over the counter medicines; $15.25 billion on vet care, $4.73 billion on pet services (e.g. grooming and boarding) and $2.19 billion on live animal sales. (Interestingly, the last figure is the only one that has recently decreased, possibly reflecting increasing acquisitions from animal shelters.) While one cannot straightforwardly extrapolate from these US figures to all the industrialised countries, it is clear that the market in goods and services for animal companions is vast, and has been growing consistently.

Food is the biggest single category here, and as the global numbers of animal companions increase, so does the demand for pet food. This raises a number of ethical issues. First, as discussed in Chapter 14, concerns about sustainability and the possible impact of pet food on the human food supply are likely to be raised (perhaps fuelling the 'backlash' against companion animals mentioned earlier). This is likely to be particularly acute at the luxury end of the pet food market, where owners are concerned that major commercial brands are of insufficiently high quality to ensure good animal welfare, and so increase demand for ultra-premium and home-made foods (and perhaps 'raw' diets). Second, there are more general concerns that pet food may contain unsuitable or toxic substances, such as melamine, aflatoxins and cyanuric acid, with serious or potentially fatal consequences for the animals. The globalisation of the pet food market makes the regulation and monitoring of the contents of pet foods even more challenging. Pet food recalls are ongoing (FDA, 2014), and further problems seem very likely, including recalls of dog and cat food for salmonella and listeria contamination (from which ultra-premium foods may not be exempt).

One further likely expansion in the food market is the growth of specialist or 'functional' foods, designed with particular health outcomes in mind – for instance, reducing obesity or promoting urinary tract health, and perhaps the addition of antioxidants to resist cognitive decline (Zicker, 2005). These do have the potential to reduce suffering in companion animals, but – as in the case of some human functional foods – there is also the opportunity for unethical marketing to gullible consumers.

Using the aforementioned APPA figures, veterinary care, supplies and medicines together account for a nearly $30 billion market, in the United States alone, one that will almost certainly grow further as more complex and expensive veterinary treatments and drugs become available. As was discussed in Chapter 12, this raises ethical questions about potential overtreatment, concerns that are likely to become more acute. Equally, though, the expansion and ready availability of veterinary care are likely to raise ethical concerns about *under*-treatment in the future, where owners do not provide animals with state-of-the-art veterinary treatment, or cannot afford to do so. Unlike the case of human health care in most Western industrialised countries, there is no state provision of any kind of health care for companion animals; it is wholly resourced by owners and in some countries by non-profits/charities (and occasionally, as *pro-bono* work by vets). Given the unsettled nature of state provision of *human* health care across the entire industrialised world, it is unlikely that this situation will change in the foreseeable future. However, there are current debates as to whether provision of adequate medical care for companion animals is an ethical, and should be a legal, requirement for owners (see, for instance, Coleman, 2005), and whether people should keep pets if they cannot afford vet bills. This is likely to become a more widely discussed ethical issue, especially as the cost of veterinary and drug treatment rises.

One way forward may be through compulsory veterinary health insurance for companion animals – though this is much more likely to be possible in countries that already have a strong tradition of pet insurance (such as the United Kingdom and Sweden) than in countries where there is no such tradition, and where any perceived imposition of insurance is likely to be strongly resisted (such as the United States). But there are future problems for veterinary insurance even in countries where it is currently popular; as the costs of veterinary medicine and drugs increase, as with human health care, either insurance premiums are likely to increase, putting them out of reach for many owners, or insurance will no longer be profitable, and therefore no longer available.

According to the Association of British Insurers (ABI), up to one in three pets needs veterinary treatment every year, with the average UK vet bill now over £300 per treatment (although complex treatments such as for hip dysplasia can cost over £4000, and ongoing conditions can cost up to £10,000). As a result, the ABI reports that £452 million was paid out in 2012 in vet bills: over £1.2 million every day (ABI, 2013). The fact that the average claim has risen by 52% (up £207) between 2007 and 2012, compared to an increase in insurance premiums of £57, makes it unsurprising that some companies, such as AXA, are withdrawing from the pet insurance market. The seemingly ever-increasing cost of veterinary treatment highlighted raises ethical questions about the future of the veterinary profession.

Increasing veterinary costs have significant effects, the most obvious being that fewer owners will be able to afford veterinary treatment for their animals, who will as a result be left to suffer, or be euthanased. The availability of advanced and expensive health care also has the potential to make many owners, who cannot afford that level of care, feel guilty and upset that they cannot take the 'best' care of their companion animals (whom they consider to be family members). As insurance companies may withdraw from an increasingly unprofitable market, the full range of veterinary care may be available only to the companion animals of the wealthy.

This raises difficulties for the veterinary profession, which, unlike the medical profession, still self-regulates to a significant degree, a matter of increasing controversy. Self-regulation allows the profession to regulate and discipline its members. However, for public confidence to be retained in a self-regulating profession, the profession needs to be trusted, in particular trusted not to put the interests of the profession, or its professionals, ahead of the things the profession was established to achieve. As Rollin comments:

> Every profession – be it medicine, law or agriculture – is given freedom by the social ethic to pursue its aims. In return, society basically says to professions it does not understand well enough to regulate, "you regulate yourselves the way we would regulate you if we understood what you do, which we don't. But we will know if you don't self-regulate properly and then we will regulate you, despite our lack of understanding."
>
> (Rollin, 2011: p. 103)

In a somewhat controversial paper, Blass (2010) takes the UK veterinary profession as an example of a profession currently prioritising its own interests, claiming that 'self-regulation allows moral integrity to be sacrificed at the expense of economic imperatives, and individual judgments to be preferred over fair process and procedure'. Blass maintains that 'This is particularly the case in professions where the practices are very lucrative', and further that the UK veterinary profession 'provides us with a perfect example of a professional body that is failing at its own self-regulation, losing the balance between integrity and economics'.

While Blass's condemnation of the veterinary profession is severe, and may not be fully justified, some of the concerns mirror those in a paper reviewing the driving forces behind recent reforms in the UK medical profession, reforms that effectively ended its self-regulation (Dixon-Woods, Yeung & Bosk, 2011). Unlike veterinary treatment, medical treatment in the United Kingdom is free at the point of use, provided by the National Health Service, so reforms were not driven so much by financial factors, but rather by concerns over the competence and conduct of some of the members, and the tendency of the profession to 'tolerate and protect' them (Dixon-Woods, Yeung & Bosk, 2011). But this may be a problem in the veterinary profession too; in both professions, the professional code of conduct dissuades colleagues from criticising each other. Dixon-Woods et al. (2011) reference the 1983 edition of the Guidance on Professional Conduct for doctors, which explicitly states that 'depreciation by a doctor of the professional skill, knowledge, qualifications or services of another doctor' could in itself amount to 'serious professional misconduct'.

How then can a profession ensure or restore public trust both financially and in other ways? Blass (2010) recommends that professional bodies undertake to audit themselves before any government or media pressure ensues, noting that it is often simply a question of time before something triggers enough of a public outcry to make the professions question their practice. Recent documentaries in the United Kingdom, such as Pedigree Dogs Exposed (Panorama, BBC 1 – see Chapter 7), have already stimulated debate about whether members of the veterinary profession always meet their ethical responsibilities towards animals, or whether, on occasion, these are overridden by the financial incentives of maintaining good relations with profitable clients such as breeders. We anticipate that in the future such questions about regulation, both from within and outside the veterinary profession, will become increasingly important.

16.5 In Conclusion: What Might an Ethical Future Life with Companion Animals Look Like?

This book has explored a range of ethical questions raised by the lives shared between people and companion animals. Some of those questions have relatively straightforward answers, where from virtually every ethical perspective, certain practices seem ethically desirable or required – such as euthanasing an animal in severe and incurable pain, and trying to reduce the instances of puppies being bred in commercial facilities with extremely poor welfare standards. However, many of the questions we have considered have much less straightforward answers. They depend on how animal welfare is interpreted, how important other human and environmental values might be judged to be, and whether we take a broadly utilitarian approach where values are weighed; adopt a rights approach where rights violations are taken very seriously even if they bring welfare gains to others; or alternatively adopt some kind of contextual approach based on particular human–animal relationships. Unsurprisingly, given so many significant differences, many different 'ethical futures' for living with companion animals can be envisaged.

For example: one important change in the way people live with companion animals has been in terms of control over their lives – in terms of diet, sex and reproduction, health, access to conspecifics and other animals, environment and access to space, and provision of training. The justification for this has been largely ethical: that out of respect for other people, the environment, and protecting the companion's own welfare, more control is better. Neutered and indoor-only cats, for instance, are not a public nuisance, do not prey on wildlife or pass on zoonoses, do not produce kittens that cannot be homed, and live more safely than cats who have outdoor access (which on some accounts of welfare can be taken as indicative of better welfare). On some versions of an ethical future, this neutered indoor life looks best, especially if combined with clicker training, complex electronic toys, and special (expensive) anti-obesity food to make indoor cats less bored, more engaged, less fat, and more amenable companions.

However, other visions of an ethical future living with companion animals look rather different, as some of the discussions in our chapters suggest. For instance, on a view that accepts that cats and dogs have some basic rights, including a basic right to liberty, or perhaps to reproduce, a future of neutered, indoor, and leashed animals looks like a future in which animals' basic rights are violated. Instead, an ethical future would involve more freedoms, especially to roam, even if this would create inconvenience and welfare compromise for others. Those who argue that 'good welfare' is about providing opportunities for animals to perform natural behaviours may propose that it is natural for dogs to bark, run and chase; it is natural for cats to hunt, climb and scratch.

Declawing, debarking, neutering, confining – all of these (it might be argued) prevent animals from performing natural behaviours. For the animals we live with to have good welfare on this view, they have to be free to perform such activities; and an ethical future life with animals would, therefore, permit and encourage this.

So, there is no single vision of an ethical future life with companion animals, but a series of contrasting visions, based on different ideas of welfare and different theoretical approaches to ethics. And of course, as we saw earlier in this chapter, from some perspectives, an ethical future with companion animals is impossible, because we should not keep them at all! However, we hope that this book has helped in clarifying, drawing out, and understanding both uncertainties about what constitutes good welfare, and the associated ethical dilemmas and disagreements that we outlined in the Introduction. We also hope that it is just one early contribution to a much more sustained discussion about the ethics of how we live with companion animals.

Key Points

- The companion animal sector is globalising, the market for companion animals and associated services is correspondingly expanding, and there are many new proposals about our lives with companion animals across ethics, policy and the law.
- We expect the development of further ethical objections to this growth in companion animals, as well as arguments that we need to recognise the social and ethical importance of companion animals more systematically.
- Challenges to the legal status of companion animals as mere property are likely to increase, and many other legal and policy initiatives are likely to be adopted (some focusing on protecting companion animals, some on protecting animals and owners, and some on general public protection).
- The already substantial amount spent on acquiring and caring for companion animals is likely to increase, especially on food and veterinary care.
- The rising costs of veterinary care will raise problems for the profession in terms of broad access to veterinary services, pet insurance, and ethical and regulatory standards in the profession.
- There are, as this book indicates, contrasting ideas of what living in an ethical way with companion animals might mean, and these may point us in different directions (especially with respect to companion animal confinement and safety vs freedom and risk).

References

ABI (2013) *Insurers pay out over £1.2 million every day to treat sick cats and dogs.* Association of British Insurers. [Online] Available from: https://www.abi.org.uk/News /News-releases/2013/06/Insurers-pay-out-over-1-2-million-every-day-to-cat-and-dog -owners [Accessed 11 September 2014].

APPA (2014) Pet Spending Higher Than Ever with an Estimated $58.5 Billion in Spending in 2014. American Pet Products Association. [Online] Available from: http://media.americanpetproducts.org/press.php?include=145057 [Accessed 12 September 2014]

Bacchi, U. (2014) French pets have feelings too. *International Business Times* 14 April. [Online] Available from: http://www.ibtimes.co.uk/french-pets-have-feelings-too-1445130 [Accessed 11 September 2014].

Blass, E. (2010) The failure of professional self-regulation: the example of the UK veterinary profession. *Journal of Business Systems, Governance and Ethics* 5 (4), 1–12.

Bressant-Kibwe, K. (n.d.) *Pet trust primer*. ASPCA (The American Society for the Prevention of Cruelty to Animals) [Online] Available from: http://www.aspca.org/pet-care/planning-for-your-pets-future/pet-trust-primer [Accessed 11 September 2014].

City of Winnipeg (2013) *By-law 92/2013*. [Online] Available from: http://winnipeg.ca/CLKDMIS/DocExt/ViewDoc.asp?DocumentTypeId=1&DocId=6054&DocType=O [Accessed 11 September 2014].

Coleman, P. (2005). Man['s Best Friend] Does Not Live by Bread Alone: Imposing a Duty to Provide Veterinary Care. *Animal Law Review*, 12, 7.

Dixon-Woods, M., Yeung, K. & Bosk, C.L. (2011) Why is UK medicine no longer a self-regulating profession? The role of scandals involving "bad apple" doctors. *Social Science & Medicine* 73 (10), 1452–1459.

Donaldson, S. & Kymlicka, W. (2012) *Zoopolis: a political theory of animal rights*. Oxford, Oxford University Press.

EU (2007) *Treaty of Lisbon: amending the treaty on European Union and the treaty establishing the European Community* (2007/C 306/01). [Online] Available from: http://eur-lex.europa.eu/legal-content/EN/TXT/?uri=CELEX:12007L/TXT [Accessed 11 September 2014].

Favre, D. (2010) Living property: a new status for animals within the legal system. *Marquette Law Review* 93, 1021–1071.

FDA (2014) Recalls & withdrawals. U.S. Food and Drug Administration. [Online] Available from: http://www.fda.gov/animalVeterinary/safetyhealth/recallswithdrawals/default.htm [Accessed 11 September 2014].

Francione, G.L. & Garner, R. (2010) *Animal rights debate: abolition or regulation?* New York, Columbia University Press.

Francione, G.L. (2012) *"Pets": the inherent problems of domestication*. Animal Rights: The Abolitionist Approach. [Online] Available from: http://www.abolitionistapproach.com/pets-the-inherent-problems-of-domestication [Accessed 11 September 2014].

Hankin, S.J. (2007) Not a living room sofa: changing the legal status of companion animals. *Rutgers Journal of Law & Public Policy* 4 (2), 315–410.

Heady, B., Na, F. & Zheng, R. (2008) Pet dogs benefit owner's health: a 'natural experiment' in China. *Social Indicators Research* 87 (3), 481–493.

Hodges, C.F. (2011). Detailed Discussion of State Emergency Planning Laws for Pets and Service Animals. Animal Legal and Historical Center, Michigan State University College of Law. [Online] Available from: https://www.animallaw.info/article/detailed-discussion-state-emergency-planning-laws-petsl [Accessed 12 September 2014]

HSUS (2014) *Pets by the numbers*. Humane Society of the United States [Online] Available from: http://www.humanesociety.org/issues/pet_overpopulation/facts/pet_ownership_statistics.html [Accessed 11 September 2014].

McLain, T. (2009) *Custody of pets in divorce*. [Online] Available from: https: //www.animallaw.info/intro/custody-pets-divorce [Accessed 11 September 2014].

Ministeriet for Fødevarer, Landbrug og Fiskeri (2013) *Hundeloven: LBK nr 254 af 08/03/2013*. [Ministry of Food, Agriculture and Fisheries of Denmark]. [Online] Available from: https://www.retsinformation.dk/Forms/r0710.aspx?id=145381 [Accessed 11 September 2014].

NHRP (n.d.) *Nonhuman Rights Project*. [Online] Available from: http://www.non humanrights.org/ [Accessed 11 September 2014].

Norwegian Animal Welfare Act (2010) Chapter 1 §3. [Online] Available (in English translation) from: https://www.animallaw.info/statute/noway-cruelty-norwegian-animal-welfare -act-2010 [Accessed 11 September 2014].

Party for the Animals (2014) *Welcome to the international website of the Party for the Animals*. [Online] Available from: http://www.partyfortheanimals.nl/ [Accessed 11 September 2014].

Podberscek, A.L. (2009) Good to pet and eat: the keeping and consuming of dogs and cats in South Korea. *Journal of Social Issues* 65 (3), 614–632.

Rollin, B. (2011) Animal rights as a mainstream phenomenon. *Animals* 2011 (1), 102–115.

Roukas, M.S. (2007). Determining the Value of Companion Animals in Wrongful Harm or Death Claims: A Survey of U.S. Decisions and an Argument for the Authorization to Recover for Loss of Companionship in Such Cases. Animal Legal and Historical Center, Michigan State University College of Law. [Online] Available from: https://www. animallaw.info/article/determining-value-companion-animals-wrongful-harm-or-death -claims-survey-us-decisions-and [Accessed 12 September 2014]

Smith, K. (2012) *Governing animals*. New York, Oxford University Press.

Together for Animals in China (2014) *TACN fundraiser 2014: shelter improvement project*. [Online] Available from: http://tacn.org/tacn-fundraiser-2014-shelter-appeal/ [Accessed 11 September 2014].

USDA (2013) *Processed product spotlight: pet food*. United States Department of Agriculture. [Online] Available from: http://www.fas.usda.gov/data/processed-product-spotlight -pet-food [Accessed 11 September 2014].

Zicker, S.C. (2005) Cognitive and behavioral assessment in dogs and pet food market applications. *Progress in Neuro-Psychopharmacology and Biological Psychiatry* 29 (3), 455–459.

Index

abandonment, 202–6 *see also* unwanted and unowned companion animals

abnormal behaviour *see* behaviour, problems

acquisition of companion animals, 43–6, 89–102, 236, 261–2

adoption, 204–9, 261–2 *see also* unwanted and unowned companion animals

affection *see* human-animal relation

aggression, 136–8, 141–2 *see also* behaviour problems

alpha roll, 137–8

American Kennel Club (AKC), 15, 92

American Veterinary Medical Association (AVMA), 8–9, 32–5, 150–1

animal rights view
  acquisition of companion animals, 99
  behaviour problems, 146
  breeding, 95–7, 110
  cat predation, 230
  confinement, 84
  convenience surgery, 178–9
  definition of, 79–82
  euthanasia, 197, 208–9
  keeping companion animals, principle of, 253–5, 265–6
  neutering, 161–3
  other companions, 245

multiple ethical approaches, 85–7

  treatment, 194

animal welfare *see* welfare

Animal Welfare Act, 92

anthropocentrism *see* human-centred view

antibiotics, 220

anti-cruelty *see* cruelty

anxiety, 141–2 *see also* behaviour problems

Aristotle, 11, 83

artificial insemination, 90, 94–5 *see also* breeding

attachment, 20–21, 41–57, 75–6, 174–5, 191–2 *see also* human-animal relation
  extreme *see* hoarding

Archer, John, 20–21

backyard breeders *see* hobby breeders

banned dog breeds, 145

behaviourism, 134

behaviour, natural
  confinement, 62–3, 68–71
  convenience surgery, 175–8
  human attachment, 51
  neutering, 158–61
  other companions, 236–41
  training, 136–8
  wild life, 229–31

behaviour problems
  behaviour therapy, 37–8, 144

behaviour problems *(continued)*
  breeding, 108–9
  commercial breeding establishments, 93–4
  confinement, 68–71
  convenience surgery, 175
  characteristics of, 133, 140–3
  'dangerous dogs', 145–6
  definition of, 140–1
  ethical theories, 144–5, 146
  human attachment, 51
  neutering, 154–5, 157
  prevention of, 142
  relinquishment, 133, 202
  training, 138–44
  welfare impacts of, 133, 142
behaviour therapy, 37–8, 144
Bentham, Jeremy, 60
biological fitness, 20–1
biotechnology, 111
birds, 10–11, 17–18, 228–31, 239–45,
    247–9
blood donation, 193–4
boarding facilities, 58
body condition score, 119–21
body mass index (BMI), 119
Boonin, David, 162–3
brachycephalic breeds *see* breeding, extreme
    phenotypes
brachycephalic obstructive airway syndrome
    (BOAS), 107–8
Brambell report, 65–6
breed clubs, 105
breeding
  artificial insemination, 90, 94–5
  behaviour problems, 108–9
  certification schemes, 100
  commercial breeding establishments,
    91–100
  designer breeds, 104–5
  ethical theories, 94–9, 109–12
  extreme phenotypes, 107–10
  health impacts of, 91–4, 105–12
  history of, 14–16, 104
  licensing, 91–2
  pedigree and purebred dogs and cats,
    14–16, 103–9
  rearing, 90–1, 94–7
  responsible, 100
  selective, 103–16
  supply and demand, 94–100, 112–14
  welfare impacts of, 91–4, 105–9

Breeding and Sale of Dogs Welfare Act, 91
British Brambell Committee *see* Brambell
    report
British Small Animal Veterinary Association
    (BSAVA), 28, 31
budgerigars *see* birds

campaigns, public, 89–90, 100
capabilities approach, 63
caring-killing paradox, 207
castration *see* neutering
casual breeders *see* hobby breeders
charities, animal, 28–30
chemical sterilisation, 152 *see also* neutering
clicker training, 139–41 *see also* training
Cochrane, Alistair, 81–2, 95, 99
commercial breeding establishments *see also*
    breeding
  ethical theories, 94–9
  internet sales, 92, 97, 100
  legislation, 92, 100
  licensing, 91, 92
  welfare impacts of, 91–4
commercial pet food *see* food, products
companion animal, definition of, 4–6
companion animals, impacts of
  on the environment, 225–8
  on human health, 52–4, 218–21 *see also*
    human, health; human animal relation
  on human welfare, 107, 174–8, 218–21
    see also human, welfare; human animal
    relation
  on resource use, 221–5
  on wildlife, 228–31
confinement, 68–71, 91–2, 204, 236–41
consequentialism, 76–9, 110–11
contextual ethical approaches *see also* ethics
    of care approach
  behaviour problems, 144–5
  breeding, 96, 111
  definition of, 82–5
  multiple ethical approaches, 87
  neutering, 163–4
  other companions, 244–5
  overweight, 126–7
  training, 135–6
contractarian view
  abandonment, 85
  behaviour problems, 144
  convenience surgery, 173
  definition of, 75–6

euthanasia, 146, 196
other companions, 243
training, 134
treatment, 191, 193, 194
convenience surgeries
debarking, 172, 175, 176, 178, 180
declawing, 172, 174–5, 176, 178, 182
ear cropping, 171–2, 174, 176, 180, 182
ethical theories, 173, 178–80
health impacts of, 173–4
preservation of dog breeds, 180–1
tail docking, 170–1, 172, 173, 176, 180–1
veterinary ethics, 181–2
welfare impacts of, 176–80
Cornish-Bowden, Captain R., 28
cost of companion animals, 9, 202, 223–5,
    263–5
Council of Docked Breeds, 170–1, 180–1
crossbreeds, 104
cruelty, 6, 19, 65
culling, 219–20, 228
'dangerous dogs', 145–6 see also behaviour
    problems

debarking, 172, 175, 176, 178, 180 see also
    convenience surgeries
declawing, 172, 174–5, 176, 178, 182 see
    also convenience surgeries
deontology see animal rights view
designer breeds, 104–5 see also breeding
Descartes, René, 11–12
Dickin, Maria, 28–9
diet see food
diseases
breeding, 108, 110–11
cat confinement, 68–71
genetic, 112, 113–14
neutering, 153–8
other companions, 238, 240, 241, 246
overweight, 121–3
treatment, 26–7, 187–9, 191–2, 194–6
unowned cats, 211–13
zoonoses, 218–21
Dogs Trust UK, 97, 210
domestication see history
dominance, 136–8, 145 see also training
Dominance Theory, 136–8
Donaldson, Sue, 254–5, 257, 259
donor animals, 188–9, 193–4 see also
    treatment, veterinary

ear cropping, 171–2, 174, 176, 180, 182 see
    also convenience surgeries
emotions see human-animal relation
endangered species, 230–1 see also wildlife
    predation
end-of-life issues see euthanasia; treatment,
    veterinary
enrichments, environmental, 59, 61, 238
ethical
judgment, 73–4
standards, 32–5
theories, 75–87
ethics of care approach
breeding, 111
convenience surgery, 179–80
definition of, 84–5
multiple ethical approaches, 85–7
neutering, 163–4
organ donation, 194
other companions, 244
euthanasia
behaviour problems, 133, 144
breeding, 97
definition of, 189–91
ethical theories, 78–9, 82, 85, 146, 196–7
other end-of-life decisions, 196–9
unwanted and unowned companion
    animals, 204–9, 213–14
veterinary treatment, 191–2
evolutionary biology, 20–21
exploitation, 95–6

Favre, David, 256–7
fearfulness, 145 see also behaviour problems
feeding see food; overweight
feral cats and dogs, 210, 211, 213, 218–20,
    229 see also unwanted and unowned
    companion animals
five freedoms, 66–7, 117, 123, 236
food
ad libitum, 121, 125
feeding strategy, 123, 127–8
food market, 262
history of, 16–17
human food supply, 221–3
products, 9, 16–17, 19, 118, 127
resource use, 225–7
Francione, Gary, 80–1, 94, 95, 161, 253–4
future of companion animals
ethical approaches, 253–5
legislation and policy, 255–60

future of companion animals (*continued*)
   products and services, 261–2
   supply and demand for companion
      animals, 261–2
   veterinary profession, 263–5

gerbils *see* small rodents
guinea pigs *see* small rodents

hamsters *see* small rodents
health *see* welfare
   insurance, 100, 263
Hearne, Vicki, 135–6
hedonism
   cat predation, 230
   convenience surgery, 176–7, 179
   definition of, 60–2
   euthanasia, 196, 207
   feeding strategy, 123
   'The five freedoms', 66
   multiple ethical approaches, 85
   neutering, 158–9
   outdoor cats, 65
   utilitarian approaches, 76, 159, 179, 207
history
   breeding, 14–16
   dog training, 17
   domestication, 10–11
   food products, 16–17
   human-animal relation, 8–15, 17–21
   other professions, 35–8
   veterinary profession, 25–35
hoarding, 50–1 *see also* human animal
   relation
hobby breeders, 90–1
House Rabbit Society (HRS), 245–6
housetraining *see* training
housing, indoor *see* confinement
human
   food supply, 221–3
   health, 52–4, 124–5, 218–21, 263
   welfare, 107, 174–8, 218–21 *see also*
      human animal relation, attachment
human–animal bond *see* human-animal
   relation
human-animal relation *see also* contextual
   ethical approaches
   attachment, 41–57, 111, 174–5, 190–2
   dominance, 136–8, 145
   history of, 8–23
   hoarding, 50–51

legal status of animals, 255–60
   role and function of companion animals, 9,
      20–21, 41–52, 252–5
human-centred view, 134, 120–1, 140–1,
      243, 254 *see also* contractarian view
Humane Society of the United States (HSUS),
      97–8
hunger, 121–3, 127 *see also* food, feeding
   strategy

illness *see* diseases
indoor/outdoor cat discussion *see*
   confinement
indoor environment *see* confinement;
   enrichments, environmental
instrumentalization of animals, 94–5
insemination, surgical and non-surgical, 95
   see also artificial insemination
internet, online selling, 92, 97, 100
invasive species, 228–9, 246–9

kennel clubs, 15–17, 105, 112–13
killing animals, 78, 81–2, 189, 196–7,
      206–9 *see also* euthanasia; wildlife
   predation
kitten mills *see* commercial breeding
   establishments
Koehler, William, 139
Kymlicka, Will, 254–5, 257, 259

law *see* legislation
legal bans *see* legislation
legal status of animals, 256–60
   citizenship, 254–5
   'living property', 256–7
   political representation, 257–8
   property, 6, 99, 256–7
legislation
   animal welfare legislation, 65–7, 256–60
   anti-cruelty, 19, 65, 256
   codes of practice, 258
   custody, 259
   evacuation, 259
   micro-chipping, 259
Lockwood, Michael, 79

malnutrition, 117, 240, 243
Mech, David, 137
mice *see* small rodents
Millan, Cesar, 139

Monash Dog Owner Relationship Scale
    (MDORS), 46, 49, 51–2
Most, Konrad, 133–6, 138, 139

Network of Relationships Inventory (NRI),
    46–7
neutering
    behaviour impacts of , 154–5, 156, 157,
        158, 159
    chemical sterilization, 152
    early, 156–7
    ethical theories, 158–64
    female cats, 155–6
    female dogs, 153–4
    health and welfare impacts of, 152–7
    male cats, 156
    male dogs, 154–5
    routine, definition of, 151
    welfare, positive, 158, 159
No Kill Movement, 208
No-kill
    policies, 213
    shelters, 208–9
non-identity problem, 109–10
North American Veterinary Technician
    Association (NAVTA), 36–7
Nussbaum, Martha, 63
nutrition see food

Obama, Barack, 89–90
obedience training, 17, 42–3, 135 see also
    training
obesity see overweight
One Health, 220–1
operant learning, 134, 138 see also training
opportunity cost of companion animals,
    223–5
organ donation, 193–4 see also treatment,
    veterinary
outdoor/indoor cat discussion see
    confinement
overfeeding, 118, 126 see also
    overweight
overhumanization, 124
overtreatment, 195–6 see also treatment,
    veterinary
overweight
    body condition score (BCS), 119–21
    definition of, 118–19
    health and welfare impacts of, 121–3
    measurement of, 118–21

obesity, 117–31
    owner characteristics, link to, 123–6
    prevention, 123, 126–8
    treatment, 126–8
ownership see human-animal relation

pain, 60–2, 76–9, 176, 179–80, 196–7
palliative care, 189–91, 196–8 see also
    treatment, veterinary
parrots, 239–42, 247–9
pedigree dogs and cats, 14–16, 103–9 see
    also breeding
Pedigree Dogs Exposed (film), 103–4
People for the Ethical Treatment of Animals
    (PETA), 59, 213–14
People's Dispensary for Sick Animals (PDSA),
    28–30
perfectionism
    convenience surgery, 177, 178
    definition of, 62–3
    feeding strategy, 123
    neutering, 160
    outdoor cats, 65
performance ethics, 245–6
pet
    definition of, 4–5
    food sector see food, products
    shops, 92, 97–9, 100
    stores, 91, 93, 99
    trade, 241–2
population (of companion animals), 9,
    17–20
    management, 211–14 see also unwanted
        and unowned companion animals
power relations see training, dominance
preference theory
    confinement, 64–5
    definition of, 63–4
    neutering, 158–60, 161
    treatment, 191
    utilitarian approaches, 76–9, 197
preservation of dog breeds, 180–1
Principles of Biomedical Ethics see
    principlism
principlism, 86–7
professions
    behaviour therapists, 37–8, 144
    veterinary, 24–40, 261–5
    veterinary nurses, 36–7
    veterinary technicians, 36–7
punishment, 134, 138–40 see also training

puppy
    classes, 135, 187 *see also* training
    mills *see* commercial breeding
        establishments
purebred dogs and cats, 14–16, 103–9 *see
    also* breeding

rabbits, 238–9, 245–6
rats *see* small rodents
rearing, 90–91, 94–7, 244–5 *see also*
    breeding
Regan, Tom, 80–82, 146, 162, 197, 208
reinforcement, 138–40 *see also* training
resource use, 221–5 *see also* companion
    animals, impacts of
relationship *see* human-animal relation
religion, 11–13, 14
relinquishment, 144, 175, 202–6 *see also*
    unwanted and unowned companion
    animals
reproduction, control of *see* breeding;
    Neutering
rescue of companion animals, 97–8, 255,
    259
rights view *see* animal rights view
Rollin, Bernard, 62, 192, 264
Royal College of Veterinary Surgeons
    (RCVS), 28, 31, 36

selective breeding *see* breeding
sentience, 80, 110, 208, 254, 256
Serpell, James, 13, 51
shelter(s) *see also* unwanted and unowned
    companion animals
    adoption from, 204–9, 261–2
    entering, number of companion animals,
        204, 209–10
    'no-kill', 208–9
    relinquishment to, 144, 175, 202–6
    workers, 207–8
shows, dog and cat, 15–16, 42–3, 108–9
Singer, Peter, 63–4, 77–9, 223
Skinner, Burrhus Frederic, 134, 138
small rodents, 237–8
small scale breeders *see* hobby breeders
sport *see* training
sterilization *see* neutering
Stilwell, Victoria, 139
stray cats and dogs, 204, 209–10, 231 *see
    also* unwanted and unowned companion
    animals

stud books, 15–16 *see also* kennel clubs
stress, 204 *see also* behaviour problems
sustainability, environmental, 225–8

tail docking, 170–1, 172, 173, 176, 180–1
    see also convenience surgeries
Thomas, Keith, 4–5, 12–13
training
    behaviour problems, 140–4
    behaviour therapy, 37
    clicker training, 139–40
    dominance, 136–8, 145
    history of, 17
    learning principles, 133–4, 138–40
    methods, 138–40
    obedience training, 17, 42–3, 135
    operant learning, 134, 138–9
    punishment, 134, 138–40
    puppy classes, 135, 187
    purpose of, 134–6
    reinforcement, 138–40
trap-neuter-return, 213–14, 231 *see also*
    unwanted and unowned companion
    animals
treatment, veterinary *see also* veterinary
    cost of, 263–5
    donor animals, 188–9, 193–4
    end-of-life decisions, 196–9
    ethical standards, 32–5
    ethical theories, 191–2, 196–9
    history of, 26–8
    medicine, modern, 187–9
    organ donation, 193–4
    overtreatment, 195–6
    palliative care, 189–91, 196–8
    prolonging of life, 194–6
    under-treatment, 263

UK Kennel Club, 15–16, 103, 105
unwanted and unowned companion animals
    see also shelter(s)
    abandonment, 202–6
    adoption, 204–9, 261–2
    euthanasia, 204–9, 213–14
    feral cats and dogs, 210, 211, 213,
        218–20, 229
    population management, 9, 17–20
    relinquishment, 144, 175, 202–6
    stray cats and dogs, 204, 209–10, 231
    trap-neuter-return, 213–14, 231
    welfare of, 206, 211, 213

utilitarianism
    acquisition of companion animals,
      98–9
    act utilitarianism, 98
    behaviour problems, 144, 146
    breeding, 95, 96
    convenience surgeries, 173–8, 179
    definition of, 76–7
    donor animals, 193–4
    euthanasia, 78, 82, 207–9
    hedonistic, 85, 179, 196–7, 207
    indoor/outdoor cat, 77, 84
    multiple ethical approaches, 85–7
    neutering, 158–61
    opportunity costs, 224
    other companions, 243–4
    preference, 76–9, 197
    rule utilitarianism, 98–9
    training, 135, 139–40
    two level utilitarianism, 99
    zoonoses, 220

vaccination, 187, 211, 213, 219–20
Veterinarian's Oath, 32–4
veterinary
    ethics, 32–5, 181–2
    expenditure, 9, 224, 263
    history, 25–35
    nurses, 36–7
    profession, 24–40, 261–5
    regulation, 263–5
    surgeries, 35, 169–85
    specialization, 30–32

technicians, 36–7
treatment *see* treatment, veterinary
Veterinary Surgeons Act, 28, 36
vets *see* veterinary
virtue ethics, 83–4, 87

welfare
    assessment of, 67–71
    behaviour problems, 133, 142
    breeding, 91–4, 105–9
    convenience surgeries, 176–80
    hedonism *see* hedonism
    indoor/outdoor cats, 59–62, 64, 68–71,
      74, 265–6
    legislation, 65–7, 256–60
    neutering, 152–8
    organisations, 19 *see also* People for the
      Ethical Treatment of Animals (PETA)
    other companions, 236–41, 242–9
    overweight, 121–3
    positive, 66, 158, 159, 236
    perfectionism *see* perfectionism
    preference theory *see* preference theory
    theories of, 60–65
    unwanted and unowned companion
      animals, 206, 211, 213
    utilitarianism *see* utilitarianism
    wildlife predation, 229–31
weight control, 126–7 *see also* food
wild-caught birds, 241–2, 243 *see also* birds
wildlife predation, 228–31

zoonoses, 218–21 *see also* diseases